DIMENSIONS IN CANCER AND PALLIATIVE CARE EDUCATION

Illuminating the Diversity of Cancer and Palliative Care Education

T0133872

DIMENSIONS IN CANCER AND PALLIATIVE CARE EDUCATION

Illuminating the Diversity of Cancer and Palliative Care Education

SHARING GOOD PRACTICE

Edited by

LORNA FOYLE
Independent Lecturer

and

JANIS HOSTAD
Lecturer/Education and Development Coordinator
Hull and East Yorkshire Hospitals Trust

Foreword by

DAVID OLIVIERE
Director of Education and Training
Education Centre
St Christopher's Hospice, London

Radcliffe Publishing
Oxford • New York

Radcliffe Publishing Ltd
18 Marcham Road
Abingdon
Oxon OX14 1AA
United Kingdom

www.radcliffe-oxford.com
Electronic catalogue and worldwide online ordering facility.

British Library Cataloguing in Publication Data

A catalogue record for this book is available from the British Library.

ISBN-13: 978 1 84619 057 5

Typeset by Pindar NZ, Auckland, New Zealand
Printed and bound by Cadmus Communications, USA

Contents

Special dedication   viii

Foreword   ix

Preface   xi

About the editors   xiii

List of contributors   xiv

Acknowledgements   xvi

1 Teaching communication skills to cancer and palliative care professionals:
  questions, challenges and debates   1
  Allie Fellows

2 *Cancer Tales*: a communication teaching tool   18
  Janis Hostad and Lorna Foyle

3 Telling stories in cancer and palliative care education: enigmatic, infinite
  mystery or trusted teaching techniques?   39
  Lorna Foyle

4 Finding human masterpieces: progressing cancer and palliative care
  education through neuro-linguistic programming   55
  Lorna Foyle and Janis Hostad

5 Treasures in jars of clay: working with critical companionship   83
  Angela Brown and Gill Scott

6 Reflective practice in cancer and palliative care education   94
  Chris Johns

7 Learning and teaching critical thinking skills   110
  Janet Holt

8 Advanced nursing practice: the potential sword of Damocles in
  education?   120
  Martin Towers

9 Integrating knowledge, skills and compassion to reconfigure a cancer
  service: a managerial perspective   133
  Sarah Bates and Wendy Page

10 Issues in research teaching and learning: what should we focus on?   155
    David Clarke

11 Memoirs from a parallel universe: Dr Who and the cybernurse –
    compassion or competence?   177
    Lorna Foyle

12 The teaching of hope and suffering in palliative care education   195
    Robert Becker

13 The challenges and importance of teaching law relating to the end of life   209
    Anne Leach

14 Diet and nutrition in cancer and palliative care education   229
    Shupikai Rinomhota

15 User involvement in palliative care education: beyond rhetoric and
    tokenism   243
    Anne Bury

16 A patient and carer course: 'I have friends in the same boat'   262
    Janis Hostad and Sally-Ann Spencer Grey

17 Climbing the mountain to self-awareness and self-care in cancer and
    palliative care education   281
    Eileen Mullard

18 Promoting leadership by education   293
    Ian Grigor

19 The ultimate challenge: a successful, productive, cohesive and dynamic
    team?   306
    Lorna Foyle and Janis Hostad

20 Managing death in a hospital context: creative approaches to teaching
    and learning about death and dying   331
    John Costello

21 'Children should be seen and not heard': ensuring that children are *heard*
    throughout loss and life-threatening illness of a loved one, via education   344
    Janis Hostad and John Holland

22 The graveyard shift: creative strategies for teaching bereavement and
    loss   364
    Janis Hostad

    Index   389

To my parents, Marie and Brian, and my daughter Crystal, for all the happy memories, love and laughter.

To my partner Trevor for suffering, tolerating, accepting and always supporting the completion of these three books. You are truly, in every way, one in a million . . . now back to the fun.

Thank you.
Janis

For Samuel, the latest arrival and the fourth of my grandsons who all illuminate my life and for Malcolm because . . .

Thank you.
Lorna

Special dedication

IN MEMORY of Julia Yeomans (known to some as Julie) whose life and personality reflected so aptly the title of this book. Julie was one of those people who walked into a room and illuminated it with her broad smile. She had an innate gift to make everyone she met feel special. She was known to both authors but was a close friend of Lorna. Aware of the creation of this book, she volunteered to write a chapter giving her perspective as a newly diagnosed breast cancer patient. Sadly that never came to fruition. Julie died and is fondly remembered as being a fun-loving, family-centred person who always saw the good in everyone. She is missed by all.

We hope that Paul (her husband), Kaye and Leo (daughter and grandson), and young Paul and Annabelle (son and daughter-in-law) will let the fireworks light up the sky and lead you to the comfort you so richly deserve.

Lorna and Janis
September 2009

AT THE BEGINNING of our endeavour to write three books about education in cancer and palliative care I lost a very special and close friend from childhood days, June Atherton. June shared her passion for life with her partner, family and wide circle of friends as she encountered the varied treatment aspects of her breast cancer pathway. The word journey is much misused in cancer and palliative care but for June and those of us who walked alongside her it was a journey, but one of self discovery, particularly for June. To while away the long hours during treatment and recovery, June was encouraged to take up painting. She found she had an inherent and creative talent which those of us who saw her work immediately recognised as exceptional but which she modestly deemed as 'average'.

Until her death her paintings were used as cards and calendars by her local hospice staff with whom she had forged a close relationship. Those of us that had one of her paintings, we treasured the gift she had left us. For me it was an important reminder of our special times together in childhood and in later years when we talked into the night sharing our joys, fears and aspirations. One month before completing this manuscript she touched my life yet again. her partner released some more of her paintings and Ralph Atherton, her brother offered me two of them. These paintings now illuminates my home as my friend June brightened my days . As I step out on another chapter of life, as does her partner and Ralph, we just need to say that though the pain of your absence is easier, you are still greatly missed and have a unique and special place in our hearts.

Lorna
September 2009

Foreword

Education is a window on the world of cancer and palliative care. This book offers a vista on a changing landscape of care and provides a comprehensive range of topics to clinicians and educationalists. It certainly illuminates a diversity of aspects and dimensions necessary for best practice in contemporary end-of-life care education. Communication is a constant theme.

The book's 'window' opens on to opportunity for enriching our learning and changing our perspectives for fresh insights and reflection. It reminds us that education is a two-way process – knowledge going out but also knowledge coming in.

Cicely Saunders started a revolution over 40 years ago. She advocated meticulous symptom control, family and community support and close liaison with all members in the patient's team of professional carers, largely based around people with cancer. It is important to continue to open up this philosophy and possibilities to increasing numbers of professionals and hence patients and carers. Education is the key. From the very beginnings of palliative care, Cicely Saunders saw the integration of that 'trinity' of care, research and education as being important, one informing the other.

The National End of Life Care Strategy challenges us to provide good end-of-life care in all contexts: hospital, hospice, home and care home, for all conditions and for a wider range of people. Building competence and confidence in the workforce is seen as an essential element for generalists and specialists alike and to promote good quality care. Specialists have a vital role in communicating with and teaching others. Education is even more challenging with the varied groups and topics in the classroom. This book contributes an important building block in the education process.

The excitement of education is in the potential for discovery, transformation and working with people's strengths and resilience, both for the learner and with the individuals, families, teams, organisations or communities with whom one works. The task for educationalists is to critically integrate the evidence base of clinical care and research findings; to understand the evidence from clinical practice and lessons learned in the field; to be realistic about the context in which the service is provided – applying to setting, demographic conditions, resource availability, legislation and policy; and basing it on service user and carer perspectives. The book provides the means to achieve such integration.

The editors have created an original collection of education ideas, teaching resources and wisdom. Each chapter's learning outcomes, key points and implications for readers' own practice, model good educational practice and are a useful aid to learning. The authors offer honest realistic accounts of their own experience in the field of education and between them present a huge range of teaching and learning methods.

This excellent volume unlocks a 'how to do it' of relevant topics, essential for the continuing professional development of colleagues as well as the service needs of the organisations for whom they work. This is vital when we are all working in rapidly changing contexts. The book demystifies the educational implications of each key aspect of service provision that underpins quality. Together with Volumes 1 and 2 in the series, Lorna and Janis present an amazing compendium of education, so much so that the message from Cicely Saunders for services still applies:

> 'Go around and see what is being done and then see how your own circumstances can produce another version; there is a need for diversity in this field.'

Saunders C (1976) *Essentials for a Hospice*

David Oliviere
Director of Education and Training
Education Centre
St Christopher's Hospice, London
September 2009

Preface

'No one has ever measured, not even poets, how much the heart can hold.'

Zelda Fitzgerald

This is the third book in the series *Dimensions in Cancer and Palliative Care Education*. The first book in the series focused on placing cancer and palliative care education firmly in its healthcare context. The second book looked at the many wonderful innovations in this field, and concentrated on the questions of 'what' to teach, 'how' to teach it, and 'to whom' it should be taught.

This third book follows on from these 'innovations'.

In this volume, the editors asked the chapter authors to look at the variety of ways in which they illuminate the diversity of cancer and palliative care education, as the title of the book describes. What is amazing is the diverse ways in which this was interpreted, with a myriad of original approaches, techniques, methods, educational strategies and imaginative innovations.

The editors asked the chapter authors to share their 'educational good practice' with the reader. All too often, educationalists, managers and clinicians find themselves reinventing the wheel when it would probably have been possible to adapt the work of others to meet the needs of their students. There is seldom time to examine thoroughly and analyse the literature relating to a topic such as communications, hope, nutrition or the law. The authors who examine these topics do so from a creative angle and often with an unusual style, adding to the interest for the reader.

The 'illumination' has certainly worked most successfully with many new topics being creatively spotlighted, such as patient and carer education, *Cancer Tales*, critical companionship, and promoting leadership.

At the heart of every author's chapter is their humanistic, compassionate and caring nature, which brings education and teaching to life, and this is interwoven with a high level of competency. There are a number of themes which run throughout the book, the main one being *communication* (which underpins the work of every educator, manager or clinician). Communication is vitally important in the field of cancer and palliative care. To reinforce this importance, communication is integrated as an essential component throughout the book, and, indeed, the first chapter focuses exclusively on the subject.

Another theme is *vulnerability*, and the open manner with which the authors share their vulnerability is touching. This is a key aspect in the 'Treasures in jars of clay' chapter, and it is implicitly (and often explicitly) in every chapter of the book.

The other theme which has emerged is that *one size does not fit all*. Interestingly, these very words have been used by many of the authors. Others have also echoed these sentiments, which illustrate how important it is to tailor education to meet the needs of specific groups and the individual. This reflects the underpinning philosophy of cancer and palliative care.

While the instructions from the publishers required the authors to use third-person, many have been rebellious and have used first-person. Where authors have done this, it has added to the impact, and suits the heart and soul of the book.

There is much for the reader to reflect on about new, inventive ways of working, which can be used or adapted to suit.

So, in summary, knowledge, sensitivity, vulnerability, compassion and know-how in equal measure are necessary to illuminate the diversity of cancer and palliative care education.

Lorna Foyle
Janis Hostad
September 2009

About the editors

Lorna Foyle MSc, BA Hons, Cert Ed, Dip HE Pall Care, NDN Cert, RGN, Cert in Counselling, NLP Master Practitioner
Independent Lecturer

Janis Hostad MSc, BA Hons, Cert Ed, Dip HE Pall Care, NDN Cert, RGN, Diploma in Counselling, NLP Master Practitioner
Lecturer/Education and Development Coordinator, Hull and East Yorkshire Hospitals Trust

The two editors' combined experience in cancer and palliative care adds up to over 50 years. The early part of their experience was firmly rooted in the clinical setting as practitioners and managers. In the latter years their focus has switched to education and research.

List of contributors

Sarah Bates
Head of Nursing, Cancer and Clinical Support
Hull and East Yorkshire Hospitals Trust

Robert Becker
Senior Lecturer
Shropshire and Mid Wales Hospice, Shrewsbury and University of Stafford

Angela Brown
Senior Lecturer
Associate Head, School of Nursing & Midwifery and Indigenous Health
University of Wollongong, Australia

Anne Bury
Independent Lecturer

Dr David Clarke
Senior Lecturer
University of Leeds

Dr John Costello
Senior Lecturer
University of Manchester

Allie Fellows
Lecturer/Practitioner
Compton Hospice, Wolverhampton

Lorna Foyle
Independent Lecturer

Ian Grigor
Senior Lecturer
University of Leeds

Dr John Holland
Chartered Educational Psychologist

Dr Janet Holt
Senior Lecturer
University of Leeds

Janis Hostad
Lecturer/Education and Development Coordinator
Hull and East Yorkshire Hospitals Trust

Dr Chris Johns
Professor in Nursing
University of Bedfordshire

Anne Leach
Independent Practitioner
West Yorkshire

Eileen Mullard
Research Nurse
St James University Hospital
Leeds

Wendy Page
Matron, Cancer and Clinical Support
Hull and East Yorkshire Hospitals Trust

Dr Shupikai Rinomhota
Senior Lecturer
University of Leeds

Sally-Ann Spencer Grey
Independent Lecturer and Consultant

Gill Scott
Independent Lecturer

Martin Towers
Lecturer
University of Leeds

Acknowledgements

The production of this book, the third in the series, has been supported by so many people with whom it has been a genuine pleasure to work.

We especially appreciate the excellent contributions made by all the authors and offer thanks to David Oliviere for writing the foreword.

To everyone at Radcliffe Publishing, thank you, especially for your continued assistance, patience and endless support.

We would also like to record our very special appreciation to those many precious patients and relatives with whom we have worked throughout the years and who shared so much. It is these individuals who enlighten, illuminate, inform, develop and improve both our care and our teaching, thank you.

1

Teaching communication skills to cancer and palliative care professionals: questions, challenges and debates

Allie Fellows

'I felt they were probably taught how to give injections and do blood pressures, but they were not taught that patients are very vulnerable. Everything they say goes straight to your heart so when they say things like, "the cancer's spread", you get very, very upset. So I think they really should be taught that patients are very vulnerable and they need to be very careful in what they say, and that we need a lot of affection and we need tender loving care almost as much as we need the drugs.'

75-year-old patient with cancer
Available at: www.healthtalkonline.org

AIM

This chapter aims to consider which are the key issues involved in planning and delivering communication skills training and to frame some of the debates, dilemmas and challenges.

LEARNING OUTCOMES

By the end of this chapter, the reader should be able to:
- discuss the context in which communication skills training has developed for healthcare professionals communicating with cancer and palliative care patients
- identify common aims and outcomes for communication skills training
- discuss the relationship between knowledge, attitude and skills
- consider modes of delivery
- identify the challenges of assessing competence.

WHAT'S THE PROBLEM?

The importance of effective communication is recognised generally in all aspects of healthcare. For patients, good communication improves the experience of care and reduces distress. For we healthcare professionals, good communication enables us to convey adequately a sense of care, to find out what patients want to know and to tailor information appropriately, to support decision-making processes and to promote adherence to treatment and lifestyle changes. This in turn reduces complaints, enhances job satisfaction and reduces stress (Maguire and Pitceathly 2002; Razavi *et al.* 2003).

However, in spite of the undoubted benefits which good communication brings to both patients and professionals, communication skills among healthcare professionals remain worryingly poor, especially as far as conveying empathy and concern and helping patients to explore their feelings are concerned (Kruijver *et al.* 2001). These skills do not improve consistently with experience alone (Cantwell and Ramirez 1997) and yet many healthcare professionals overestimate their own communication skills, underestimate patients' levels of distress and do not take up opportunities for further training (Ford *et al.* 1994).

Since the importance of communication skills has undoubtedly become better recognised as an essential part of pre-qualifying training for many healthcare professionals, it might be argued that over time, communication with patients will improve anyway as these newly qualified professionals begin to practice. However, there are a number of problems with the assumption that a greater emphasis on communication in pre-qualification training will, in time, lead to better communication in practice.

First: too often, communication on pre-qualifying courses is still taught at a fairly theoretical level, to large cohorts of students and by educators without specialist skills or knowledge in teaching communication. As has been argued elsewhere, 'knowing how to' is not necessarily an indicator of 'being able to do' (van Dalen *et al.* 2002), certainly in a complex area such as human interaction.

Second: even if it is the case that pre-qualification training in communication has improved, working with cancer and palliative care patients confronts the healthcare professional on a daily basis with extremely delicate and difficult situations requiring a high degree of skill and sensitivity. Student nurses and doctors still report feeling inadequately prepared to talk with families about subjects like death and dying (Barclay *et al.* 2003; Hjorleifsdottir and Carter 2000) and may therefore still require additional post-qualification training and support.

Finally: the transfer of knowledge and skills from the classroom to the clinical environment is mediated by a number of factors, including the prevailing workplace culture (Eraut 2005). Newly qualified professionals may find it difficult to implement and develop the skills and attitudes they have been taught if these are not valued or supported by the senior staff with whom they are working.

It therefore seems that there is a continuing need to address communication skills deficits in post-qualified staff and that questions of what to teach, how to teach it, how to assess it, to whom it should be taught, by whom and in what format are complex. Addressing these issues in an ever-changing health service requires ongoing research and dialogue. Readers searching for a definitive answer on 'how to do it' may be disappointed.

THE CHALLENGE OF ADDRESSING THE PROBLEM THROUGH EDUCATION

Educational quality generally resides in the appropriate alignment of teaching and assessing activities with the desired learning aims and outcomes (Biggs 2003). Put simply: What is it that trainees should be able to do? What are the best methods for helping them learn to do it? How can success be measured? However, this process does not take place in a political vacuum. 'Desired outcomes' are equally dictated by service requirements, political imperatives and resources as by patients' and professionals' needs.

Notions of what constitutes 'best practice' are subject to interpretation. The dominant discourse in healthcare research remains positivist and closely allied to the medical model. A hierarchical approach to research methods generally deems large quantitative studies as 'valid' while smaller scale qualitative studies are likely to be dismissed as 'anecdotal'. When developing healthcare education in the UK, it is therefore likely that courses drawing from a positivistic evidence base may be viewed by fund holders as more 'credible' and therefore more likely to attract resources.

The inherent danger in bowing to this demand for 'evidence-based' teaching on purely positivist terms is that it has a tendency to produce a 'one size fits all' approach to education. Many quantitative studies, by their very nature, struggle to capture the complexity and uniqueness of individual processes. While recognising that qualitative studies may be less generalisable, let's also recognise that they have potential to offer greater insights into these qualities. Education generally has a tradition for multi-method approaches to research, indeed good educators could be described as pursuing ongoing action research, responding to and evaluating the diverse needs of individuals and groups from moment to moment and course to course. This does not mean that teachers should not take account of current research and political imperatives but rather that good teaching demands a healthy and critical approach to the evidence coupled with the ability to be reflective and reflexive to the needs of individuals and groups.

When deciding what to teach and how to teach it, educators attempting to adopt a critical approach to the evidence base may find that this involves compromises between educational quality, pragmatism and political expediency. Educators need to consider what is ideal, what is possible and what is likely to be recognised and supported by those who decide the priorities, hold the purse strings and allocate the study leave.

WHY IS COMMUNICATION WITH CANCER AND PALLIATIVE CARE PATIENTS SO DIFFICULT?

Communicating with patients facing a serious or life-threatening illness involves balancing a number of potentially conflicting and complex processes.

Healthcare professionals often report feeling undertrained and undersupported to step into this difficult arena (Maguire and Pitceathly 2002).

At a relational level, being confronted with an anxious, distressed or angry individual may empathically raise feelings of anxiety and distress in the healthcare professional. The concept of 'traumatic' or 'vicarious' countertransference, in which the worker experiences feelings of helplessness and incompetence when working with a traumatised patient, is well recognised in the psychotherapeutic field (Herman 1992) but may not be so familiar in other areas of healthcare. Similarly, issues of loss, grief and mortality may, through identification, evoke actual or feared issues for the worker. As a defence against these difficult feelings, the health professionals may feel compelled to avoid issues which are personally painful or threatening or to act in ways which enable them to feel more adequate but which may inadvertently distance them from the patient (Maguire 1985; Rosenfield and Jones 2004).

At a functional level, communication with patients and their families requires that health professionals balance their own agenda with that of the patients. Kruijver *et al.* (2000) have defined this as an 'open two-way communication in which patients are informed about the nature of their disease and treatment and are encouraged to express their anxieties and emotions'. This seemingly straightforward process can raise all kinds of problems for the healthcare professional. It is no easy task to ascertain the information needs of an individual, when these may change from moment to moment, conflict with needs of other family members and with the amount of information the healthcare professional may need to give to gain informed consent or to plan treatment.

Effective communication therefore requires the integration of a variety of skills, used intentionally and in response to the unique circumstances of that interaction, and all this in what may be an emotionally charged consultation.

WHAT IS IT WE WANT HEALTHCARE PROFESSIONALS TO BE ABLE TO DO?

The obvious answer to the above question is, of course: to communicate better. Common aims and outcomes for communication skills training tend to include:

➤ identifying patients' psychosocial and spiritual as well as physical concerns
➤ communicating with empathy
➤ finding out patients' informational needs and tailoring information appropriately
➤ increased self-awareness about blocks to communication
➤ handling difficult situations, such as breaking bad news and dealing with distress.

However, each of the above aims is open to interpretation and debate, just as what is meant by 'good communication' itself varies. Some writers have used the term 'counselling skills', implying an emphasis on relationship building, emotional support and psychological assessment (Maguire and Faulkner 1988). More recently the terms 'communication skills' or 'advanced communication' have been adopted, reflecting a wider set of skills including assessing, information-giving, collaborative decision-making as well as listening and supporting. What seems fairly consistent through the literature, however, is that the majority of patients prefer a patient-led or patient-centred approach while recognising that a significant minority prefer a 'doctor'-led consultation (Dowsett *et al.* 2000). The term 'patient-centred' is, of course, itself open to interpretation and debate. A useful way of conceptualising patient-centredness is as diametrically opposed to a disease-oriented or doctor-centred approach in which the patient's experience, knowledge and preferences are viewed as being less important than the doctor's interpretation of the evidence base (Bensing 2000).

Surely, true patient-centredness requires that the health professional values the unique experience of the patient as a whole person rather than as a collection of symptoms or a problem to be solved *and* that health professional has the ability to find out what that particular patient wants at that particular moment (which may be for the health professional to take the lead). This fits with the definition offered by Laine and Davidoff ((1996) quoted in Heaven *et al.* 2003): 'an approach which is closely congruent with and responsive to patients' wants, needs and preferences'.

DOES EFFECTIVE COMMUNICATION MEAN BETTER RELATIONSHIPS OR BETTER SKILLS?

> 'As a patient, I tend not to be very concerned with the mechanics of communication, only that I feel understood.' (Epstein 2006)

Studies addressing patients' experiences consistently show that qualities such as care, compassion, being 'treated like a human being', dignity and respect are prioritised by patients (DoH 2000). This suggests the need to address attitudes in healthcare professionals and, in particular, potential blocks to empathy, care and compassion. However, a change in attitude by itself will not necessarily lead to a change in behaviour (Hulsman *et al.* 2002). Indeed, arguably many blocking behaviours arise from a misplaced sense of care in which it is feared that more open and honest communication will 'damage the patient' (Maguire 1999) or in which the healthcare professional is unable to endure witnessing the emotional distress experienced by the patient (Omdahl and O'Donnell 1999).

Conversely, if healthcare professionals are purely taught skills and strategies to explore psychosocial concerns, promote patient autonomy and choice, give information appropriately and effectively and are made aware of behaviours that block communication. These newly acquired skills and behaviours are unlikely to translate into a change in practice if the professional retains underlying beliefs and attitudes which do not value them (Jenkins and Fallowfield 2002).

There seems to be a consensus in the literature that developing healthcare professionals' communication skills requires that we address skills, knowledge and attitudes. In short, professionals need to *know* 'how to', to be able to *show* 'how to' and to have the *intention* to do so in practice (Hulsman *et al.* 2002; Parle, *et al.* 1997). So far, so good, however what is not clear is the exact nature of the relationship between attitudes, knowledge and behaviour. Less apparent still in the literature is the significance of self-awareness or emotional intelligence and the part this may have to play in enabling health professionals to recognise their own needs and anxieties and to adopt appropriate strategies to manage these in order to more appropriately identify and address the needs and concerns of their patients.

WHAT DO PROFESSIONALS NEED TO KNOW IN ORDER TO COMMUNICATE BETTER?

> 'Experience does not gather merely with the passage of time but rather through a "clinical dialogue with theory" in which existing ideas, theory and past experience are challenged or confirmed.' (Benner 1984)

Empirical knowledge

A great deal of research evidence on the information needs and preferences of patients, on behaviours which enhance or block communication and on the impact of communication on both patient and professional has amassed over the past thirty years (*see* references for a list of relevant studies). Much writing on the teaching of communication skills advocates inclusion of this evidence base as a rationale for the need to change practice (Maguire and Pitceathly 2002).

The types of behaviours and skills and the empirical and ethical rationale for a more patient-centred way of relating are also compatible with the core qualities generally recognised within the psychological literature as essential to forming therapeutic relationships. Some courses may also cover the evidence base in relation to broader psychological theory – for instance utilising person-centred or humanistic theory. For courses attracting university credits, this has the advantage of enabling students to engage in a critical evaluation of the relationship between the empirical evidence and 'grand theory'. Either way, from a motivational perspective it seems clear that if they are to learn, healthcare professionals need to be presented with the opportunity to consider the evidence for *why* they should change their practice.

The question to consider is whether this kind of knowledge alone is sufficient to change practice or whether other kinds of knowing are necessary as well. As Carper (1988) points out, real life situations are often too complex and messy to apply 'scientific' or 'technical knowledge' to and, in order to deal with situations characterised by 'uncertainty, uniqueness and conflict', a more holistic conception of knowledge may be necessary.

Self-knowledge

Much of the literature written about communicating with cancer patients comes from medical, nursing or psycho-oncological perspectives. While the impact of the professional's own 'emotional mixture' upon his or her ability to communicate effectively is recognised, generally this has been linked to issues about self-efficacy, i.e. the professional's own perception of his or her competence and effectiveness (Fallowfield and Jenkins 1999; Maguire and Pitceathly 2002) or attitudes and intention (Jenkins and Fallowfield 2002). However, what is noticeably absent in the literature is the impact of the professional's own history, experience and personal coping style on his or her ability to communicate, deal with difficult feelings or questions. Even where the above is acknowledged, the emphasis still tends to remain upon skills development rather than personal self-awareness (Kurtz *et al.* 1998).

What is meant by the term 'self-awareness' is not always clear, neither is the role this plays or how it can best be developed. Consider a typical example from a facilitated skills practice.

Example from a facilitated skills practice session

It is week eight of a 12-week course. Participants have covered the research on facilitating and blocking behaviours and in particular the impact of premature reassurance. They have discussed how the urge to reassure may arise from a need to manage their own anxiety. They have received detailed feedback on a recorded interaction and have had opportunities to practise skills in small group role-play sessions each week.

Role-played patient: . . . Yes, I've been referred for a lump in my breast and I'm worried that it might be cancer.

Nurse: Well, we don't know that yet, that's why we need to do some tests.

Role-played patient: The thing is, my friend had breast cancer last year and she's been really ill . . . *[Looks distressed.]*

Nurse: I can understand how you feel, but let's see what the tests say first.

Facilitator: OK let's stop there. *[Plays back recording of interaction. Directs question to the nurse.]* How do you feel it's going?

Nurse: Good. I'm showing empathy and listening to her concerns.

Facilitator: Anything you're not so sure about?

Nurse: No, I think it's going really well.

[Facilitator takes feedback from observers who note attentive non-verbal behaviour and a warm and caring tone of voice but identify that the nurse is blocking rather than showing empathy.]

Nurse: Yes, but she's really scared and needs reassurance.

[Facilitator reminds her of the research and challenges this.]

Facilitator: Do you think your reassurance will stop her being scared?

Nurse: Well, no . . .

Facilitator: What might it stop her doing?

Nurse: Telling me about it?

[Facilitator checks out how the 'patient' is feeling.]

Patient: I feel you're not listening to me. I'm really scared and you just keep telling me not to worry until I've had the tests. Now I feel stupid as well.

Nurse: *[Sounding really frustrated.]* I knew that, I *knew* it and now you've pointed it out I can hear myself blocking. But I couldn't hear it at the time and I still couldn't hear it when you played the recording back! If I know intellectually that reassuring doesn't help, why can't I stop myself from doing it? I don't even realise I'm doing it!

There follows an exploration of what thoughts and feelings are evoked in the nurse when she is in this situation. What emerges is that she struggles personally with uncertainty and that she copes with this by 'not worrying about things until she has to'. Additionally she finds other people's anxiety almost unbearable to witness and experiences an overwhelming compulsion to placate and reassure.

The example described will no doubt be familiar to anyone teaching communication skills and most facilitators will generally accept the need to explore intrapersonal as well as interpersonal processes. What is still subject to debate and may be worthy of more research is the significance of self-awareness in how skills are developed and the value or otherwise of including content explicitly designed to promote reflection and introspection on areas such as personal values, attitudes, motivation and anxiety.

It is interesting that implicit in training for supporting the bereaved, which tends to have evolved from a counselling or psychotherapeutic perspective, is the notion that the development of self-awareness is central to effective communication. This approach suggests that to develop empathic skills one needs to have examined and addressed the personal experiences, attitudes and defences which may block one from relating to others at any depth beyond the purely superficial (Mearns 1997) or, conversely, may lead to an over-identification or over-involvement with the client. The types of issues which tend to be addressed in training bereavement supporters and counsellors are identified below.

➤ To what extent has the healthcare professional addressed existential issues about death and dying, spiritual beliefs, own losses and experiences of bereavement?
➤ What is the professional's own preferred coping style and to what extent are they aware of this? Do they impose it on others?
➤ How comfortable are they with strong feelings of anger, distress, guilt and blame?
➤ What is their motivation? Are they aware of their own desire to be 'needed' or viewed as competent or to find solutions?
➤ Have they explored their own value base? How much does this impact on their attitude to others?

It could be argued that nursing and medicine are separate endeavours from counselling and that the values of counselling cannot be applied. However, it could equally be argued that the shared values of care, empathy and patient-centredness require similar training and development in one's capacity to critically reflect, drop barriers and defences and separate one's own needs and issues from those of the patient. If one accepts the necessity of exploring one's personal attitudes to death and dying as a prerequisite to working with the bereaved, then it is equally necessary to explore them in training to work with the life-limited and their families. The issues around motivation, loss and ability to relate to the distress of others are similar if not the same.

Of course if self-awareness, attitudes and values were proved to be a pre-requisite for effective communication skills, this raises an interesting ethical dilemma. Those embarking on a career as counsellors will be aware from the start that development of self-awareness is an explicit part of the training and personal therapy is generally a course requirement. For healthcare professionals undertaking communication skills training as part of service framework requirements, this is not currently the case. How fair is it to ask participants to engage in this kind of introspective reflection? (And how likely is it that they will do it?) What implications might this kind of introspection have for people with concurrent life crises, losses and the equivalent? NICE (2004) does, however, recommend that psychological support for patients be underpinned with suitable support for the healthcare professional. Most educators will be well aware that provision of clinical supervision is still patchy, not accessed by everyone to whom it is offered and may be facilitated by staff whose own training and skills in psychological aspects of care are minimal. Unless there is a culture in the health service of assessing motivation and emotional 'fitness' for working with other people's trauma and distress, and unless appropriate support is available for whatever issues it raises, should it be the educationalist's place to address this?

Experiential knowledge

Research suggests that communication skills (in any context, not just health) are best taught (and learned) by providing opportunities to explore factors facilitating and hindering communication, to practise, reflect, and give and receive constructive feedback in a supportive learning environment. Typically, participants are given the opportunity to discuss situations in which they find communication difficult and to generate scenarios on which they wish to work. Video clips, demonstrations and exercises are used to promote discussion on aspects of communication, to build a safe learning environment and to utilise the experience of the group in accordance with adult learning principles (Chant *et al.* 2002; Inskipp 1996).

While there is a reasonable consensus on experiential methods, one area which may be worthy of further exploration is that of the relative merits of use of actors versus teaching course participants to role-play patients for practising skills. The use of actors in teaching communication skills is discussed further in Chapter 2 and there are certainly strong arguments that actors playing 'standardised patients' offer great benefits in terms of the range of emotions and situations they are able to portray. However, to return to the idea of experiential knowledge, it has been my experience that participants regularly cite the experience of 'being the patient' as having the most impact on learning. Arguably, 'knowing' in a theoretical sense that premature reassurance is unhelpful is very different from 'knowing' from experience how angry and dismissed one felt by the healthcare professional's (well-meaning) attempt to placate.

LENGTH AND ORGANISATION OF TRAINING

I earlier stated that the development of communication skills training involves a compromise between what is ideal, pragmatic and politically acceptable. Nowhere are the tensions between these forces more apparent than in the organisation of delivery of training. Consider the comparison in Table 1.1 between recommended skills levels for healthcare professionals and the equivalent number of hours training recommended by the largest national counselling skills qualification awarding body.

On this basis, a 30-hour course would be required to train health professionals up to a basic level of competence. A 90-hour course would be needed for advanced (Level 2) skills. Studies on format and delivery of training have varied in their recommendations from 10 to 15 two-hour or three-hour sessions to a three-day to five-day residential course (Faulkner 1993; Heaven and Maguire 1996). More recently it has been suggested that a three-day model is both sufficient and effective (Fallowfield *et al.* 2004; Wilkinson *et al.* 2002). However, it should be noted that the courses in the above studies were delivered by expert facilitators to willing participants. For participants whose attitudes are more entrenched or who are less motivated to attend and change practice, a longer training period may be necessary (Heaven *et al.* 2006).

In an applied discipline, expertise develops through the combination of theoretical knowledge and experience in real practice situations. Competence, proficiency and expertise therefore lie on a continuum in which the practitioner increasingly draws on past experience and critically tests out theoretical knowledge and hypotheses in practice. Through this process, the practitioner becomes increasingly able to interpret clinical situations, assessing which aspects are important and which are irrelevant to long-term care aims.

One of the criticisms levelled at counsellor training is that it neglects the context in which students will apply their skills. Similarly, if the values, attitudes and practices learned on communication skills courses are not supported by workplace culture and by colleagues, it may be extremely difficult to sustain these in practice. Heaven *et al.* (2006) suggest that while end of course evaluations show an initial improvement in skills, these are much more likely to be fully integrated into practice if opportunities for further support and critical reflection (in this study, through clinical supervision) are created.

DOES EVERYONE HAVE THE SAME TRAINING NEEDS ANYWAY?

Since this book is aimed at palliative and cancer care education, generally, potential trainees will be post-qualification and from a variety of disciplines. This raises several questions.

➤ Is there a set of core skills transferable across all situations or do different situations and/or disciplines require different sets of skills? For example, are the communication skills needed by a clinical nurse specialist in palliative care the same as those needed by a consultant in oncology?
➤ Do junior staff need the same training as senior staff? If not, what are the differences?
➤ Each professional group has its own culture, its own 'traditional' approach to learning, which may need to be supported or challenged in different ways. Should a uni-professional or a multi-professional approach be employed?
➤ Do patients want different things from different professionals? While there appears to be a consensus on core issues such as patient-centeredness, being treated with respect and dignity and the importance of acknowledging psychosocial concerns and feelings, there seems to have been little or no research on this specific question.

All the above suggest the possibility that different professionals' training needs may converge and diverge along several dimensions:
➤ professional agenda and work context
➤ previous experience of education and preferred learning style
➤ patient-led expectations of each professional group
➤ service-led expectations of professional groups and according to seniority.

WHO SHOULD TEACH IT?

> '*Communication skills teaching is different . . . it has its own subject matter and methods. Knowing how to teach cardiology does not equip you to teach communication skills. Knowing how to communicate in normal conversation is not the same as understanding the specific skills of communicating with patients.*' (Kurtz et al. 1998)

Until relatively recently, healthcare professionals received little or no training in communication skills. For this reason, many educators in healthcare have found themselves teaching a subject in which they themselves may have received little or no formal training. Conversely, practitioners who are highly trained and skilled communicators may have little formal knowledge or experience of teaching, learning and assessment. Ideally, for any subject teachers need:

➤ a clear grasp of and much practice in the skills they are trying to teach
➤ a conceptual framework in which to place the skills if they are to be used intentionally and purposefully
➤ knowledge and experience of teaching and learning.

Additionally, as communication is increasingly recognised as an essential skill and deficits in this area become less acceptable, facilitators are likely to experience an increase in reluctant participants 'sent' to meet service requirements. Biggs (2003) argues that motivation is a 'product of good teaching not a prerequisite for learning'. Finding out what students want to learn, especially when they feel resistant to learning, requires skilled and confident facilitation. Finally, experiential teaching and learning demands an appropriate safe learning environment. So further additions to the list may be required:

➤ sufficient knowledge of the relevant research base to appear credible and to be able to respond appropriately to challenges and criticism
➤ highly developed listening and facilitation skills which encourage participants to share rather than act out anxieties
➤ asssertiveness skills to maintain a safe learning environment for participants and to hold professional boundaries
➤ confidence to engage other professionals whose perceived knowledge and/or status may feel higher than one's own
➤ flexibility and willingness to adapt teaching methods if this will help the participants to engage with the learning process.

The tensions between keeping up with research, maintaining a practice base for credibility alongside teaching commitments will be a familiar challenge to many healthcare educators. However, nowhere is it more essential to meet this challenge than in an environment in which participants may be anxious or even hostile and in a subject which is so key to good care.

TABLE 1.1 Comparison of NICE (2004) recommended skills level and equivalent counselling skills qualifications*

NICE Guidance: recommended model of professional psychological assessment and support		Counselling and Psychotherapy Central Awarding Body: definition of service levels and associated qualifications.		
Level / group	Should be able to	Service level	Definition	Qualification / minimum guided learning hours
Level 1 (All health and social care professionals)	Recognise psychological needs. Demonstrate effective information giving and compassionate communication. Show general psychological supportiveness.	Informal 'helping work'	'Using counselling skills to work with the personal concerns and distress of others' 1 During interactions which arise as part of a broad range of helping work.	Certificate in Initial Counselling Skills. (QCA no. 100/2521/2 30 hours
Level 2 (Health and social care professionals with additional expertise)	Screen for psychological distress. Apply psychological interventions such as anxiety management.		2 Within professional helping relationships.	Certificate in Counselling Skills (QCA no. 100/2520/0 90 hours
Levels 3 and 4 (Trained and accredited professionals)	Assess psychological distress and psychopathology. Offer counselling, psychotherapy and specialist psychological and psychiatric interventions.	Formal psycho-therapeutic work/ therapeutic counselling	Preparation for psychotherapeutic work. Working therapeutically with life events such as loss and bereavement. Working with mental health and other psychological issues.	Advanced Certificate in Counselling Skills 90 hours + Certificate in Counselling Studies 90 hours + Advanced Diploma in Therapeutic Counselling + Further specialist qualifications

* The shaded area represents the training needs of medical staff, nursing and associated health and social care professionals (qualified and unqualified).

WHAT ARE THE CHALLENGES IN ASSESSING COMPETENCE IN COMMUNICATION?

> '[I]t is a formidable task to develop modes of evaluation which are, at one and the same
> time, sensitive to the trustworthiness of the trainees, the insight and experience of the
> trainers and the interests of future clients.' (Dryden and Thorne 1991)

The related subjects of assessment and competence are huge and complex. For a full discussion on the use of competencies in palliative care education, *see* Chapter 2, Book 2 of this series Dimensions in Cancer and Palliative Care Education (Becker 2007).

The specific challenges which relate to devising assessment strategies and defining competence in communication skills training reflect, more or less, the areas of dilemma and debate discussed throughout this chapter. In the field of human relating, components of communication such as warmth, care, empathy, genuineness, trust, confidence and emotional intelligence are notoriously difficult to define and assess. And yet it is these qualities over (perhaps) more readily observable skills or behaviours which are prioritised consistently by patients (Dowsett *et al.* 2000; Wright *et al.* 2004; Epstein 2006). Instruments designed to evaluate patients' experiences of doctors' communication and relating skills are often based on the patients' perceptions rather than on a set of specific skills or behaviours. Yet such skill and behaviour sets can be specified using questions, such as those given by Mercer *et al.* (2004):

how was the doctor at . . .
- being interested in you as a whole person (not just treating you as a number) or
- showing care and compassion (seeming genuinely concerned, connecting with you on a human level)?

Examples of questionable patient-centredness

Using subjective judgements based on the above, how might the following be assessed?
- The student uses paraphrases, checks understanding and gives information appropriately, thereby ticking every box, but exudes not a whiff of warmth or caring. She reflects, 'You are very shocked by this news', in the same tone of voice in which she might say, 'You have sat on my hat' (to borrow an example from Carl Rogers).
- The student prematurely reassures, asks too many closed questions but somehow you forgive him because, beyond his lack of skills there is evidently a warm and caring human being and if the patient were asked, she would prefer the second (arguably less skilful) individual.
- The student demonstrates both caring and appropriate skills in a specific context but seems unsure about how or why these work. She cannot articulate how she might transfer these principles across to other situations.

By contrast, 'objective' instruments designed to test the outcomes of training courses were generally intended to measure changes in behaviour and the effectiveness of the training rather than to assess the training *per se*. The difficulty with this approach is that while some robust and objective ways of assessing interview behaviours have been developed, arguably, researchers have measured what is most readily observed rather than what is most relevant.

The difficulty with this is that without the same means of assessing the appropriateness and responsiveness of the intervention, a 'block' could be labelled as a 'facilitating behaviour' and vice versa (Heaven *et al.* 2003).

Examples of different blocking/facilitating interactions

Patient: I'm really worried about what'll happen when they discharge me.
Healthcare professional: And how are you feeling about the chemotherapy?

In the example above, the question is open, directive and has a psychological purpose. Yet it is nevertheless a block because it assumes that the healthcare professional knows what the patient means and potentially switches the subject.

Patient: My family have all been so worried so I thought if we all saw the doctor together we could just get some reassurance you know . . .
Healthcare professional: And did it help?
Patient: Not at all. She was so graphic about it all, my wife was just in pieces . . .

Strictly the healthcare professional's question above is both closed and leading. However, because it is responsive to what the patient is saying and motivated by a genuine desire to listen, it is facilitating rather than blocking.

The challenge in assessment terms, and what characterises the most expert practitioner, is her ability to grasp intuitively the situation as a whole. In attempting to articulate and break down each step of the performance, the very nature of the expertise is lost and communication is reduced to a procedural rather than a holistic endeavour. On this basis, arguably assessment of competence requires both subjective and objective measures, and interpretive and qualitative evaluation strategies are required to supplement any quantitative methods.

KEY POINTS

■ Short courses in communication skills by themselves are only a beginning to improving patients' experience of care and meeting their information and support needs. Lasting changes in healthcare professionals' attitudes and ability to communicate need to be supported in practice.

■ The core values of care, respect and compassion should be central to all aspects of healthcare. Educationalists are ideally placed to ensure that a patient-centred approach and good communication skills are explicit in all courses and not sidelined as a 'specialist subject'.

▪ With its tradition for action research, education can make a significant contribution to both challenge and complement the dominant positivist evidence base. Educationalists need to engage in dialogue and be willing to share their practice and research through networking and publication to further knowledge in this area.

CONCLUSION

Compassionate and effective communication is arguably the cement which holds together all other aspects of care. Without it, the experience of care and caring is seriously diminished for patients, carers and healthcare professionals. There is now an extensive body of research which highlights communication issues and identifies how these can be addressed through training. There is also a reasonable consensus that training needs to address knowledge, skills and attitudes and that it should be delivered by trainers with appropriate specialist skills and experience.

This training has been largely aimed at post-qualified senior staff to address identified deficits. While short, intensive training courses may offer a pragmatic solution to improving skills in the short term, there are legitimate concerns that they may have limited impact on entrenched attitudes and in further developing skills in practice unless there is a workplace culture and resources to support such change. And of course the broader question this raises for healthcare education is this: How acceptable is it in the first place for healthcare professionals to qualify in any discipline without having received sufficient, appropriate training and demonstrated competence in communicating with vulnerable and distressed people in potentially difficult situations?

IMPLICATIONS FOR THE READER'S OWN PRACTICE

1   How good a role model are you?
   a   When did you last get some feedback on your own communication skills?
   b   How self-aware are you and what steps have you taken to actively improve your self-awareness?
   c   To what extent do you model the principles of good communication in your relationships with your students?
2   How up-to-date is your knowledge on communication theories and current evidence on 'best practice'?
3   How do you rate your facilitation skills and would you consider a peer review of these?
4   How do you get your own support and do you 'practice what you preach'?
5   How do you let others know about the materials you develop and evaluate? Where are your networks for sharing information and ideas?

REFERENCES

Barclay S et al. (2003) Caring for the dying: how well prepared are general practitioners? A questionnaire study in Wales. *Palliat Med.* **17**: 27–39.

Becker R (2007) The use of competencies in palliative care education. In: Foyle L, Hostad J (eds) *Innovations in Cancer and Palliative Care Education.* Oxford: Radcliffe Publishing.

Benner P (1984) *From Novice to Expert.* California: Addison-Wesley.

Bensing JM (2000) Bridging the gap: the separate worlds of evidence-based medicine and patient-centered medicine. *Patient Educ Couns.* **39**: 17–25.

Biggs J (2003) *Teaching for Quality Learning at University.* Buckingham: Open University Press.

Cantwell B, Ramirez A (1997) Doctor–patient communication: a study of junior house officers. *Med Educ.* **31**: 17–21.

Carper BA (1998) Response to 'Perspectives on knowing: a model of nursing knowledge'. *Sch Inq Nurs Pract.* **2**: 141–4.

Chant S et al. (2002) Communication skills training in healthcare: a review of the literature. *Nurse Educ Today.* **22**: 189–202.

Department of Health (2000) *NHS Cancer Plan.* London: DoH.

Dowsett SM et al. (2000) Communication styles in the cancer consultation: preferences for a patient-centred approach. *Psychooncology.* **9**: 147–56.

Dryden W, Thorne B, editors (1991) *Training and Supervision for Counselling in Action.* London: Sage.

Epstein RM (2006) Making communication research matter: what do patients notice, what do patients want, and what do patients need? *Patient Educ Couns.* **60**: 272–8.

Eraut M (2005) Continuity of learning. *Learning in Health and Social Care.* 2005; **4**: 1–6.

Fallowfield L, Jenkins V (1999) Effective communication skills are the key to good cancer care. *Eur J Cancer.* **35**: 1592–7.

Fallowfield L, Maguire P, Ramirez A et al. (2004) *NHSU/NHS Advanced Communication Skills Training (ACST) Development Project.* Cancer Research UK: Marie Curie Cancer Care, NHSU/NHS.

Faulkner A (1993) *Teaching Interactive Skills in Healthcare.* London: Chapman and Hall.

Ford S, Fallowfield L, Lewis S (1994) Can oncologists detect distress in their outpatients and how satisfied are they with their performance during bad news consultations? *Br J Cancer.* **70**: 767–70.

Heaven C, Clegg J, Maguire P (2006) Transfer of communication skills training from workshop to workplace: the impact of clinical supervision. *Patient Educ Couns.* **60**: 313–25.

Heaven C, Maguire P (1996) Training hospice nurses to elicit patient concerns. *J Adv Nurs.* **23**: 280–6.

Heaven C, Maguire P, Green C (2003) A patient-centred approach to defining and assessing interviewing competency. *Epidemiol Psichiatr Soc.* **12**.

Herman J (1992) *Trauma and Recovery.* London: Harper Collins.

Hjorleifsdottir E, Carter E (2000) Communicating with terminally ill cancer patients and their families. *Nurse Educ Today.* **20**: 646–53.

Hulsman RL et al.(2002) The effectiveness of a computer-assisted instruction programme on communication skills of medical specialists in oncology. *Med Educ.* **36**: 125–34.

Inskipp F (1996) *Skills Training for Counselling.* London: Cassell.

Jenkins V, Fallowfield L (2002) Can communication skills training alter physicians' beliefs and behaviour in clinics? *J Clin Oncol.* **20**: 765–9.

Kruijver IP *et al.* (2001) Communication skills of nurses during interactions with simulated cancer patients. *J Adv Nurs.* **34**: 772–9.

Kruijver IP *et al.* (2000) Evaluation of communication training programs in nursing care: a review of the literature. *Patient Educ Couns.* **39**: 129–45.

Kurtz S, Silverman J, Draper J (1998) *Teaching and Learning Communication Skills in Medicine.* Oxford: Radford Medical Press.

Maguire P (1985) Barriers to psychological care of the dying. *BMJ.* **291**: 1711–13.

Maguire P (1999) Improving communication with cancer patients. *Eur J Cancer.* **35**.

Maguire P, Faulkner A (1988) Improve the counselling skills of doctors and nurses in cancer care. *BMJ.* **297**: 847–9.

Maguire P, Pitceathly C (2002) Key communication skills and how to acquire them. *BMJ.* **325**: 697–700.

Mearns D (1997) *Person-centred Counselling Training.* London: Sage.

Mercer SW *et al.* (2004) The consultation and relational empathy care measure: development and preliminary validation and reliability of an empathy-based consultation process measure. *Fam Pract.* **21**: 699–705.

National Institute for Clinical Excellence (NICE) (2004) *National Guidance on Cancer Services. Improving Supportive and palliative care for adults with cancer.* London: NICE.

Omdahl BL, O'Donnell C (1999) Emotional contagion, empathic concern and communicative responsiveness as variables affecting nurses' stress and occupational commitment. *J Adv Nurs.* **29**: 1351–9.

Parle M, Maguire P, Heaven C (1997) The development of a training model to improve health professionals' skills, self-efficacy and outcome expectancies when communicating with cancer patients. *Soc Sci Med.* **44**: 231–40.

Razavi D *et al.* (2003) How to optimise physicians communication skills in cancer care: results of a randomised study assessing the usefulness of posttraining consolidation workshops. *J Clin Oncol.* **21**: 3141–9.

Rosenfield PJ, Jones L (2004) Striking a balance: training medical students to provide empathetic care. *Med Educ.* **38**: 927–33.

van Dalen J *et al.* (2002) Predicting communication skills with a pencil and paper test. *Med Educ.* **36**: 148–53.

Wilkinson S, Gambles M, Roberts A (2002) The essence of cancer care: the impact of training on nurses' ability to communicate effectively. *J Adv Nurs.* **40**: 731–8.

Wright EB, Holcombe C, Salmon P (2004) Doctors' communication of trust, care, and respect in breast cancer: qualitative study. *BMJ.* **328**: 864.

FURTHER STUDY

The reference section above includes a number of studies on patient needs and preferences and the development of communication skills courses and resources for teaching and assessing communication skills.

2

Cancer Tales: a communication teaching tool

Janis Hostad and Lorna Foyle

'You, the audience have a special responsibility in the way you listen to the stories and engage with them. It is important not to become a voyeur, distanced or cocooned from what is here. Relate the stories to yourself, and your own life. Learn from them.'

Nell Dunn (2002)

AIM

This chapter aims to illuminate the work of Nell Dunn and a European working party funded by Mundipharma International Ltd. This is an effective method using dramatic techniques to stage illness and subsequent communications teaching as part of the patient's journey.

LEARNING OUTCOMES

By the end of this chapter, the reader should be able to:
- explore the ways that the *Cancer Tales* workbook can be used in teaching to facilitate enjoyable learning (providing advantages and disadvantages for each method)
- identify the strengths of using stories as a 'performance' to teach healthcare professionals
- focus on the power of this approach when health professionals play patients and their loved ones allowing them to connect with the craft of empathy
- identify the precautions teachers need to put in place to ensure participants' safety and involvement
- discuss the use of actors in simulating patients, performing in relevant live theatre dramas.

INTRODUCTION

This chapter is very different to the previous one. Allie Fellows has done a sterling job of reviewing and reflecting on the communications research to date. However, this chapter is designed to complement the first one and avoid duplication in that it is a practical guide to teaching communication skills. The chapter authors have identified and addressed one specific approach to developing improved communication skills. They believe there are many methods of teaching communication effectively and efficiently, but this focuses on just one of the ways of achieving success. It will be useful to all those who teach communications, as an extra tool in their tool bag.

Often the terms 'communications', 'counselling' and 'therapeutic communications' are used synonymously. When the authors use the word 'communications', they are looking at it from the therapeutic stance.

> 'Therapeutic communication is the conscious, deliberate, and purposeful use of verbal and non verbal communication skills within the interaction, to assess problems, attend to emotional cues, and elicit patient concerns.' (Pollard and Swift 2003)

Over two years, a British writer undertook a series of interviews with people who were affected by cancer, some improving and some dying, and this produced a wealth of material. Nell Dunn tells how she was affected by a personal loss, and how she became frozen in a lonely world. She then started to write *Cancer Tales*, and get on 'the trail', finding out what people could do for one another in such traumatic circumstances.

> 'I had many long conversations with doctors and nurses and ordinary people in the front line, who told me what it was like. I wrote it all down, and, taking five very special women, I made this play.'

During her conversations, she discovered the difference that it made to patients and their family to be listened to, or sometimes ignored. She began to realise what people could do for one another. *Cancer Tales* was originally prompted by her father's death from cancer twenty-five years ago – a 'pretty appalling experience', worsened by failures of communication. As she explained:

> 'They – the doctors – didn't talk about it. And we didn't talk about it. I spoke to no one. My lips were sealed. It was a case of: 'Don't come here for help – nobody home'. I didn't know what it was for one person to support another through a crisis. I didn't know how to help those numb feelings of no man's land. In those days, there wasn't a language to talk about anything bad that was happening, and it's still difficult to talk about painful things. It was sad we couldn't discuss it.'

So, in order to develop *Cancer Tales*, Nell had many long conversations with doctors and nurses and 'ordinary' people in the front line, who told her what it was like, and she captured it all on paper. Nell's investigative work eventually became a series of five female monologues, and was converted into an inspirational play, produced by Nell herself and Trevor Walker.

A senior manager from *Mundipharma International Ltd*, was so moved by the production (which he saw in Italy) that he tracked Nell down to seek permission to develop a communication skills resource book for healthcare professionals working in cancer and palliative care. The workbook was developed under the auspices of the European Association for Palliative Care (EAPC), the European Oncology Nursing Society (EONS), the Lance Armstrong Foundation (LAF) and OpenMinds, with assistance and guidance from an editorial board consisting of palliative care, pain and communications experts. A team of dedicated communication skills experts came together to adapt the play, using the experiences of the characters in *Cancer Tales*, and to provide commentary and learning points from the text in the form of a highly individualised workbook. It highlights some of the communication issues that are faced when caring for cancer patients. It is an excellent resource for anyone who teaches different aspects of cancer care, and uses original ways of improving communications. Mundipharma International Ltd sponsored this work, and produced thousands of workbooks, to be given to healthcare professionals working in cancer and specialist palliative care areas, to cascade communications skills training into their own areas of clinical practice. The plan was that this workbook would be utilised by health professionals across the whole of Europe. However, such wonderful pieces of work can end up consigned to library shelves or nurses' stations if not supported effectively.

THE STATE OF PLAY

Within healthcare at present, there have been many drivers working towards improved communications, some of which are:

➤ Department of Health Cancer Plan (2000)
➤ NICE Supportive and Palliative Care Cancer Service Guidance (2004)
➤ The Audit Office (2005)
➤ Health Service Ombudsman Report (2006)
➤ Cancer Reform Strategy (2007)
➤ *High Quality Care for All* – NHS Next Stage Review report from Lord Darzi (2008)
➤ End of Life Care Strategy (2008)

Effective communications is an essential part of caring for patients with cancer. At the moment the main approach nationally is the well-publicised advanced communications initiative (as mentioned in the previous chapter). 'Connected' is the new name for this national communication skills programme, which incorporates the best of a number of previous communications skills training programmes, but specifically from three similar 'variants'. It is a three-day programme, based on experiential learning, using actors to enable intensive role-play. The national programme is managed by a team based within the *National Cancer Action Team* (NCAT). It is delivered through the local *Cancer Networks*, where they develop a local base of course facilitators. This has been developed in accordance with the NICE Supportive and Palliative Care Guidance (2004). While this initiative goes some way to solving the problem, it will take many years to ensure that all senior health professionals have attended.

The effectiveness of communication skills training is not in doubt, and is widely accepted. However, as Fellows (2009) points out in the previous chapter, the inherent danger in acquiescing to this demand for 'evidence-based' teaching in this way is that it has a tendency to produce a 'one size fits all' approach to education. Much of this training, like the 'Connected' initiative, has been largely aimed at post-qualified senior staff, to address identified shortfalls in their skills. However, this means that junior staff's communication skills deficits tend to go largely unaddressed. This Cancer Tales approach is different, and it might be particularly useful for these junior staff who, in the main, are the ones who spend the most time by the bedside. As the reader is aware, poor communications can have serious costs for the patients and their relatives (DoH 2000), something that has to be avoided in the future. Communications have now been accepted as a core element of care, but the growing body of evidence suggests that communications remain problematic for health professionals (Kelsey 2005). In keeping with this, the number of evidence-based training programmes continues to increase, but according to Fallowfield *et al.* (2001), nurses' communications have *not* improved in recent decades.

If this is to be accepted, then new approaches to teaching the topic should be welcomed and encouraged. Appropriate research that does not just measure confidence levels (as described in the previous chapter) needs to be developed, to find different means of achieving success. Also, if inadequate training in communication is a main factor in contributing to stress and lack of job satisfaction in these individuals (Fallowfield and Jenkins 1999), there needs to be a comprehensive plan to rectify this.

THE *CANCER TALES* APPROACH

The workbook is titled *Cancer Tales: communicating in cancer care*. The editorial board said that the workbook was developed in association with clinicians, patients and communications experts as a tool to support clinicians involved in the management of cancer.

> It aims to build upon the themes arising from each scene of the play, to stimulate the reader's consideration of the areas in which communication could be improved, and provides guidance and practical exercises to help develop a sense of empathy with the emotions of patients and their families, and to expand skills to address these.

The *Cancer Tales* workbook contains the full text of the *Cancer Tales* plays, alongside additional information, to enable easy cross-referencing, and all evidence-based. The chapters each contain questions related to communications issues, as well as the use of discussion tips, practice points, and literature on the topic under consideration. It is likely that the reader already has excellent teaching packages and other resources on many of these topics found in the book. However, it is hoped that they can creatively integrate parts of their own packages, along with different elements from this workbook.

One of the most pleasing aspects of this approach is its flexibility. The editors encourage the facilitator to use and adapt the resource to fit their own personal

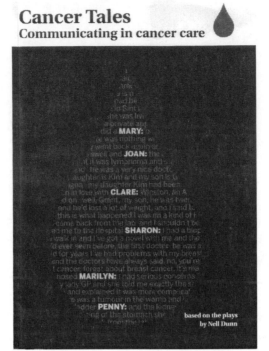

FIGURE 2.1· *Cancer Tales* cover image

requirements. They are aware that health professionals are very busy individuals, and by providing this approach allow them to use it from cover to cover without adaptation, to save time. However, it can also be used in many different ways with little effort. It covers so many important issues, from breaking bad news to dealing with different emotions, addressing sexuality, end-of-life issues, managing pain, saying goodbye, and many more.

The next section will discuss the ways in which the book could be used as part of a course for more junior qualified health professionals, as part of an action learning set. This approach has much to offer, in that it could be accomplished by weekly sessions over ten or up to twenty weeks, depending on how often the health professionals are available, and whether two chapters can be covered in one meeting. It could be possible to complete two chapters in a half-day, four in a full day depending on the time available. This offers a chance to change some of their deep-rooted attitudes, by revisiting their approaches to communications in different ways, and incorporating self-awareness exercises. As Fellows (2009) states: 'short, intensive training courses may offer a pragmatic solution to improving skills in the short term, but there are legitimate concerns that they may have limited impact on entrenched attitudes'. Macmillan nurses, other specialist cancer and palliative care nurses, managers and educationalists might find this an appropriate mode of delivery, and decide to work through the book using an action learning set. This is an excellent way of learning, but does require a skilled and disciplined facilitator.

WHAT IS ACTION LEARNING?

Using action learning to facilitate *Cancer Tales*:

> *'Action Learning is a continuous process of learning and reflection, which happens with the support of a group or a 'set' of colleagues, working on real issues with the intention of getting things done. The voluntary participants in the group or 'set' learn with, or from, each other, and take forward an important issue with the support of the other members of the set.'* (McGill and Brockbank 2003)

Action learning is a process for bringing together a group of people with varied levels of skills and experience, to analyse a mutual work problem or issue, and develop an individual action plan which allows each member to identify their own learning needs. These groups that are brought together are known as *action learning sets* (ALS). In the *Cancer Tales* context, a clinician who is skilled in communication training (as mentioned above) can initiate an ALS which can integrate the varied aspects of communication, as detailed in the workbook, with members' own unique communication issues.

What is an action learning set?

Action learning sets are an approach which can be used to foster learning in the workplace. The emphasis is on learning from experience, and then acting on that learning. The size of a learning set is usually a minimum of six, to a maximum of eight. The set size is small in order to ensure a high quality of learning. The ALS can vary in composition. One ALS could include eight individuals from different disciplines, such as a multi-disciplinary team working in the same area – for example, a hospice. Another group of ALS could consist of eight members from the same discipline, for example nurses from six different specialist clinical areas, such as hospices. There are several roles available within the set. These roles comprise that of presenter, set member (not presenting) and facilitator.

Role of the presenter and set members

The presenter brings their issue, or problem or project, to the rest of the set. He or she describes their issues of concern through a narrative account. This should include a description of how it really is 'in the here and now'. Issues from the real world of practice ensure that the learners learn best when they actively participate (McClimens and Scott 2007). The presenter receives questions from others in the group.

This person takes and addresses *only* those questions with which he or she is comfortable at this time. An example of this process is outlined below.

Example of interaction between set presenter and other members

Set presenter: I was washing Alice's face yesterday. She knows she's dying. The consultant had told her earlier in the day. Tears started rolling down her face, so I asked her what was going on for her. Well, she looked at me, then turned towards the wall and blanked me out.

Other member 1: What did you do next?

Other member 2: How did you feel? How do you think she felt?

Other member 3: Do you think your question was formed appropriately? If you could re-run that again, what would you say and do?

Other member 4: Whereabouts were you when this happened? Who else was nearby?

This would fit in particularly well with the chapter on end-of-life issues (Chapter 20), aspects of which could relate back to the above discussion. This would add to the richness of the conversation, with underpinning guidelines and useful literature. Also, the set might take the option of using this part of the play, if it had anything of value to add to the session.

The presenter then decides on action points to take forward and commit to, and shares this with the group. He or she will be expected to report back on ensuing events at a subsequent meeting of the group.

The facilitator's role

The facilitator's role is to oversee the process, ensuring that everyone is able to participate and that necessary elements (such as ground rules) are dealt with appropriately. It is important in this role to 'keep things on track', although it is also important not to become a 'back-seat driver'. As a teacher, it can be difficult letting the group run the session and organise the issues in ways that suit them, when the natural instinct might be to take over.

The facilitator's role when formulating action learning sets is to do much of the initial organisation. However, as the groups become familiar with the process, they usually start to take on much more of this themselves. The group can select a communication issue that relates to an appropriate chapter in the *Cancer Tales* workbook. For example, they might try using the chapter on respecting patients' privacy and dignity. The group might need to be encouraged by the facilitator to bring supplementary information on this topic at first, but very quickly they will establish a format of who will do what for the next meeting. Each set member may have different issues to present on respecting patient privacy and dignity, or there may some similar issues emerge within the set. It is vital that each set member has the opportunity to present their issue or perspective in their own words. Once all set members feel that all aspects have been explored on that specific communication issue, and individual action plans have been devised, a new communication issue can be identified from the *Cancer Tales* workbook for the next meeting. The set facilitator will support set members to work on their communication issues.

This role of facilitator will involve 'creating conditions' to enable each 'issue' presenter to concentrate fully on their issue, and to get the salient support from the other set members. When the facilitator becomes more familiar with this role, he or she can find it very rewarding, observing the individuals in the group grow in self-confidence and ability.

As part of a similar venture (Royal College of Nurses Pilot Palliative Care Action

Learning Set), one of the authors (who acted as a facilitator) was very pleased and proud of the group's dynamic approach and excellent achievements. At the end of the course, all the managers of the local community and hospital NHS trust and hospices came to a grand formal project presentation and evaluation. The group actually ran the action learning set on stage, in front of all these notable people, confidently, competently and *without* the facilitator!

Action learning cycle

Action learning sets have been heralded as fostering a thorough and individualised approach to learning and improving interpersonal skills. The emphasis is on learning from experience, and then acting on that learning. This is shown in the learning cycle (Figure 2.2) which is fundamental to this approach to learning.

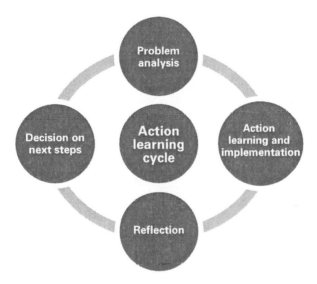

FIGURE 2.2 Action learning cycle

Running an action learning set

Before the meeting, each set member will think about the communication issues which they wish to bring to the set.

At the first meeting, ground rules should be set that apply to this and all subsequent meetings. Members should allocate the necessary time for these meetings. Over a designated period, each set member will be given an opportunity to explore their issues, and will be asked to report back to the set on their actions at the next meeting.

At the end of presentation time, the person presenting their communication issue will give feedback on how they experienced the process and what learning may have taken place. Set members may also comment on their observations, and the learning, on both the process and content.

The process of presentation time will be repeated for as many set members as is possible in the time available.

Establishing ground rules

In order to enable set members to work on real communication issues, it is important that the set facilitator gets them to establish ground rules to adhere to at every meeting. Here are some that you may wish to ensure are created. Confidentiality should be respected within the group, and nothing should be discussed outside the set, unless permission has first been negotiated from within the set. Everyone should make a commitment to attend the meetings, and meetings should start and finish on time. Only one person at a time presents an issue. No personal issues are to be brought to the set meeting, and set members are to ask appropriate questions, and to allow the presenter time to reflect on their issue.

Action learning sets can explore issues specific to a set member, or can select a communication scenario highlighted in the *Cancer Tales* workbook.

Advantages

➤ Working with small sets allows everyone an opportunity to share experiences.
➤ Everyone participates in the learning process.
➤ The set generates an ethos of reciprocity and support.
➤ Set members can identify workbook chapters specific to their communication issues.
➤ Set members learn to relate to others more effectively and improve communication skills via the process as well as from the workbook.
➤ Set members learn a more disciplined way of working.
➤ Self-confidence of set members is improved.
➤ Networking is encouraged.
➤ Set members learn about themselves, and the way they work and interact with people.
➤ In-depth learning about group processes takes place.
➤ The course runs at a pace dictated by set members.

Disadvantages

➤ Set work is labour intensive.
➤ Set members are required to commit to attend meetings, and the time-consuming nature of this commitment can impact on their lives. Some people may not enjoy working in such an intensive way, or in groups.

This method of learning can be liberating, as it emphasises the need for change and is a continuous process, involving reflection and supported by colleagues with a specific outcome in mind.

CHAPTER MEETINGS

Chapter meetings are a wonderful way of using this material. It might be productive to take the reader through the first chapter, 'Breaking bad news', which is a very familiar topic to everyone working in cancer and palliative care.

This chapter starts with a dialogue between the doctor and the patient. Clare, the patient, is actually a psychologist working in a cancer unit. The dialogue brings to life the issues relating to breaking bad news, and helps the participants to recognise the problematic behaviours and attitudes of health professionals. It can be useful to read the dialogue to the participants, with facilitators playing each part, so that the participants can listen more attentively. However, it can also be most worthwhile to have the participants read the parts, to empathise more effectively with the patient, and this is often the best approach.

The workbook provides questions for the reader, for example:

> How will you respond when a patient asks you:
> - Do I have cancer, what does this mean?
> - What tests will I have to have?
> - Who will my doctor be?
> - Can I see my records?

These are issues which could be discussed after the short excerpt from the play, together with what went well, what could have been done differently, and what might be other effective ways of dealing with this situation. When the authors run chapter workshops, they invite the participants to take it in turns to 'have a go', using their ideas, and role-playing it with Clare. If this approach is used, it obviously requires detailed ground rules, as identified and described in the last section. It can be most effective to run and re-run different parts of the excerpt, depending on the participants' ideas, agenda and the learning outcomes of the session.

The book describes the salient points involved in breaking bad news, how to most effectively construct appropriate questions, and how, depending on the response of the patient, the health professional might structure their conversation. There are also specific phrases that often help, which the participants could try out. The editors of this *Cancer Tales* workbook have provided excellent practice points throughout this and all of the chapters, which a facilitator could use in many different ways to stimulate learning and generate discussion.

One section is titled 'Ensuring support is provided following a diagnosis', and it offers different approaches to providing support and then provides a quote from Clare: 'I sat there propping up my face with my hands . . . I am all alone.' This quotation can generate much discussion. The workbook then provides the flowcharts (Maguire *et al.* 1993) which many readers will already use when teaching this topic. Most teachers will utilise other models and approaches at this point, and will ask the participants to discuss the merits of each. The participants could also be asked to bring along their trust's (or organisation's) standard statement, or local guidelines, on breaking bad news, and then debate how they can make them specific to their own 'local' area of work, using the information in the book.

The 'Breaking bad news' chapter concludes by answering the four questions from the beginning of the section.

This has not covered all aspects of this first chapter, nor has it identified all the different approaches that the facilitator could take with this material. This is one of 41 chapters, which illustrates the detail and richness of the workbook.

How to run chapter meetings

It is essential to organise the meetings to ensure maximum attendance, to fit with when it is easiest for the attendees to be available.

When the groups are convened, it is important to keep the same dates throughout, so that each participant knows which chapter meeting they are attending, and can complete any preparatory reading. Each teaching session should always relate strictly to each chapter, so, remembering the great detail in each chapter, this does require strict time-keeping. These chapter meetings can be effective as part of a rolling programme. (If possible, repeat the chapter's sessions for maximum through-put.) Participants can then come to the chapter meeting as and when they require. This means individuals might attend the meetings which match their learning needs, which have been identified as part of their personal development review (PDR) or other appraisal system. However other individuals will attend all the chapter meetings, but may take a year or more to access them all.

The facilitator's role

The facilitator can utilise any of these above approaches to facilitate the participants' learning, or can find other more creative methods of using this book. If the facilitator belongs to a team, they could choose different members to facilitate different chapters. However, some continuity tends to increase the participants' comfort during the meetings and, as a result, their learning. The *Cancer Tales* editors intended that the facilitators would include their own material, which can only add to its richness. The workbook is meant to be flexible enough to accommodate this.

In most cases, using an actor at these meetings is sadly probably not possible, as, due to cost, it is often not an option. However, having the participants or other colleagues read the stories, as described above, does work most effectively.

Another plus for this approach is that if the facilitator is a clinical nurse specialist, a teacher-practitioner, a practice development nurse (or performs a similar role), ongoing support might be possible. In between sessions, the facilitator might be able to work with (or observe) some of the participants in practice, to gauge how much they have learned.

General advantages

➤ Working with a large group is less labour-intensive.
➤ Cross-fertilisation of ideas can occur.
➤ Working through the book as a group is easier than working through it as an individual.
➤ Participants can be encouraged to bring their own information, which means more resources for the whole group (and more learning materials).
➤ Group work can generate an ethos of reciprocity, e.g. sharing protocols, documents, literature.
➤ Larger groups tend to discuss a wider variety of issues. (Individuals working on their own seldom see as many facets and dimensions to the problems or solutions.)

General disadvantages
➤ Not everyone might get a turn to speak or share.
➤ The sessions may not be run at everyone's ideal pace.
➤ Some individuals are less comfortable in groups, and as a result they are not likely to fully participate.

The authors believe that this approach, taught in this style with much discussion, sharing, self-awareness exercises and role-play with feedback, can change attitudes and entrenched beliefs. As Egan (1977) said, 'in order to understand communications, it is important to be self-aware, and to value other people's emotions.'

THE WORKBOOK AS A SELF-LEARNING TOOL
The health professional could work though the book from cover to cover, reading each chapter in turn. Alternatively, they might only choose chapters which are appropriate to their workplace, or they could start with the ones they need to improve their skills the most. The authors would advise having a 'reflective diary', which can be used to answer the questions and practice points from the book. It would also be useful for the learner to reflect on their own present skills level, relating to each chapter. Perhaps they could rate themselves at the outset, considering what they think is their present competency level, and again at the end of the course as a rough guide to their learning. The learner could also write an action plan as to how they might improve these skills. It would be useful for them to revisit the action plan later, at a time they have previously identified, in order to check their continued development.
     The facilitators might be involved in the following ways:
➤ by assisting someone who is working through the book on their own, perhaps by having periodic tutorials to check on their progress (and discussing specific issues which the learner has identified in their reflective diary)
➤ by discussing the learning points, questions and practice points, making suggestions on how the learner might improve their skills
➤ by observing them in practice, and then writing a short report, providing useful evidence for their Knowledge and Skills Framework (KSF) portfolios (or other similar evidence-based portfolios).

Advantages of the self-learning approach
➤ It allows the participant to work through the workbook at their own pace.
➤ They can work on the specific chapter and topics which suit them the most.
➤ They can access resources as and when they require them.
➤ This approach requires only minimum input from the facilitator.

Disadvantages of the self-learning approach
The participant misses out on the learning which is gained by:
➤ being involved in group debates, discussion and analysis of the stories
➤ sharing ideas and approaches

➤ observing the 'actors' role-play, acting out the story and feeling that strong sense of empathy
➤ receiving the feedback with which to gauge how much they have really learnt if the majority of the learning has been done on their own.

Facilitating short, problem-based learning sessions, on an *ad hoc* 'needs' basis, can be a compromise between the above two approaches. This would bring together a few individuals who are working on their own. They could get together to discuss their specific issues and problems. All group members contribute their ideas as to how to solve each specific problem.

CANCER TALES INTEGRATED INTO ROUTINE TEACHING SESSIONS

As already mentioned, most readers are likely to have teaching packs on most, if not all, of the topics found in *Cancer Tales*. Another opportunity to use this workbook is when you are running a session on breaking bad news, or pain and symptom control, or general communications. At that point, you could use an extract from the book which fits in with the topic and the learning outcomes.

The following ideas are just a few options for using this approach with the reader's existing teaching packs.
➤ Use a passage to read to them as a story, and ask for comments.
➤ Encourage them to act out key issues, and then get feedback.
➤ Choose a number of different sections from the workbook which fit the specific topic.
➤ Utilise some of the excellent questions and learning points, alongside your own material.
➤ Ask the group to read a story prior to the next session, with specific questions which you pose, to be answered at the next meeting.

For example, one of the authors regularly teaches sexuality, using her own previously prepared teaching material. However, she now integrates extracts from four out of the five women's stories in *Cancer Tales*. Each extract is carefully chosen because it illustrates an aspect of sexuality which relates to the session and the expected learning. While the book has no specific scene or chapter on the topic of sexuality, much can be extracted from the different stories to meet the teacher's requirements. For example, the 'Sharon' chapter illustrates how stoic the patient was about her tests, her fight against cancer, the loss of her breast, and her treatments, but how she found that losing her hair was different. This was, she said, because 'I have always been a person who is very much my appearance, and how I look to people'.

The whole of this section is read to the students (not just this extract), usually followed by this short diary extract from Roy Castle's autobiography *Now and Then* (1993).

> *'Mouth is rotten. Throb-throb . . . Pain . . .*
> *Is it worth it?*

> *I couldn't play the trumpet because of the ulcers, and tap dancing was disappearing*
> *off into the sunset.*
> *A few strands of hair on my pillow.*
> *Here we go . . . I wonder what I will look like.*
> *As my hair became very straggly, I decided to shave it off.*
> *I was amazed how it changed my appearance, from sadly pathetic, to fiercely*
> *threatening.*
> *My relatives all remarked how I resembled my father.*
> *Each time I caught sight of myself in a mirror or shop window, it startled me.*
> *It was in this stark, bald state, that I tried one of my rare visits up to the village, as my*
> *energy level seemed sufficient . . .*
> *The reactions of friends, acquaintances and shopkeepers were all vastly different.*
> *Some would see me, blush and hurry past, as if they didn't know what to say.*
> *I identified with an "Oh dear, it's him! What can I say?"*

This can create much discussion in the classroom about how, for some individuals, losing one's hair may be one of the more traumatic events. For others, it matters much less. Often, there are gender differences, or, as in Roy's case, it seems to be about the symbolism of what it meant, and about how it affects others and changes their behaviour towards him. After this, the excerpt using Sharon is often role-played, with the participants using different approaches.

An excerpt from Mary and Rebecca (scene 7) looks at a similar aspect of body image:

> **Rebecca:** There is no one else in the world I can talk to about having hairy legs, except for you, Sara. To think two months before I got sick, I was thinking if only I could lose every single hair on my body.
>
> **Mary:** And there was Rebecca and Sara. Sitting on her hospital bed, Rebecca bald and without a single bit of hair anywhere, and they both started to laugh.

This then leads to discussion about how to broach the topic, and what is (and should be) written in the patient's notes.

In scene 16, there is a short (but very powerful) extract which looks at an aspect of love and intimacy, and this poignant extract really brings the session to life.

> **Joan:** One morning I went in, and he was sitting on the bed, just sitting on the edge all alone. He said 'My back is aching', so I go round and I sit at the other side with my back against his to ease him, so we were back to back, me and Grant, and I could feel the heat of his body going through me . . . we stayed like that for ages.

The Penny and Marylyn story is very useful in sexuality sessions, to explore how the partner can best be supported, and explores the participants' views on homosexuality, and can challenge them appropriately.

Penny: When Marylyn died, there was a rainbow in the room. There was no rush at the hospice. I stayed with her a long time. I lay on the bed next to her. I felt her love. Then my mum came and fetched me.

 . . . Before I met Marylyn, I had a lot of love affairs.

Marylyn: *(a voice in the distant background)* But after she met me, she only wanted me. Penny went to Fortnum and Masons and bought the wine for the funeral.

Penny: She was a very stylish woman, was Marylyn.

The above section illustrates that it is relatively easy, having become conversant with *Cancer Tales*, to find appropriate extracts from the different dialogues to illuminate a teaching session. Both the authors of this book use this approach very frequently.

USING HEALTH PROFESSIONALS AND ACTORS TO ROLE-PLAY

Using *Cancer Tales* in this way allows the patients and their families to, as Speigel (1994) terms it, 'speak the unspeakable'. The participants can respond to 'the unspeakable' in a safe environment, and prevent themselves from answering inappropriately with actual patients.

Health professionals in role-play

Health professionals can gain a great deal from participating in the role-play. It allows them to see the issues from the patient's point of view, and to empathise more effectively. To be empathic is crucial to building rapport in a relationship. Burnard (2005) concurs with this, suggesting that entering the client's frame of reference accurately is one of the most important aspects of the therapeutic relationship. Reynolds, Scott and Austen (2000) stress that literature identifies that the main barriers to showing empathy are lack of trust, lack of privacy and lack of time.

 Role-play is often labelled as false and contrived, and some assert that in the clinical setting, the patient and carer would respond differently (Relf and Heath 2007). However, role-play provides a safe environment where clinicians can tackle pressing communication issues, without impairing patients. During the role-play, these issues can be discussed, particularly the lack of trust. If you use health professionals in role-play, be very mindful of their feelings and anxieties. They may have had experience of previous role-play sessions, which has left them with negative attitudes towards the activity. They may be self-conscious and wary of participating. The outcomes in teaching in this experiential way are that students not only improve their communication skills, but gain insight into their client's experiences, and gain unexpected insight into their own culture and value system. Always set ground rules before starting any sessions.

 When conducting a role-play teaching session (whether it is with a health professional or an actor), the same guidelines apply. There are many more aspects to consider, but the list below begins to illustrate how much preparation and planning is necessary.

➤ Ensure that the health professional knows that they can stop whenever they wish.

➤ Ensure that *positive feedback only* will be given initially, no matter how hard that might be.

➤ Make sure that the group do not feed back any negative points.

➤ Only after the positive points have been covered, allow the group to share other ways that the interaction might have been completed.

➤ Be careful at this point, because negatives will often emerge when you look at different ways of addressing the issues.

➤ Stop and start the session after only short intervals – when there are useful learning points.

➤ Ensure that the emphasis is on the group, and not the role-players, to find different approaches and recognise the skills.

➤ Never have a participant play the opposite gender, as it is not possible to ask an individual to act credibly as someone of the opposite sex. (Always adapt the story, not the person!)

➤ Ensure that you notice all the non-verbal communication, including body language and paralanguage.

➤ Notice how much the listener is talking, and how much the 'character' is talking, and feed this back.

➤ Encourage the group to offer feedback, using the appropriate methods such as paraphrasing, summarising, understanding hypotheses, open questions, challenges, and so on.

➤ Have they picked up all the cues? What have they missed?

➤ Get the group to help to redirect the session (if necessary).

➤ Provide your feedback when the entire group has finished discussions.

These techniques need a great deal of skill and knowledge to be applied well, so it is important therefore to co-facilitate with someone who is clearly skilled in this approach. Also, have a supervisor (or a mentor) until you feel skilled and confident in teaching in this way.

As already mentioned, in many cases using actors is not possible, especially for those working in the NHS, where finding the money to pay actors is very difficult.

However, occasionally, and being very creative, you might find the money to show-case a special event, using actors to illustrate the effectiveness of this approach. The use of role-play and actors is also discussed in Chapter 20 (by Costello).

If using an actor for the first time, remember

● Actors, while able to act proficiently, must also be able to offer feedback appropriately.

● Do not assume that they can do this, because in many cases they cannot.

● Make sure that they are already trained, or gain their willingness to train them appropriately. (If they don't want to do this, do not use them.)

● The appropriate training is very important and usually time consuming. Don't forget that they will expect to be paid while doing this.

● If you are using actors, you must spend considerable time in briefing them. This includes briefing them regarding their role, the character's background, and also informing the actor if and when you expect them to ad-lib.

● Make sure they have comprehensive written briefing notes. (This is different to the 'Connected' initiative, because in 'Cancer Tales' they are playing a scripted part. However, later in the role-play, using the participants' agenda, they can move from scripted to unscripted acting.)

● Often actors are expected to be 'simulators', meaning that they respond (without a script) as a patient to what they receive from the professional. They still need a great deal of preparatory work to act in this way.

● Only ever use actors with a facilitator who is already skilled in using this approach.

● Ask a facilitator to supervise (or mentor) those who are new to these techniques, until they gain confidence and skills in using role-play and actors effectively.

Using actors and role-playing with health professionals are both ways in which the characters and the stories in *Cancer Tales* can be changed and developed further.

In *Cancer Tales*, it is probably easiest to use the group participants to read the stories and, if it becomes necessary, develop the stories further with short role-play scenes with different group members. The role-play is most helpful in developing the participant's skills, as well as focusing on important learning points for all the group members.

Advantages

➤ These methods are safe, because they allow practice away from the patients.

➤ If they are set up and facilitated effectively, they offer safe environments in which to learn.

➤ They allow maximum empathy, especially when health professionals participate in role-play.

Disadvantages

➤ For some participants, this approach produces a very high level of stress.

➤ It requires highly skilled, fully trained facilitators.

➤ If not run effectively, it can de-skill the participants.

MARKETING AND SHOWCASING *CANCER TALES*

'Only our kind of art, soaked as it is in the living experiences of human beings, can artistically reproduce the impalpable shadings and depths of life. Only such art can absorb the spectator, and make both understand and inwardly experience the happenings on the stage, enriching his inner life, and leaving impressions which will not fade with time.' (Stanislavski 1989)

Many aspects of patient care assume particular importance near the end of life – such as the experience of suffering, the need for human connection and non-verbal and emotional means of communication – and these are difficult to convey via traditional teaching methods. Unlike these approaches, drama can afford access to the personal dimensions of illness, demonstrating realistic complexity in relative safety (Lorenz *et al.* 2004).

The quotation from Stanislavski embodies the essence of a *Cancer Tales* perform-ance, which emotionally engages the audience and highlights the impact of poor communication skills and care delivery in the cancer care setting. *Cancer Tales* as a theatrical production lends itself particularly well to humanistic teaching.

It is vital to gain the backing, support and interest from managers, colleagues and 'would be' students. This type of venture is not always seen for the benefits it could provide, but more often as entertainment which leads to learning – but then who said learning should not be fun? So, perhaps the first step is to get people curious. If it is possible to market a one-off session, where people can come along and really see for themselves the power of the story and the effects it has on health professionals, it might enthuse them and galvanise them into action.

This approach has been a positive experience for the authors, and for others who have also used this route. The photos shown in Figures 2.3 and 2.4 are taken from one of these workshops, where three actors were used to bring the material to life. They played the various characters from *Cancer Tales*, and as they bring the characters to life, there is seldom a dry eye in the room.

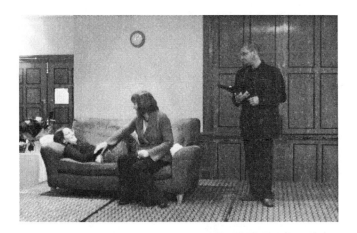

FIGURE 2.3 Actors bringing the *Cancer Tales* material to life

Inviting all interested parties, and introducing *Cancer Tales* by explaining its back-ground and the planned approach, is the first step of an action plan. The second is to truly engage healthcare professionals by using these types of professional actor. This might be achieved by gaining sponsorship for a one-off event. The company who sponsored the development of *Cancer Tales* is committed to supporting this com-munications training initiative and is usually very generous in this manner. It is also beneficial to use the same actors as other facilitators in the area or network. This will keep the cost down, by having only once to invest in the actors' learning of their lines, and having rehearsals. Once the actors know the general approach, they are usually quite adaptable. If the facilitator is going to use actors for role-play, ensure that these actors are trained and conversant in giving constructive feedback. This approach it is always well received, and could even be used with patient groups.

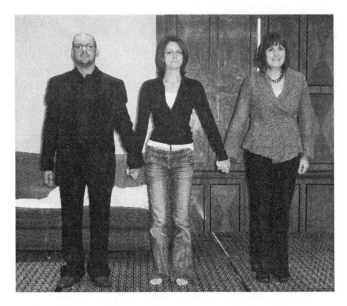

FIGURE 2.4 Having appropriately prepared actors is always well received

KEY POINTS

■ A variety of methods for the delivery of communications training must be available to meet the needs of different learning styles and levels of staff, and to begin to address changing participants' attitudes.

■ Appropriate research has an important part to play in examining the benefit of new initiatives such as *Cancer Tales*.

■ The national perspective on communications training needs to incorporate the different creative approaches (like *Cancer Tales*) that are being run by experienced facilitators around the country.

■ When new creative approaches have been found to be successful (audited and researched), a database could be set up which illustrates good practice.

■ A variety of teaching methods can be used in conjunction with *Cancer Tales*.

■ Highly skilled facilitation is crucial in the delivery of this exciting new educational venture.

CONCLUSION

The authors were asked by Napp Pharmaceuticals to help to develop a project which would assist in the *Cancer Tales* book being brought to life by experienced health professionals, and in creating a proactive learning strategy that would *not* be consigned to dusty shelves. The authors have run workshops for those experienced in communications and teaching, to explore and share ways that they might enrich their teaching by using *Cancer Tales*. It is hoped that this chapter has gone some way to further that same goal.

The main emphasis of this chapter has been, as stated at the outset, to illuminate the *Cancer Tales* workbook as a tool for teaching communications skills. Researchers, educators and national strategists all need to connect and 'communicate' effectively. There is a need for that 'joined-up thinking' at a much higher level. By continued research, auditing and engaging in productive dialogue, the solutions might already be there. So, there is a need for re-energised reciprocity, networking and the cascading of new knowledge in this area. Finally, combining all the expertise, commitment and compassion, initiatives such as *Cancer Tales* will be 'illuminating', demonstrating diversity in educational approaches and making a difference to practice.

IMPLICATIONS FOR THE READER'S OWN PRACTICE

1   How might you utilise *Cancer Tales* in your working practice?
2   To what extent do you use drama in your 'existing teaching tool bag', and how might you develop this for the future?
3   What new creative approaches can you take away from this chapter and adapt?
4   Which excerpts of *Cancer Tales* can you use as part of your existing portfolio?
5   Analyse the possible barriers to introducing this package to your own environment, and how you might over overcome them.

REFERENCES

Burnard P (2005) *Counselling Skills for Health Professionals*. 4th ed. Cheltenham: Nelson Thornes.

Castle R (1998) *Now and Then: an autobiography*. London: Robson Books.

Department of Health (2008) *High Quality Care for All: NHS next stage review final report*. London: DoH.

Department of Health (2008) *End of Life Care Strategy: promoting high quality care for all adults at the end of life*. London: DoH.

Department of Health (2007) *Cancer Reform Strategy*. London: DoH.

Department of Health (2000) *The NHS Cancer Plan: a plan for investment, a plan for reform*. London: DoH.

Dunn N (2002) *Cancer Tales*. Cambridge: Mundipharma International Ltd.

Egan G (1977) *You and Me: the skills of communication and relating to others*. Monterey, CA: Brookes/Cole.

Fallowfield L, Saul J, Gilligan B (2001) Teaching senior nurses how to teach communication skills in oncology. *Cancer Nursing*. **24** (3): 185–91.

Fallowfield L, Jenkins V (1999) Effective communication skills are the key to good cancer care. *Eur J Cancer*. **35** (11): 1592–7.

Fellows A (2009) Teaching communication skills to cancer and palliative care professionals: questions, challenges and debates. In: Foyle L, Hostad J, editors. *Illuminating the Diversity of Cancer and Palliative Care Education*. Oxford: Radcliffe Publishing.

Kelsey S (2005) Improving nurse communication skills with the cancer patient. *Canc Nurs Pract.* **4** (2): 27–31.

Lorenz KA, Steckhart M, Jilisa M, Rosenfeld KE (2004) End of life using the dramatic arts: the Wit educational initiative. *Acad Med.* **79** (5): 481–6.

Maguire P, Faulkner A, Regnard C (1993) Handling the withdrawn patient: a flow diagram. *Palliat Med.* **7**: 333–8.

McClimens A, Scott R (2007) Lights, camera, education!: the potentials of forum theatre in a learning disability nursing program. *Nurse Educ Today.* **27**: 203–9.

McGill I, Brockbank A (2003) *Action Learning Handbook.* London: Kogan.

National Audit Office (2005) *Tackling Cancer: improving the patient journey.* London: NAO.

National Institute for Clinical Excellence (2004) *Improving Supportive and Palliative Care for Adults with Cancer.* London: NICE.

Pollard A, Swift K (2003) Communication skills in palliative care. In: O'Connor M, Aranda S. *Palliative Care Nursing: a guide to practice.* Oxford: Radcliffe Publishing.

Relf M, Heath B (2007) Experiential workshops. In: Wee B, Hughes N, editors. *Education in Palliative Care: building a culture of learning.* Oxford: Oxford University Press.

Reynolds W, Scott PA, Austin W (2000) Nursing empathy and the perception of the moral. *J Adv Nurs.* **32** (1): 235–42.

Speigel D (1994) *Living Beyond Limits: new hope for people facing life threatening illness.* New York: Random House.

Stanislavski C (1989) *An Actor Prepares.* New York: Routledge.

FURTHER READING

• *Cancer Tales: communicating in cancer care workbook.*

Copies of the workbooks are available online at www.cancertales.org

ACKNOWLEDGEMENTS
The authors of this chapter wish to thank Nell Dunn and Trevor Walker, the European Association for Palliative Care (EAPC), the European Oncology Nursing Society (EONS), the Lance Armstrong Foundation (LAF), Open Minds, the European working party and of course Mundipharma International Ltd. Without their creativity, hard work and generosity this excellent communications workbook would not be available to enrich the teaching and learning of those working in this specialist field.

3

Telling stories in cancer and palliative care education: enigmatic, infinite mystery or trusted teaching techniques?

Lorna Foyle

'Storytelling is fundamental to the human search for meaning. The past empowers the present, and the groping footsteps leading to this present mark the pathways to the future.'

Mary Catherine Bateson (2001)

AIM

This chapter aims to capture the impact, influence and power of storytelling in cancer and palliative care education.

LEARNING OUTCOMES

By the end of this chapter, the reader should be able to:

- explore the concept of storytelling and its relationship to cancer and palliative care education
- explore the range of uses for storytelling in healthcare, cancer and palliative care education
- identify similarities and differences between storytelling and narrative discourses
- identify the potency and disadvantages of using stories in delivering cancer and palliative care education
- discuss the craft of storytelling and its relevance to cancer and palliative care educators
- stimulate their own creativity in using stories as an educational tool in cancer and palliative care settings.

INTRODUCTION

No story sits by itself. Sometimes they meet at corners and sometimes they cover one another completely, like stones beneath a river (Albom 2003: 8). This description of a story provides a concise summary of a tale which does not unfold in isolation but sits alongside or within other stories and, perhaps more significantly, is a constituent part of a far greater, ultimate story. The metaphor of stones on the riverbed can be likened to the unique experiences that each individual encounters within their life which are influenced and moulded by their contact with other people's stories. The human quest for meaning can be compared to how their story relates to the force and flow of the river; that is, pondering what their unique contribution to life and mankind might be. This is my own unique interpretation of the opening metaphor in this chapter. In neuro-linguistic programming terms, it can be whatever the reader chooses it to be. This chapter will be written in the first person. This is done purposefully in order to eliminate the constraints and rigours of academic writing and illuminate the power of storytelling. The use of the first person can be useful in many contexts (Webb 1992).

In everyday life, stories and metaphors abound. Each of us can recount stories in which we have been involved or that have been passed on to us from our circles of family, friends and colleagues, and even fleeting encounters with passing strangers can become the substance of personal legend. From the stories we tell and hear told, new stories evolve or emerge from exposure to varied experiences on a daily basis. This later may be repeated and integrated into individual present and future life biographies. The stories that each of us relates have the capacity to convey information, provoke profound emotion, stimulate humour, motivate and initiate great change along with other equipotent effects. These powerful reactions can be induced in a more focused way by relating specific stories that are designed to connect with the listener. Most people ingenuously regale their stories to those who will listen, oblivious of the potential responses that may be evoked. There are professions that deliberately utilise storytelling as an inherent part of their professional and personal development and such activity is considered a core constituent of their education processes. The healthcare professions are a prime example of where storytelling is consciously and unconsciously utilised during training and continuing professional development.

Stories and metaphors form a large part of the activities of educationalists from the caring professions, which include nursing, medicine, allied medical practice, counselling, psychotherapy, social work and volunteer caregiving. These stories tend to include patients' experiences but are quite definitely recounted from the professional's perspective. They are generally selected because of their impact on professional practice and the level of personal connection and involvement felt by the storyteller.

Patients and carers have their stories, too. These stories will reflect the individual's experiences of illness and their exposure to the prevailing healthcare service provided. These narratives can be heard often in public arenas or in the remotest and quietest of places.

Whatever their role in a healthcare story, each person involved will have their own unique perspective on the events and may describe them differently. Stories about healthcare and illness are arguably the most frequently related topic in contemporary society.

Similarly, cancer stories where patients go on to recover tend to be one of the most popular subjects to reach the public domain and are usually recounted by those who have undergone the illness and treatment experience. In contrast, individuals affected by the diagnosis of a life-limiting illness and who face imminent death are less likely to reveal their experiences quite so publicly; they are more selective about divulging their story, choosing the audience, time and place to do so. These types of narratives are often recounted by professionals who work in close proximity to dying people and who have been involved in the provision of their care.

Stories have more specific applications in the provision of healthcare. These applications can include the therapeutic use of storytelling in psychotherapy (Banks-Wallace 1998) or, as is more relevant to this chapter, as a teaching tool in the delivery of formal or informal healthcare education. Although this chapter does not consider the therapeutic use of stories in the care of patients and carers affected by a diagnosis of cancer or life-limiting illness, it is worthwhile to note that while stories cannot heal the body they can often bring some elements of comfort and meaning to the lives of those individuals who face death. The therapeutic use of story may provide the opportunity to acquire a new skill or resurrect a discarded ability by healthcare professionals delivering highly sensitive support and care to an extremely vulnerable population. Surely, it is an ambition worth pursuing.

The specialities of cancer and palliative care education particularly benefit from the propitious use of stories by clinicians and teachers. Like all clinicians and educationalists, I have produced this chapter as a result of my encounters with patients, carers, colleagues, students, family, friends and acquaintances as they have contributed to my unfolding story.

The subjective nature of this material is crucial for gaining meaningful insight into these stories. The stories may then become an itinerant part of the reader's own learning and narrative journey.

BACKGROUND

According to *Chambers Dictionary* (1998), 'story' is defined as a legend, a narrative of incidents in their sequence, a fictitious narrative, a tale, anecdote, legend or history. The definitions of 'narrative' that appear in the same dictionary are as follows: that which is narrated, a story; a written or spoken account or a series of events in the order in which they occur. According to this source, one apparent difference between these two definitions appears to be that stories can recount fictitious events whereas narratives can outline personal and actual events. While this is a tenuous distinction, it will not be extensively explored in this chapter. Metaphor is usually an integral part of storytelling. 'Metaphor' is defined as a word or phrase, story or action which literally denotes one thing but by analogy suggests another (Cade 1982). Metaphor is very personal and individual and, in the context of healthcare, seems to be common in relation to illness (for example, cancer) (Spall *et al.* 2001). The metaphor is used by patients to cope with illnesses with incapacitating effects (Sontag 1978), subsequent treatments and impending death. Metaphors are routinely used as part of a therapeutic process enabling patients or clients to explore, express and understand problems from a personal perspective (Spall *et al.* 2001). Metaphors are intricately woven into the fabric of stories and have similar enabling processes in the provision of education.

Frank (2000) proposes that stories can be delivered in either of two ways – that is, oral tradition or written narrative – or in both. Story and narrative are often used interchangeably, however, people do not tell narratives, they tell stories. 'Let me tell you a narrative' sounds strange (Frank 2000). For the purpose of this chapter, this interpretation will be used to distinguish between the written word (narrative) and oral delivery (story). This poses a paradox for me, in that, in order to explore the nature of oral storytelling, I am required to discuss the issues through the medium of the written word. The range of definitions surely depicts the numerous perspectives that are held on the subject of storytelling. Edwards (1997) suggests that all narrative can be viewed as story.

Storytelling remains an age-old tradition that continues to serve many purposes in the world today and is gaining recognition as an important tool utilised in the provision of healthcare and healthcare education. Storytelling can be differentiated from everyday communication as having three components: the story itself, be it real or imagined; the process, that is the telling of the story; and finally the oration, the way in which the story is told (Rosen 1985). The articulation of stories is an important facet in the conveyance of information. It is not enough to just read a story (ibid.). Reading of the printed word eradicates many spontaneous qualities such as tone, pitch, variation of pace, eye contact, gestures, mannerisms, facial expressions and other subtle personal characteristics (Rosen 1988).

The creation and telling of stories has been used universally by individuals, groups, communities and cultures to provide meaning, hope, purpose and understanding in life. The word 'story' derives from the Greek and means knowing, knowledge and wisdom (Yoder-Wise and Kowalski 2003). This is the intended outcome that storytellers aspire to in the educational setting.

Written narratives used in educational provision can include the case study, history-taking and reflective practice. Reflection is used as a teaching strategy to promote experiential learning and to integrate theory and practice (Padmore 2007). Teaching reflective practice will be discussed in more detail in Chapter 6.

Another way of using stories that has gained popularity in twenty-first-century teaching and is more often considered a therapeutic tool in healthcare is described as bibliotherapy. It requires clients to have reading and writing abilities. Bibliotherapy consists of a selection of reading that has relevance to a person's life and the issues they may be facing. The recommended literature and stories tend to connect with our innate ability to identify with others and may often prompt a cathartic episode or a release of inner emotions. Bibliotherapy has been used by therapists to promote inner healing. Teachers often provide students with lists of appropriate novels, biographies and poetry so that they may gain insight into the impact that illness has on individuals and their carers. This relies on the student's being committed to reading the appointed text, although cancer and palliative care educationalists may read selections of these works in the classroom setting. This type of literature often transfers to the media of film and television and can become yet another valuable resource for cancer and palliative care teachers. Healthcare educationalists will recommend biographies and novels that give particular perspectives to their speciality. In cancer and palliative care, such books are in abundance. Not all patients suffering from cancer will be cured physically, but poetry can bring about a sense of healing that gives patients and carers an opportunity to reflect and experience spiritual growth (Robinson 2004). Bibliotherapy is now used by a number of people who are recommended to it by their general practitioners and the designated reading is housed in the local library (Morrison 2008). It is used by local health authorities so that individuals may experience an element of healing, by the alleviation of either suffering or mental anguish. There is a paucity of research as to the effectiveness of bibliotherapy but it is certain that most stories will stimulate some response, be it negative or positive.

The types of stories that are common in healthcare education include real life stories, which later become case studies. These can include stories which may or may not include real people and the occasional hypothetical story – for example, made-up scenarios. It has been observed that students prefer real or true stories rather than hypothetical stories (Fairbairn 2002).

Case stories can become case studies from the experiences of healthcare practitioners and are used in teaching students from all backgrounds, both in the clinical and more formalised educational institute settings. Stories that examine case management can epitomise logical deduction, judgement, decision-making and clinical practice knowledge and understanding; sharing the constituents of these develops expertise with students (Cox 2001). During a teaching session the teacher may notice some topic worth bringing to the students' attention, perhaps when it becomes apparent that it relates to something not yet experienced or witnessed by a member or members of that group. Case studies based on a patient's story and the teacher's involvement may be formal and prepared prior to a teaching session. This form of teaching tool invites participation from all the students as appropriate; diagnostics, decision-making, case reasoning and clinical skills are developed by drawing knowledge and understanding from previous cases which in turn can be used for planning best care in future scenarios. This perspective is reinforced by nurse teachers who perceive that the term 'case study' is viewed as safe and is expected of a good teacher in a university (Hamer 2004).

In nursing, stories have deliberately been used to teach topics such as ethics, cultural sensitivity and communication skills (Davidhizar and Lonser 2003). Other stories often emerge spontaneously during a teaching session in response to a student's participation or their demonstration of a deficit in specific knowledge. These stories are often categorised as anecdotes, which can be used in a variety of ways.

Anecdotes can relate the beliefs of specific societies, by elucidating the obstacles and barriers that confront heroes and heroines and subsequently how these can be overcome. These stories may contain subtexts of warnings of excessive overconfidence or mistaken assumptions and impulsive judgements (Cox 2001) and are often delivered by the teacher as an antidote to similar characteristics exhibited in the current batch of students. However, in contrast to the case study, anecdotal stories are viewed by nurse teachers as carrying an associated risk of inappropriateness, including inappropriateness of tone (Hamer 2004).

Clinicians are constantly using the oral format of storytelling, whether by expressing their part in a patient's story at a case presentation or recounting it as part of a clinical teaching session.

A major part of any clinician's training includes listening to each patient's stories by eliciting from them their perspective of events at the time the clinician encounters them. This is described by medical practitioners as history-taking and by nurses as nursing assessment. This task is crucial to future interpersonal relationships and interactions between healthcare professionals and patients and carers. Individuals live their stories and in sharing them will modify them, reaffirm them and produce new ones. Interpretations of experience are constantly changing. Healthcare professionals, by attentive listening, are provided with an opportunity for active participation in each individual's unfolding story and can demonstrate interest by asking appropriate questions. Some of these questions may be pertinent to the assessment process. Other questions may not have relevance to the assessment process but may offer an opening to connect with patients at a deep and profound level. The knowledge gleaned from these types of questions will extract different facets of patients' and carers' stories. These differences may be infinitesimal but can eventually have significant impact on the quality of care and support they will receive.

> 'Story has a powerful capacity for revealing the significance of the trivial.' (Livo and Reitz 1984: 108)

Equally importantly, there is a unique opportunity to formulate a rapport and develop an empathetic understanding of their unique and unfolding situation. Although story-telling is applicable to all sectors of healthcare provision and education, the specialities of cancer and palliative care are awash with stories and anecdotes.

STORYTELLING IN CANCER AND PALLIATIVE CARE EDUCATION

Storytelling is the perfect vehicle to illustrate some of the key features that embody the delivery of high standards of oncology and palliative care. After all, we live and die in story (Stanworth 2004). It enables oncology and palliative care educators to illustrate complex case management and issues around dying that require sensitive communication. Furthermore, it is an opportunity to encourage students to participate in listening to their patients' stories. It can be a powerful and enjoyable way for teachers to teach and students to learn about issues in oncology and palliative care (McNeilly *et al.* 2008). Different spaces invite the exploration and telling of different stories (Jennings 2005). Generating deliberate opportunities within an educational curriculum is one way of appealing to learn through the process of storytelling (McNeilly *et al.* 2008).

Storytelling addresses the needs of students with different learning styles and can facilitate the development of higher-level thinking skills. It provides an opportunity for productive interaction between learners and teachers while developing knowledge, understanding and insight into the speciality of palliative care. Storytelling has the potential to build intrinsic motivation, self-esteem and curiosity, even in healthcare professionals who find palliative care a difficult area to work in. In cancer and palliative care education, it is important that the implications of working in this sensitive area are responsive to the needs of each group of healthcare learners.

Storytelling is the ideal medium to generate individualised and group learning. You cannot know what goes on in the learner's mind but, if you perceive the 'pattern' of a story and understand that it could be useful to them at this specific point in their learning, then that is reason enough to tell it (Deikman 1982). The learner's unconscious, creative imagination will seek and find the 'meaning' relevant to their learning situation. No explanation, no direct statement of a story's meaning can substitute for the way it impacts on the hearer's perceptions. Stories can help learners to adapt their views about caring for dying patients by enhancing their flexibility of thought. Similarly, by suspending routine healthcare provision constraints, stories can help heighten student awareness and fuel their imagination with the energy necessary to attain their learning outcomes.

As somebody who has employed this strategy in clinical and educational settings, I have been aware of how storytelling attracts students' attention and engages them in the learning process. I have always been enthralled by how stories can help people to grow and change. There are individuals who weave a story into their teaching which leaves you constantly reappraising the issues and reviewing the slightest nuances, long after the story has been told, and their special skills have similarly inspired me. Like most teachers, I want to give my students the best experience possible and want to improve my own storytelling skills so that my stories are deemed memorable.

I recently embarked on a specific project to attain a master practitioner certificate in neuro-linguistic programming (NLP) which focused on modelling excellence (more information on this topic is available in the next chapter). The aim of this project was to improve my storytelling skills when teaching topics specific to cancer and palliative care. As the project progressed, there developed a realisation that many of the skills required to tell stories can apply to other, more generic topics in the delivery of healthcare education.

However, there are special considerations in telling stories about death and dying. These include age, prior experiences of the learners and their existing knowledge and understanding. The main aim of this project was to identify a model of excellence in the art of storytelling. In order to acquire these skills and teach others to tell suitable stories in their teaching, I approached two nationally recognised palliative care lecturers who have a reputation for delivering a good story and connecting emotionally with their audience. I observed their teaching and conducted interviews after their teaching sessions. The next section of this chapter outlines some of the findings.

RESULTS OF STORYTELLING STUDY IN PALLIATIVE CARE EDUCATION

The palliative care teachers identified worked in two different areas of England and from henceforth will be referred to as Bob and Jan. I negotiated to observe them in their own institutional settings. The sessions that I observed of both teachers were on specific palliative care subjects. Although these sessions focused on palliative care, they dealt with completely different topics. Bob's session was about nursing dying patients and being near to death while Jan's session focused on breaking bad news to patients who are not fully aware that they are dying.

I interviewed both teachers after completion of their scheduled session. One of the key pieces of information I wanted to find out was whether they used the same stories for particular palliative care sessions and what influenced them in using their selected stories.

These teachers admitted to having specific sessions where they used 'tried and tested' specific stories to set the scene and make appropriate learning points. Other stories in their repertoire would be accessed on a spontaneous basis in these sessions if certain group or individual reactions necessitated this. However, the original story remained a constant feature.

My observation records focused on stories that were a regular feature in these specific sessions and the follow-up interviews honed in on the choice of these stories. There were similarities in each orator's story. Particularly noteworthy was that the story they told recounted their own experiences in the provision of palliative care. Strikingly, each educator related an incident within their story that exposed their own vulnerabilities.

The teacher who is able to self-disclose may bring to students certain insights which they may not otherwise have gained about the uncertainty of real-life practice (Cox 2001) and the self-disclosure makes the teacher appear far more human. This discovery reflected the results found by Hamer (2004), whereby nurse teachers who told stories which included self-disclosure were seen as taking on a level of personal risk.

The stories that I heard from Bob and Jan were delivered in a humble and self-effacing way. By using stories in which they owned to not being able to cope initially in a clinical setting, the teachers demonstrated bravery and courage (Hamer 2004). This vulnerability of the teacher sets the scene and seems to establish a rapport with the group members almost instantaneously. Each facilitator explored their vulnerability in relation to a patient they had worked with and then adapted the process of telling the story to match or respond to the learning needs and emotional state of the individuals and group. At the two educational events I spoke to, a sample of students after each session observed. The size of the two groups was between 20 and 30. One group consisted of pre-registration students and the others were qualified oncology and palliative care nurses. Without exception, all the students I spoke to gave the impression that they thought the teachers were talking directly to them, indicating a high level of connectivity.

There were many other features in the delivery of the story that were critical to creating the right atmosphere. My observations of the teachers noted that they mainly used eye contact, body posture, gesture, facial expression, voice tonality and modulation. Even movement in front of the group across the floor space appeared to have significance and ensured that the story connected with each individual. Jan and Bob responded and adapted their stories to individual and group reactions. Both storytellers related their stories in such a way that I felt that they had unconsciously met the students' representational states and learning styles (*see* Chapter 4). Other aspects of the story content and delivery clearly provoked emotional responses. These included compassion, sadness (identified by the facial expression of the students) and association (nodding in agreement) in both sessions. The sadness was often lightened by Bob and Jan as they interspersed their stories with humour (identified by ripples of laughter). These humorous moments were deliberately introduced to lighten the mood as Bob and Jan identified their students' diminishing spirits (Morris and Page 2004).

Interviews with the lecturers provided useful information about the intention behind the stories and the delivery of the stories within the session. The observation and interviews stimulated me to develop a couple of models. The first model was to assist me in visualising the dynamics and interface between the group and teacher when stories are told. This model is outlined in Figure 3.1.

The second model was created to develop excellence in storytelling as part of an NLP master's project and as such is written with NLP concepts in mind. I now use that model to teach other healthcare professionals to improve their storytelling skills in one-day workshops.

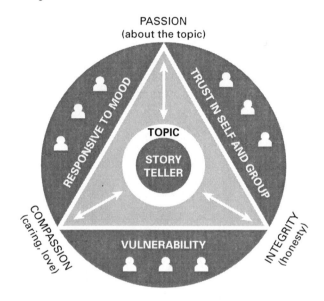

FIGURE 3.1 Model illustrating the interface between teacher and students when stories are delivered in a palliative care teaching session
© Lorna Foyle 2009

In the first model, as given in Figure 3.1, aspects represented can be explained as follows.

➤ The inner circle represents the storyteller's preparation. This includes purposively matching the story to the group, the learning outcomes and the group composition.

➤ The three points of the triangle represent the three qualities that need to be amalgamated to start and complete the process of storytelling. They are passion, integrity and compassion.

➤ Passion focuses on the story topic and the process of storytelling.

➤ Integrity builds on the relationship that is developed between the group and the teacher and the association they all feel with the story. This establishes a connection to the story as well as a connection between students and storyteller which is unique to the moment. Compassion is felt by the storyteller as he or she reconnects back into the scenario that is the essence of their story and relates it to the group. Consequently compassion is engendered in the students for the storyteller as well as for the individuals who reside within that story as the story unfolds.

➤ The outer circle represents an outer shield that is responsive to the needs of the storyteller and the group (ensuring self and group protection). Palliative care educators have to ensure individual, group and their own safety as stories may often unwittingly connect with people who may be experiencing distressing personal issues in their own lives. (Both teachers were keen to stress that the individual and personal safety and comfort were paramount to the success of the story and the session.)

➤ The people symbols represent the group as individuals and as a collective unit.

Observation and interviews with Bob and Jan seem to emphasise that the content and the style of delivering the story were of equal importance. So in palliative care storytelling, it appears that the content and process of telling the story have equal value.

SIGNIFICANCE OF THE STORYTELLING MODEL

At the heart of the model shown in Figure 3.1 is the storyteller.

The purpose of Bob's and Jan's stories was to get across some of the difficulties that the students might encounter in the palliative care setting and some of the qualities they may need to care for dying people appropriately. The purposive intention that these two storytellers illustrated in their stories was this: when caring for dying people, humility, flexibility, endurance and an ability not be judgemental are all crucial. Most importantly, the message that Bob and Jan conveyed was that healthcare providers need to demonstrate caring, humility and compassion during their interactions with the dying. Their own brand of humility was expressed by sharing how they had coped with dying people and broken bad news, not as competently as they would have liked, at the outset of their nursing careers. Their skills have clearly developed over time with a high level of training and extensive experience (Hostad 2004). The aforementioned qualities should be evident in caregivers to the individuals who are facing death. Expertise and knowledge will develop over time for those inexperienced in delivering palliative care but caring should be inherent in all caregivers. These qualities should translate into the provision of care and the way in which we communicate. This is something to which we all aspire but do not always achieve.

Stories have the potential to change people's perceptions and generate ideas and they can be a great form of communication. The use of stories can be the means by which an organisation creates a common identity by providing examples of good or bad behaviour or both (Snowden 1999). Putting these teachers' stories into context, their purposive stories contained both elements, good and bad, and created a common bond between teachers and students.

Stories with a purpose can be very powerful. There are likely to be common elements in stories used in the palliative care teaching context.

➤ They should be able to capture and hold the attention of the students. They should have relevance to the learning outcomes. They should stimulate curiosity and evoke responses in the students.
➤ Good stories perpetuate themselves and, although linked with an original storyteller, they should transfer to other palliative care educational settings where other storytellers can stamp their own identity on them.
➤ The stories should contain common characteristics and there should be some inherent values of the storyteller within the story.
➤ A good story can be told to all audiences regardless of educational background, role or experience, and all healthcare students should gain meaning from it at different levels.
➤ Stories and the metaphors they contain can provide new forms of understanding and should be relevant to most students in the learning group.

After observing and interviewing Bob and Jan, I realised that they both used purposefully selected palliative care stories which were delivered with fervour and immeasurable integrity. Most nurse teachers perceive telling stories as a performance to gain a reaction from the audience (Hamer 2004), but they should closely scrutinise their motives as they may be focused on entertainment rather than on the learning outcomes (Weimer 2002).

Stories evolve from a need to communicate our experience with other human beings. When educators teach, they need to talk not only about the subject at hand but also about their personal experiences related to that specific subject. This is how emotions are shared and how students become inspired to learn more about these topics.

When stories are heard we can be transported, together, outside of the present moment to another time and place. We live the experience of the storyteller through the use of our imagination and senses. Good storytellers inject emotion and meaning into the content. Stories bring the teller and listener together, via a personal connection to both the speaker and the topic. Storytelling is an experience to be shared by storyteller and story listeners; it is the interaction between the two that makes a story come to life!

Most palliative care nursing stories are based on true life experiences, as demonstrated by the palliative care educationalists I observed. My own stories certainly are. I relive the story outlined below with pre-registration and post-registration nursing students every time I tell it.

> 'As a newly appointed hospital Macmillan nurse, I can recall visiting a lady, Ethel, aged 74, who had a diagnosis of breast cancer with metastatic spread to her bones. She had been referred to me and this was my first visit. I went to talk to her about her future care after treatment in hospital. As I entered her room, she appeared distracted and somewhat confused. She pointed abstractedly round the room saying:
> "There they are", then looking at me. "Surely you can see them?"
> "See what?", I asked.
> "The dogs, the dancing dogs, just look at them; aren't they wonderful?"

I could not see the dogs and concluded that she was confused. I looked at her notes and checked her results and found that her recent blood results indicated high calcium levels. Diagnosing hypercalcaemia and after discussions with her multi-disciplinary team, I recommended that she be commenced on biphosphonates and fluids. It was agreed I would return when she was less confused. I did return later that week and the nursing team reported that she appeared a lot less confused.

I walked into the room she was in and started to initiate discussions around future care. As a throwaway line after I had introduced myself, I said:

"I did come before, but you weren't feeling very well because you could see dancing dogs all around the room."

Ethel gave me a knowing look, became quite agitated and demanded that I get her handbag out of her bedside locker. I did so immediately and she spent a couple of minutes rooting around what was a voluminous black bag. Then I heard a triumphant "Aha, take a look at these then" and she thrust towards me a packet of old black and white photographs. Each of the photographs showed a picture of dogs. All of the dogs had frilled collars and pointed hats. As my face started to portray some understanding she looked at me again and said, "My dogs are always with me."

As our discussion progressed, it emerged that Ethel in her youth had been a dog trainer and she had toured with a circus for many years with her renowned dancing dogs.'

I use this story to discuss the fact that however confused patients may seem, often the hallucinations they describe are embedded in reality (Stedeford 1994) and the patients need psychosocial understanding whatever their cognitive state and our belief state.

Returning to Bob and Jan, it was evident that these teachers were accomplished in the process of delivering a story. It seems that several factors are important to ensure a captivating presentation which engages the audience with the story. From feedback from these presenters, it was clear that they felt it important to prepare the session well and to ensure the story had significance to the student group. Some of the skills that were witnessed are outlined below.

➤ Modulation of voice tonality was used to create an atmosphere as the story progressed. This can have a great impact on how students connect with the teacher and the story.

➤ The use of gestures and facial expressions adds to the students' ability to associate with the story but must be congruent to the story. It is important to try to ensure that these gestures and expressions are appropriate and natural.

➤ Pacing is essential and involves both the volume and rate at which you speak, and consequently the progression of the story. In telling palliative care stories, silences were managed with great composure. Silence was used to emphasise a key point while allowing time for the students to connect with the stories and absorb the finer subtleties of the tale.

➤ Finally, once the story is finished it is important to stop! Do not digress but rather leave the students to their thoughts. Let them dwell over the story. Not everything has to be explained, or tied together. Allow loose ends. Let the students go away thinking about what has been said and not said, and let them draw their own meaning from it. They will approach you if they require clarification on any points.

Being passionate about the process of telling the story does warrant an investment in preparation time for the student and teacher to reap some hidden rewards and establish an almost intangible connection. The outcome should be worth all the hard work that is put into the preparation.

Disadvantages of using storytelling in teaching

Conversely, some teachers would see preparation time as a disadvantage (Rosen 1988), as it takes them away from other responsibilities. Thinking about the proportion of time that will be dedicated to stories in a session (Woodhouse 2007) can leave teachers feeling stressed and indecisive. Students can perceive the topic as threatening if it threatens their personal values (Fairbairn 2002), and they may feel vulnerable. As storytelling can be a powerful medium, the practice of storytelling should be pursued reflectively and with a critical eye (Strathie and Holmes 1996). The response of students may depend on their previous exposure to stories: they may love them or hate them (Woodhouse 2007). It may not complement every student's learning style. How stories are received is reliant on the commitment of the lecturer (Weimer 2002). The success or failure of storytelling does rest with the teacher as they aspire to command their audience's attention with the artistry of an accomplished craftsperson.

KEY POINTS

- Storytelling is inherent in all societies and cultures at a macro and micro level.
- In the literature, story and narrative are interchangeable.
- In healthcare, stories are used in a variety of ways including the clinical setting, psychotherapy, research and education.
- Metaphors are integral within stories.
- Oncology and palliative care educationalists utilise pre-determined stories for pre-planned teaching sessions. Other stories may be accessed in response to student participation.
- Planning the session is important to match the story to the needs of the student group and its context within the session itself.
- The story should be congruent for all and the technique of delivering the story is pivotal to its success and the students' learning.
- Storytelling can be used universally and is a simple and straightforward way of illuminating key issues in the specialities of oncology and palliative care.

CONCLUSION

This chapter has explored the advantages of storytelling in healthcare provision, more specifically in cancer and palliative care education. It has described the differences and similarities between narrative, metaphor, bibliotherapy, reflective writing, case study and storytelling. The planning of sessions with stories embedded in them is crucial.

Encouragement and training in the delivery of stories can enhance the experience for students and teachers and can generate lifelong memories. Stories are a powerful tool (Hamer 2004; Wee 2007) in the cancer and palliative care teacher's repertoire and understanding how to use then more effectively can produce a more meaningful and edifying response in the students we teach. They can be used to illuminate teaching or to set a scene and can provide a building block for active learning (Wee 2007).

Effective storytelling can be a great and exquisite art. A well-developed and presented story can cut across age barriers and experience and will hold the interest of its listeners as well as reaching out to them. Stories may well be remembered long after other teaching techniques. Knowing and applying the basics of storytelling will strengthen your stories. Most importantly, stories can give a voice to patients when they are no longer able tell their own stories and may go on to transform healthcare provision. Truly, it is possible to capture the enigmatic and infinite mystery of storytelling and it should be a trusted technique in the educationalist's portfolio.

> 'My story is important not because it is mine . . . but because if I tell it anything like right, the chances are you will recognize that in many ways it is also yours.' Frederick Buechner (1991)

IMPLICATIONS FOR THE READER'S OWN PRACTICE

1 What do patient stories mean to you?
2 How embedded are stories in your teaching practice?
3 How can you develop opportunities for students to use their stories in the classroom?
4 What skills do you need to acquire to feel confident in delivering stories in your teaching?
5 How would you motivate other healthcare professionals to use stories in their teaching?
6 How will you identify the impact your stories will have on your students?

REFERENCES

Albom M (2003) *The Five People You Meet in Heaven*. New York: Little Brown.
Banks-Wallace J (1998) Emancipating potential of storytelling in a group. *J Nurs Scholarsh.* **30** (1): 17–21.
Bateson MC (2001) *Composing a Life*. New York: Grove Press.
Bowles N (1995) Storytelling: a search for meaning within nursing practice. *Nurse Educ Today.* **28** (6): 1182–90.
Buechner F (1991) *Telling Secrets*. San Francisco, CA: Harper.
Cade BW (1982) Some uses of metaphor. *Aust J Fam Ther.* **3** (3): 135–40.
Chambers Dictionary (1998) Edinburgh: Chambers Harrap Publishers.
Cortazzi M (1993) *Narrative Analysis*. London: Falmer.
Cox K (2001) Stories as case knowledge; case knowledge as stories. *Med Educ.* **35**: 862–6.

Davidhizar R, Lonser G (2003) Storytelling as a teaching technique. *Nurse Educ.* **28** (5): 217–21.

Davidson MR (2003) A phenomenological evaluation: using storytelling as a primary teaching method. *Nurse Educ Pract.* **3**: 1–6.

Deikman A (1982) *The Observing Self.* Boston, MA: Beacon Press.

Edwards D (1997) *Discourse and Cognition.* London: Sage.

Fairbairn GJ (2002) Ethics, empathy and storytelling in professional development. *Learn Health Soc Care.* **1**: 22–32.

Frank AW (2000) The standpoint of storyteller. *Qual Health Res.* **10**: 354–63.

Frymier AB, Thompson CA (1992) Perceived affinity seeking in relation to perceived credibility. *Comm Educ.* **41**: 389–99.

Hamer S (2002) Telling stories. *Pract Dev Health Care.* **1** (1): 158–60.

Hamer S (2004) *Nurse Teachers' Perspectives of Their Use of Storytelling in the Teaching Context* [unpublished Ed.D thesis]. University of Leeds: Schools of Education and Continuing Education.

Hostad J (2004) An overview of hospice education. In: Foyle L, Hostad J, editors. *Delivering Cancer and Palliative Education.* Oxford: Radcliffe Publishing.

Jennings S (2005) *Creative Storytelling with Adults at Risk.* Milton Keynes: Speechmark Publishing.

Kelly B (1995) Storytelling: a way of connecting. *Nursingconnections.* **8** (40): 5–11.

Livo NJ, Reitz SA (1986) *Storytelling: process and practice.* Littleton, CO: Colorado Libraries Unlimited, Inc.

Maguire P, Faulkner A, Regnard C (1993) Handling the withdrawn patient: a flow diagram. *Palliat Med.* **7**: 333–8.

McNeilly P, Read S, Price J (2008) The use of biographies in paediatric palliative care education. *Int J Palliat Nurs.* **14** (8): 402–6.

Morris S, Page W (2004) Humour in cancer and palliative care: an educational perspective. In: Foyle L, Hostad J, editors. *Delivering Cancer and Palliative Education.* Oxford: Radcliffe Publishing.

Morrison B (2008) The healing power of reading. *The Guardian.* 5 January.

Padmore S (2007) Case study: a stilted tool or a useful learning and teaching strategy. In: Woodhouse J, editor. *Strategies for Healthcare Education: how to teach in the 21st Century.* Oxford: Radcliffe Publishing.

Relf M, Heath B (2007) Experiential workshops. In: Wee B, Hughes N, editors. *Education in Palliative Care: building a culture of learning.* Oxford: Oxford University Press.

Robinson A (2004) A personal exploration of the power of poetry in palliative care, loss and bereavement. *Int J Palliat Nurs.* **10** (1): 32–9.

Rosen B (1988) *And None of It Was Nonsense: the power of storytelling in school.* London: Mary Glasgow Publications.

Rosen H (1985) *Stories and Meanings.* Sheffield: National Association for the Teaching of English.

Schmidt-Bunkers S (2006) What stories and fables can teach us. *Nurs Sci Q.* **19**: 104.

Snowden DJ (1999) Story telling: an old skill in a new context. *Bus Inform Rev.* **16** (1): 30–7.

Sontag S (1978) *Illness as Metaphor.* Harmondsworth: Penguin.

Spall B, Read S, Chantry D (2001) Metaphor: exploring its origins and therapeutic use in death, dying and bereavement. *Int J Palliat Nurs.* **7** (7): 345–53.

Stanworth R (2004) *Recognising Spiritual Needs in People Who Are Dying.* Oxford: Oxford University Press.

Stedeford A (1994) *Facing Death: patients, families and professionals.* 2nd ed. Oxford: Sobell Publications.

Strathie L, Holmes CA (1996) Story as a reflective process for nurses. *Int J Nurs Pract.* **2**: 99–104.

Vezeau T (1993) Story telling: a practitioner's tool. *Am J Matern Child Nurs.* **18** (4): 193–6.

Weimer M (2002) *Learner-Centred Teaching: five key changes to practice.* San Francisco, CA: John Wiley and Sons.

Webb C (1992) The use of first person in Academic writing. *J Adv Nurs.* **17** (6): 747–52.

Wee B (2007) Teaching large groups. In: Wee B, Hughes N, editors. *Education in Palliative Care.* Oxford: Oxford University Press.

Woodhouse J (2007) Storytelling and narratives: sitting comfortably with learning. In: Woodhouse J, editor. *Strategies for Healthcare Education: how to teach in the 21st Century.* Oxford: Radcliffe Publishing.

Yoder-Wise P, Kowalski K (2003) The power of storytelling. *Nurs Outlook.* **51**: 37–42.

FURTHER READING

• Owen N (2001) *The Magic of Metaphor: 77 stories for teachers, trainers and thinkers.* Camarthen: Crown House Publishing.

USEFUL WEBSITES

www.patientvoices.org.uk
www.pilgrimprojects.co.uk
www.rbkc.gov.uk/libraries/bibliotherapy
www.timsheppard.co.uk/story

4

Finding human masterpieces: progressing cancer and palliative care education through neuro-linguistic programming

Lorna Foyle and Janis Hostad

'Some people say they haven't yet found themselves. But the self is not something one finds, it is something one creates.'

Thomas Szasz

AIM

This chapter intends to explore the basic tenets of neuro-linguistic program-ming (NLP) in context with contemporary healthcare provision, and more specifically to demonstrate its versatility in the speciality of cancer and palliative care provision and the education of healthcare professionals who provide patient care. This will include its application in the clinical settings and in educational processes to train staff.

LEARNING OUTCOMES

By the end of this chapter, the reader should be able to:
- gain knowledge and understanding of the principles of NLP in cancer and palliative care
- explore the applications of NLP in the delivery of cancer and palliative care across a range of healthcare settings
- explore how the teacher might use NLP techniques to be more eloquent and effective in the training of a cancer and palliative care workforce
- discuss how different NLP approaches can improve cancer and palliative care provision via education.

INTRODUCTION

In writing this chapter, the authors have set out to present an overview of NLP and its specific application in the execution of best practice in cancer and palliative care. Alongside this goal, it is intended to explore some of the NLP techniques that can be creatively employed as teaching tools to educate those healthcare professionals that provide that care.

For those of you already acquainted with NLP, this chapter will not explore the complete range of techniques but select those that the authors have experienced success with, both in the classroom and in clinical setting. The concept of NLP may be completely new for some readers. To all of you, they (Janis and Lorna) ask only that you embrace and work with the concepts and ideas in this chapter in the spirit that they are intended. The chapter will focus on NLP concepts of representational systems, rapport, reframing and well-formed outcomes, with the inevitable foray into other NLP topics. Most of the areas covered here are written about extensively, and are widely available in other books. Unique to this chapter will be discussions by one of the authors (Janis) on developing an NLP model. This model was created to meet oncology healthcare professionals' supervisory needs. The main purpose of the project was to train clinical supervisors to facilitate group supervision. This project was developed so that all grades of staff have access to supervision in a modern cancer centre. This NLP model was designed as part of the project to help supervisors establish and maintain trust during a supervisory session. The details of this rapport model will be explored in greater detail later in the chapter.

Teachers in the speciality of cancer and palliative care generally know what they want to pass on, what they consider is important for them and their students. Most of us involved in education in this speciality generally connect unhesitatingly with our own moral code, ethical beliefs and values in the conveyance of knowledge. The purpose behind our teaching should incorporate these values. The inclusion of essential information is of paramount importance, but more often it is our ability to influence learners that is neglected. Developing highly visible and caring approaches to communicating with patients and carers should be uppermost in the teacher's mind and behaviour, and should be imperceptibly transmitted to the students. The use of NLP in a teaching environment empowers teachers to persuade students in a creative and illuminating way and enhances interpersonal and intrapersonal effectiveness of student and teacher alike.

BACKGROUND

In order to understand the benefits and limitations of utilising NLP in cancer and palliative care provision, this section of the chapter will focus on providing a description of NLP. The acronym 'NLP' refers to neuro-linguistic programming. NLP has been described as a theory, methodology and ways of thinking. It has been suggested that NLP can be pragmatic, practical and can initiate an innovative approach to improving communication to clients and consequently the development of professional and interpersonal relationships. NLP was first developed in the 1970s by Richard Bandler, a mathematician and psychologist at the University of California, Santa Cruz, and the then Assistant Professor of Linguistics, John Grinder. At the suggestion of the anthro-pologist Gregory Bateson, also a writer on cybernetics and communications theories, they decided to analyse the work of the leading communications experts of the time, which included Milton Ericson, Fritz Perls and Virginia Satir. Bandler and Grinder studied these and other communicators and therapists who had achieved consistently good results with clients who had formerly been labelled 'difficult'. These experts were then 'modelled' and specific patterns of thinking, language and behaviour were iden-tified as making a profound difference in the context of communication and change. These patterns of thinking, language and behaviour are easily taught, and are believed to enhance effectiveness across a variety of contexts. NLP is used in diverse areas to allow people to develop new levels of competence. It is used internationally in fields such as sports, business, healthcare counselling and education.

NLP draws upon many different disciplines and ways of thinking in addition to the original contributions from the early research. It has been described as advanced common sense, and people who encounter it in its purest form for the first time have been reported as recognising elements of NLP that are familiar to them already.

Today NLP is used in many different contexts, including management, leadership, communication, relationships, negotiation, education, managing change, conflict resolution and psychotherapy. Yet little research has been conducted into the specific outcomes of using NLP in some of the aforementioned areas. Additionally, the generic nature of NLP skills has meant that little is published in a way that is made directly rel-evant to healthcare professionals. One exception is a brief series of papers and debate in the *British Medical Journal* by Walter and Bayat (2003). Further peer-reviewed research is required to assess whether NLP may be of any benefit in the specialities of cancer and palliative care, although there are signs that more research within these areas is emer-ging. Claire Rushworth, who died unexpectedly, was an early pioneer and author in utilising NLP techniques with patient and carers in a cancer centre in Leeds. She then moved on to educating and helping healthcare professionals who provided care.

An exploratory study undertaken by Sargent *et al.* (2004) looked at a living with cancer project. The study sought to evaluate the delivery of a cancer patient and carer peer support group facilitated by NLP trainers who gave education and interventions when appropriate. In addition, a four-day NLP training course for healthcare profes-sionals designed to improve their communications skills was evaluated. Despite the overwhelming positive response in the peer support group, particularly about com-munications skills and relaxation training, many of the patients remained sceptical about NLP interventions (Sargent *et al.* 2004). Adapting NLP training to make it more relevant to the issues of cancer patients and carers would be one way of surmount-ing this problem, while another would be to use NLP trainers who are also oncology healthcare professionals, as the authors of this chapter indeed are. Janis and Lorna have run many NLP workshops for cancer and palliative care staff across the country and have found that being able to contextualise the NLP to this speciality has been imperative. Having the same background as the staff you are teaching is vital, to *pacing*, *matching* and gaining *rapport* quickly. While it is not impossible to teach these skills without this background, it is so much easier to be able to apply NLP in the context of healthcare, where there is a shared philosophy and baseline of knowledge. Being aware of the techniques and approaches which are most likely to work best with cancer and palliative care patients is undoubtedly a bonus.

NLP is just one of a multitude of approaches to communications skills acquisition. It provides a model for understanding the processes of communication and aims to provide options for developing flexible communications approaches. The characteristics of NLP include the encouragement of an adaptable, reflexive and outcome-focused approach to communication. NLP includes specific tools and techniques that aim to build rapport. These techniques seek to promote the fast creation of empathetic connections, to establish trust and understanding, while simultaneously promoting the management of internal emotional states. NLP also aims to provide strategies for releasing negative emotions, overcoming trauma and phobic responses and increasing control over emotional states (Rushworth 1994). Furthermore, NLP is characterised by a focus on language and aims to promote the use of specific and purposeful language patterns in particular contexts. In contrast to traditional counselling approaches, which assume weeks and months to produce gradual improvements, NLP tries to produce change much faster. The potential for a rapid response can prove useful for patients and health professionals alike in the increasingly time-pressured environment of the health consultation. This potential to speed up interpersonal communications and connect at a meaningful level with the client population is particularly salient in the speciality of palliative care, where time is limited as impending death approaches.

NLP is the study of the structure of the subjective experience. According to NLP, everything that people think, say or do – behaviours of excellence, talents and skills, all of this – has an underlying, recurring pattern. NLP implies that there is an underlying template which, when brought to a person's notice, can be changed, rearranged, even taught to someone else.

NLP looks at exploring how people do what they do. NLP challenges individuals who maintain their problems by repeating them over and over again. NLP is also about equipping people to perform differently, competently, in familiar and unfamiliar situations. This is emulated by reproducing inherent skills that some people have that help them to cope well or even excel. These skills can be extracted and put into a format that can be easily acquired by others.

The methodology that is used to do all this is called modelling. NLP builds cognitive and behavioural models of how successful people do what they do – how they behave, how they say what they say, how they think, and how their beliefs and values fit together in an enabling way (Walker 2002). NLP aims to enhance subjective awareness of interpersonal relationships and has been described as an 'operational epistemology' when employed in a robust ethical framework as it has several hallmarks that can contribute to clinician–client and educator–student interaction (Turnbull 1999).

WHAT IS NLP?

Neuro-linguistic programming as a concept is quite confusing. By dividing NLP into its component words helps to explain it.

➤ The *neuro* aspect is all about the mind and how it takes in and processes information.

➤ The *linguistic* element is all about how we use our language and how we label ourselves.

➤ *Programming* is a word left over from the days of the personal computer which has mirrored NLP's dramatic rise in usage over the years. Patterning might be a better word. Having taken in outside information (*neuro*), and talked to ourselves or others about what to do (*linguistic*), we then run a series of actions or behaviours designed to achieve our particular goal in that situation (*programming*). Our behavioural programmes may stem from the skill of excellence, doing things really well. However, we may run a negative pattern over and over again that leads to depression, or worse. This patterning element of NLP is the *order and sequence* of internal representations that lead to that particular behaviour – good or bad, liked or disliked, wanted or unwanted. If you know the sequence, you can change the order and thereby change the behaviour and the emotions accompanying them (Walker 2002).

REPRESENTATIONAL SYSTEMS AND RAPPORT

As the early researchers of NLP observed their 'subjects', they noticed that people tend to give away information about their unconscious processing in their eye movement patterns as well as in changes in their body posture (Dilts *et al.* 1980). Similarly gestures, fluctuating voice tone and breathing shifts were linked to sensory-based language: '*I see that clearly*', '*I hear what you are saying*' or '*let's remain in touch*'. These observations finally concluded that the foundations of all our experiences are composed of what we see, hear, feel, smell and taste – our five senses. The topic of NLP tends to use the words visual (V), auditory (A), kinaesthetic (K), olfactory (O) and gustatory (G) instead (VAKOG). Information coming from the outside world can reach us only in this way. Once inside, it passes through the various *internal filters*, such as our beliefs, values, memories and life experiences, among other things. This is our internal representation, which is how internal images, sounds, feelings, smells and tastes are constructed about outside events. The internal imagery that is triggered by our sensory experiences can produce real effects in our bodies and affect our capabilities in the real world. Patients, carers and healthcare professionals have their own style of speaking, their own unique way of selecting words and phrases that make up their verbal communications. When you can 'speak their language', it allows you to connect with them at a deeper level.

In the classroom or with teams it can be most enlightening to get them to fill in a predicate questionnaire and find out what their predominant predicates (senses) might be. When looking at team dynamics, it is interesting to see who works together best, based on whether they are mainly visual or kinaesthetic or whichever other predicate dominates.

Much discussion ensues as a result of participating in this exercise, on things that irritate them about colleagues, patients' relatives and even their own partners! As an example of this, one of the authors (Janis), who tends to wear 'very noisy, dangly earrings' does not hear them *at all* (she is predominantly kinaesthetic) although everyone else does, particularly her partner (who is predominantly auditory) who finds them most annoying!

While there are many factors which influence the words we use, one of the most significant relates to the five senses, although in NLP the three that are most likely to be used are visual, auditory and kinaesthetic. The visual modality contains a further sub-modality – that of associated and dissociated – which is very important and refers to whether or not you can see yourself in the picture (visual internal representation).

You are associated if you see the world through your own eyes. If you can see yourself in the picture, then we say you are dissociated.

If you are associated in a memory, then your feelings (happy, sad, fearful) about that memory will be more intense. It can be seen that being associated means you are fully aware of yourself including all of your personal values, emotions and feelings. Often you can see people smiling in a faraway trance-like state, and when you ask them they say that they are remembering a good experience; they might say 'I could almost feel the snow' or something similar. 'I could smell the sea air.' This would indicate that they were associated.

If you are dissociated, then you are seeing the world from the perspective of a dispassionate observer. This is more like watching a movie of your life rather than being there and any feelings will be less intense or not at all. This can be a helpful place to be when we are making logical decisions or dealing with conflict or challenges.

In the clinical setting, an example of this might be that a patient who is frightened of radiotherapy can learn to '*dissociate*' from the experience for the duration of the treatment. Patients can also be taught to do this when they find it too painful to be '*associated*' with their present experience – so much so that it prevents them from sharing their deeply troubling feelings. They can be taught to talk about these issues in a '*dissociated*' way, which makes it easier to share and does not feel quite so raw. It is important that students know this is possible, but also that it is imperative to undertake the proper training in order to become competent at this technique prior to working with patients.

This technique is not dissimilar to the techniques used by Kearney (1996) in *Mortally Wounded* when getting his patients to do image work and tell stories associated to the pictures that allow them to deal with their problems but in a 'dissociated' way. He describes their soul pain as 'the experience of an individual who has become disconnected and alienated from the deepest and most fundamental aspects of himself or herself'. For these individuals, being 'dissociated' can work effectively at 'reconnecting' them with themselves in a way that is acceptable to work through their pain.

This can also be a useful technique with nurses who are too involved and 'cannot see the wood for the trees' – to 'dissociate' from the situation may help them to be more objective and realistic about the situation.

The authors have used these techniques in many different ways, including as a relaxation technique where the patient is so associated to the experience that it allows them to truly relax and be free of the difficult, agonising and painful psychological issues related to their illness.

In an exercise in the final chapter in this book (Chapter 22, Exercise 1), Janis uses this technique but not labelled as such. It is an exercise where the participant is encouraged to '*associate*' into the loss situation in order to meet the outcome of the activity, empathising, understanding and contextualising the feelings and behaviours of loss.

In the domain of NLP, the way a person is thinking is revealed in the language they use. By paying close attention to a person's eye movements, you are able to determine which representational system they are using to access information. Once you are aware of which system your patients, carers and students are using, you can speak to them using their language patterns. Eye movements can be very useful in determining how our clients represent their world and will generate our response in any given interaction. Although much discussion abounds about NLP eye accessing cues, there are numerous anecdotal reports about its effectiveness. Unfortunately as yet there is insufficient evidence to support the claims made about it, though it is to be hoped that this will be rectified in the future with appropriate research. Eye movement cues assist us in accessing information and stored memories (*see* Figure 4.1). While the ensuing information does not hold true for all people, it can be applied to the majority of the population.

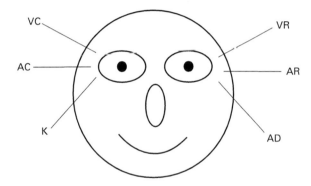

FIGURE 4.1 Eye accessing cues

These are the usual meanings of lateral eye movements – the illustrations assume that you are facing the other person (so that their left is your right).

Key

VR = **Visual Remembered**: Eyes up and to the left usually mean that a person is remembering something visually – 'Can you picture how your body was before your surgery?'

VC = **Visual Constructed**: Eyes up and to the right usually mean that a person is imagining (constructing) something visually. 'Can you just imagine what it's going to be like when chemotherapy is finished?'

- When eyes move up right or left, the individual tends to stand straight erect, and they can appear tense. They tend to use jerkier movements. Their breathing can appear shallow and be higher in their chest. They tend to speak more rapidly and their voice sounds higher pitched. The language they use will include words such as 'see', 'look', 'view', 'appear' and 'regard'.

AR = **Auditory Remembered**: Eyes left side (horizontal) usually mean a remembered sound – 'This pump is the one that makes the irritating buzzing sound when the chemotherapy is delivered.'

AC = **Auditory Constructed**: Eyes right side (horizontal) usually mean an imagined (constructed) sound – 'You will hear my voice though an intercom when you are in the MRI scanner.'

- When eyes are across the midline, the individual's posture and gestures are likely to include head tilted at an angle and rhythmic movements. Their breathing tends to be mid-chest and even. Their voice can sound melodic, rhythmic and medium paced. The language they use will include words such as 'hear', 'listen', 'sounds', 'cries', 'speak' and 'tell'.

K= **Kinesthetic**: Eyes down right usually mean that a person is accessing a bodily feeling or emotion – thinking and feeling about 'what having a cancer diagnosis means to them'.

- When eyes are looking down, usually to the right, the individual's posture may be more rounded and they tend to use flowing movements. Their breathing can be deeper, extending to their lower abdomen. The pitch of their voice will also be lower, deeper and sometimes slower. Some of the words they are likely to use can include 'grasp', 'concrete', 'firm', 'handle' and 'feel'.

AD = **Internal Dialogue – or sometimes classified as Auditory Digital**: Eyes down left usually means that a person is accessing internal dialogue. This is stimulated by questions such as 'What's going on in your mind at the moment?' This may generate a wealth of inner dialogue which can be detected by the healthcare professional by observing the eye moments and is typical at times of stress.

- When eyes are looking down, generally left, the individual is likely to fold their arms, have their head up and hold themselves erect. Their breathing may appear tighter and more restricted. Their voice may have a monotone timbre and their words may sound clipped. The words they are likely to use 'include', 'decide', 'understand', 'consider' and 'ponder'.

Sometimes, we may pay more attention to the commentary being conducted in our heads rather than to the interaction with patients, possibly to the detriment of both participants.

As with all generalisations, there are exceptions to the eye accessing cues process outlined above. Some left-handed people and a few right-handed people may have their cues reversed.

The more familiar clinicians and educationalists can become with eye accessing acuity and the words that people use, then the more clearly they will notice the way people are changing from one sensory system to another.

The representational system and sensory words that someone is favouring from moment to moment are part of their unique process of communication, while the subject they are talking about provides the content. As people tend to get engrossed in the content of their conversation, they are generally unaware of the processes they are using. This information will enable you to start getting into harmony with patients, carers, colleagues and students more readily. By operating at the process level, the healthcare professional can have a powerful unconscious effect by establishing a deep sense of rapport with their clients.

Having taught this in the classroom, we cannot expect that the students will walk away with this high level of skill, however, creating this awareness does seem to encourage many participants to carry on learning more, so that they can hone their skills later. The authors encourage the participants to at least learn to notice when the patient or loved one looks down during a sensitive conversation, so that an appropriate question can be posed and rapport maintained.

Examples of appropriate questions that maintain rapport

Say after bad news has just been broken and the health professional is trying to show empathy, he or she might say:

'That was an awful lot to take in and sadly not what you were hoping for.'

If the patient looks down right, the nurse having noticed this might ask:

'Your emotions must be all over the place, right now. Tell me about some of those feelings?'

Alternatively, if the patient looks down left, the nurse might ask:

'Your thoughts must be all over the place, asking yourself all sorts of questions, all sorts buzzing about in your head. Tell me some of what is going on in your mind right now?'

There is only a subtle difference, but a significant one if you are on the receiving end. It does not take long to acquire this skill through practice; this ability will eventually become second nature. Some individuals have much more obvious eye movements than others do; with the less obvious ones, it does take some time to see the more miniscule movements.

It can be useful to ask the students, having tried it in the classroom, to go away and practise this with family and friends and come back and report on their success. It is always important to prepare and focus prior to a significant conversation, when it is likely that this skill might be useful.

Rapport

The capability to match and synchronise on several levels of thinking and behaviour is the key to building rapport (Laborde 1998). The three main areas to concentrate on when building rapport are physiology, voice qualities and the words that people use (Walker 2002). There are two basic patterns for creating rapport; matching and mirroring. The term 'matching' is used to describe the precise duplication of an aspect of another's behaviour – for example, when crossing the right leg over the left leg. However, if this action is replicated by the left leg crossing over the right, it is described as mirroring. This matching and mirroring can occur at an unconscious level between two people when they are connected; they will stand in the same way, with posture and gestures either matching or mirroring each other. This is a natural and instinctive type of connection, although Turnbull (1999) suggests that in sustaining and establishing interpersonal relationships, rapport that appears instinctive can be attributed to substantial experience in the clinical setting and these subtle skills have moved into unconscious competence.

When matching, you should generally focus first on body language, then voice and finally the person's words. It was discovered that 55% of the impact of a presentation is determined by your body language, 38% by your voice and only 7% by the content or words that you use (Mehrabian and Ferris 1967). Body language includes body posture, facial expressions, hand gestures, breathing and eye contact. You should start by matching one specific behaviour and, once you are comfortable doing that, then match another and so on.

One exercise which is most effective for raising the group's awareness of non-verbal mirroring or matching is to ask two individuals to stand opposite each other and move their arms and try to stay synchronised. Then ask them to do the same with their eyes closed. They are usually very surprised by the results, with some couples amazingly being able to stay in synchrony with their eyes closed. This always leads to much discussion as to how that might happen (*see* Figure 4.2 photo).

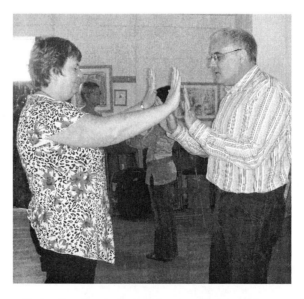

FIGURE 4.2 Non-verbal mirroring being maintained even with eyes closed

For voice, you can match tonality, speed, volume, rhythm and clarity of speech. All of us can vary aspects of our voice and we have a range in which we feel comfortable. If someone speaks very fast, much faster than you yourself do and at a rate at with which you would not feel comfortable, match this person by speaking faster while still staying within a range that is comfortable for you.

For words, match predicates. If the person you are communicating with is using mainly visual words, you should also use mainly visual words and similarly for auditory, kinaesthetic and auditory digital words. To some extent, you should also use the same words as the other person, although paraphrasing can be used. However, it should be remembered that individual interpretations of some words can be different. For example, someone might say that going to visit the hospice was 'tremendous'. In your model of the world, you may interpret 'tremendous' as meaning 'outstanding', implying an enjoyable experience, whereas the person saying 'tremendous' might have meant that visiting the hospice was for them a formidable and frightening experience. In this case, you would not be matching but mismatching the words.

Some people find the idea of matching another person artificial and contrived, and attempting to do so makes them feel uncomfortable. To overcome this uneasiness, it is useful to understand that mirroring and matching are a natural part of the rapport-building process and that you are doing it unconsciously every day with your close family and friends. Each day gradually increase your conscious use of matching, at a pace that is comfortable and ethical for you. Matching done with integrity and respect creates positive feelings and responses in you and others.

Rapport is the ability to enter someone else's world, to make them feel that you understand them and that there is a strong connection between the two of you. In the highly specialised areas of cancer and palliative care provision, the ability to swiftly establish a rapport with the patient and their carers is crucial. Different purposes require different degrees of rapport (Argylle 1983) – for example, intimate questions require a deeper rapport than simple information-gathering questions which can be undertaken at a superficial level.

Building and maintaining rapport in the classroom is axiomatic to a successful outcome. As Spohrer (2007) suggests:

> 'Keep building your rapport skills – aim for a symbiotic relationship with your pupils – you need them as much as they need you.'

Most readers will at some time, we are sure, have experienced a teacher who completely failed to connect with their group. When time is taken to establish rapport with the students, to truly get into the way they are thinking and behaving, it pays off. Communicating with them and leading them through learning, becomes so much easier.

The exercise below could be used with students learning how to get into rapport with their patients.

Exercise 4.1 Building rapport
Please work in threes to complete this exercise.

You (A) will try to match and mirror your non-verbal and verbal behaviours to your partner (B) and the third person (C) will act as an observer. The observer will use the observation sheet below and provide positive and constructive feedback to (A) before the triad members change places. On completion of this exercise, the whole group will feed back on the commonality and the differences in successful matching behaviours (or lack of them) in the triads. The whole group will discuss how they might overcome these difficulties to try to achieve the required outcome.

RAPPORT OBSERVATION SHEET

Behaviour or technique (matching and mirroring)	Tick or cross	Comments
Bodily movements, mirroring or mismatching		
Size of information chunks		
Volume of voice		
Pitch and tone of voice		
Pacing of voice		
On the same wavelength; tuned in; common ground		
Topic interest and context (situation and issues)		
Predicates (e.g. visual or hearing etc.)		
Breathing rates		

This form can also be used effectively as part of an educator's peer review, as mentioned above. However, the observer will then be looking for more eclectic abilities illustrating that they can pick up the general behaviours as well as being able to utilise a number of different techniques. For instance, regularly swapping to different predicates to ensure mass appeal, and the teacher showing that when students ask questions or comment, they can hone in on any student's specific behaviours by subtly matching and mirroring them.

Another NLP technique related to rapport is pacing. Bavister and Vicker (2008) define it as *'gaining and remaining in rapport with someone, by matching their map of the world through language, behaviour, beliefs and values'*. So pacing is the sum of these techniques plus the ability to continue to maintain rapport with the other person.

Example of using pacing techniques

O'Connor and McDermott (1996) illustrate pacing by telling a short story.

O'Connor's daughter was given a camera for Christmas and she spent many happy hours taking photos, however, when they were developed none of them was in focus and the young girl began to cry. He proceeded to tell her that it was her first attempt and it would be better in the future and, after all, the photos had all been taken indoors. This did not console the girl; in fact, she just cried and cried. Then he realised that he was not pacing her and he stopped and changed his approach. He said something along these lines:

> *'You spent so much time and effort in taking all those special photos. You must be so sad that you cannot see them now.'*

The little girl stopped crying and said;

> *'Yes, Daddy, I am sad I cannot see them, but now I know what went wrong. I can try to get it right when I take lots of them outside next time.'*

The conversations are similar, but one was pacing and one was not; in the second one, O'Connor really did match his daughter's map of the world.'

This is a useful way to illustrate to students what we mean by pacing, and then it can be contextualised to the healthcare setting. Sadly many complaints are received in the NHS, largely because a health professional has not taken the trouble to see the patient's or their relatives' map of the world. When health professionals say something like 'I understand exactly how you feel', when clearly they can not, they are failing to pace. The importance of empathy has long since been recognised (Wiseman 1996) and more recently it has been suggested that health professionals' ability to empathise remains poor (Kruijver *et al.* 2001). Rapport skills help health professionals to gain the empathy they require, and as a consequence to continue 'pacing'.

In the classroom it can be valuable to provide learners with questions that patients often ask or statements that they often state (related to their life-threatening illness). In groups they can provide responses to each of these, which they believe will pace the patient and show empathy. An appropriate answer can then be shown to the students and compared to theirs, thus helping to increase their awareness of this important technique. The next section focuses on a meta-frame for clinical supervision and a model for establishing and maintaining rapport within the clinical supervision context.

CLINICAL SUPERVISION

Janis has spent some time developing a comprehensive clinical supervision programme. This was developed as a result of a survey of all existing nursing staff prior to a move to a purpose-built cancer centre.

The findings from this survey were interesting:
➤ 150 were sent out
➤ 47 were not returned.

Of those returned:
➤ 71 stated that they had no supervision
➤ 32 stated that they had some form of supervision.

This survey illustrated that the staff were in the main receiving no supervision. The 32 who thought that they were receiving supervision identified mentorship, ward meetings, educational support and general team meetings with peers as being examples of formal clinical supervision. Clearly there was a lack of understanding as to what clinical supervision is. However, when given the definition, they *all* felt that it would be of benefit to have this type of 'help'. As a result of this survey, a system for clinical supervision was developed to meet the staff's identified needs.

The importance of this type of support has been widely reported and known for some time (DoH 1993; Butterworth 1994; Johns 1995). Hawkins and Shohet (2000) talk about how vital 'Pit head time' is, during which the staff can wash off their 'emotional grime' during working hours. Timpson (1998) suggests that the setting-up of such structures illustrates management's belief in the contributions of staff, and this might in time lead to unrealised potential in terms of patient care.

Much clinical supervision can be accomplished using NLP – for instance, the metaphors used in the above paragraph can be most useful in working with members of staff in gaining rapport. Jones (1997) recommends that the rich symbolism of language and metaphor should be employed as a potential therapeutic tool in clinical supervision. Calish (1994) supported this, discussing the benefits of 'artistic metaphor' and how metaphors can enhance supervision by providing a means to express aspects of the therapeutic relationships.

Winstanley and White talk about the usefulness of group supervision and the fact that an organisation should have established formal guidelines for conducting such sessions. However, they also postulate that within this approach there should not be too many hard and fast rules, but that the catchword should be 'flexibility' (Winstanley and White 2003). This flexibility fits with the responsive nature of NLP.

The group approach was acknowledged by Janis; along with the feedback from the survey, it meant that much of the supervision would be carried out in groups. The staff who worked in groups (wards, teams) – which was the majority of staff – requested that the supervision be carried out in groups, with the option to have individual supervision (over and above this) should they require it. The implications from this survey meant that many vital training needs had been identified.

To meet the needs of the staff, many 'new supervisors' would need to be identified and trained. While there were a number of senior staff members with good communications skills, who were keen to learn, they had little or no experience of facilitating groups. The aspect of group supervision that most individuals new to working with groups in this way find generally to be most difficult is establishing and maintaining rapport. Therefore Janis decided to observe three practitioners who were considered experts in this area. By observing them and watching their behaviour and actions in detail – what they did, and how they did it – and asking relevant questions, she accumulated much rich data to analyse and find common patterns in order to construct an NLP model.

From these data a very useful meta-frame emerged. A meta-frame is provided when you step back and, looking from a distance, comment on a process (Walker 2002). An unexpected surprise was that when this was developed into a diagrammatic format, it spelt the word 'rapport'! The meta-frame as seen in Figure 4.3 starts at the top pinnacle, with these two aspects considered by the experts to be essential to establishing initial rapport.

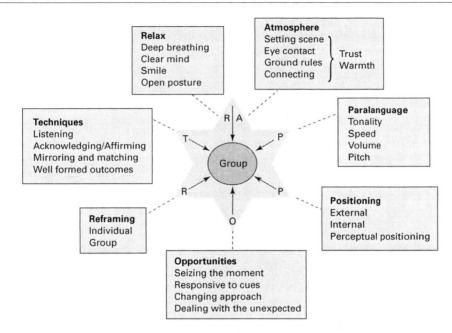

FIGURE 4.3 Meta-frame for establishing and maintaining rapport © 2009 Janis Hostad

The opposite point on the star is opportunities, which is another key attribute of rapport. Opportunity may use any one of the other points, or indeed a number of them (depending on the type of opportunities which present themselves). This element does seem to set aside those who demonstrate excellence in clinical supervision. This skill was both conscious and unconscious at different times during the sessions, as was evidenced by comparing the observations with the feedback from the supervisors.

Sometimes the skill was shown by helping an individual, and sometimes by helping the whole group. The 'opportunity skills' were often different but showed in a high level of flexibility, responsiveness and an ability for immediate analysis. This flexibility has already been described above by Winstanley and White (2003) with regard to its importance.

In terms of NLP, these individuals illustrated a knack of answering at the appropriate 'logical level' with who, why, how, what or where questions. As they were not familiar with NLP, this again illustrates mastery of these skills at an unconscious as well as a conscious level. The other points of the rapport star are used either together or separately, depending on what is happening at that moment. Each of the elements of this frame is important but, due to space constraints, they cannot be discussed further here.

The second diagram was devised to teach the 'opportunity' technique by using an NLP model, so that others, too, could learn to master this ability. Ensuring that individuals learn this is best achieved via an acquisition process which can be used in the classroom to aid the participants to acquire this skill. (This might be useful to others who are teaching this topic.) The model could be taught as part of a three-day course covering all aspects of the meta-frame. It has been piloted with good feedback from the participants, who had fun and much laughter as they tried it for the first time. They did find it to be most helpful in gaining this skill, which up until then they said had seemed difficult to 'pin down' let alone acquire! (*See* Figure 4.4 below, and the accompanying acquisition exercise.)

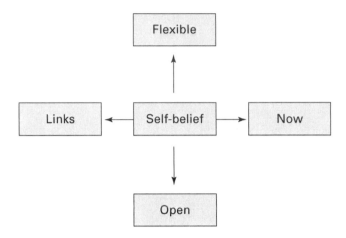

FIGURE 4.4 Model for using 'opportunity' as a group clinical supervision supervisor © 2009 Janis Hostad

---

Exercise 4.2 Acquisition of opportunity skills

This is a very useful exercise in the classroom and time must be given so that everyone can participate. In the first instance it will be carried out with one 'willing' volunteer so that everyone understands the process. Then the participants will work again in triads, with one member observing, one instructing and one acquiring the skill. This will work as follows:

A card each with a different aspect of the model will be placed on the floor mirroring the model above. The participant will then be asked to 'step on to' the central card – Self-belief.

Self-belief

While the participant is standing on the card, ask them to think of a time when they know they made a difference with a patient and family member with whom they truly 'connected'. Allow the positive feeling to reinforce their belief in self. (Techniques can be used to ensure that they are able to *associate* with this experience.) When they have achieved this, ask them to move off the 'Self-belief' card and, when ready, to move on to the 'Now' card.

Now

As this is about being in the moment, ask the participant to look around and view the group experience – what are they noticing? Ask them to vocalise their observations. (Encourage and reinforce their comments.)

When they feel they have achieved that, get them to move off the 'Now' card and to move to 'Open'.

Open

First, ask them to think of a time when they were completely in rapport with another person.

Second, ask them to think of a time when they dealt with something unexpected and it felt good.

Use senses to ensure that they *associate* with the experiences. 'Anchor' each experience so they can resource them when they need to. Check that they feel they are open to the unexpected, being accepting of whatever might come, seeing, hearing and feeling the message. Ask them to move on to the 'Links' card when they are ready.

Links

Tell them to again remember that time when they made a difference with a patient and to trust that they can use their skills to connect and link with the group. They need to know that they will find useful ways to link the different members of the group when they need to. Tell them that when the opportunity presents itself, they should trust that they will also know how to link relevant topics. And they will be able to link what they are noticing now with what has gone before, just as they did for the patient. When they are comfortable with this, ask them to move on to the 'Flexible' card.

Flexible

Ask them to notice how flexible they have already become during this acquisition process. They should also notice how good it feels to use so many different skills and to be this flexible. And they should know that being flexible in approach will help them to be successful in using opportunity in building rapport during clinical supervision.

When every one has had a turn, the participants will be given opportunities to use 'opportunity' with a larger group, two groups together, and a further three to observe and feed back. (They may have a copy of the model in front of them initially.)

The acquirer(s) will be given feedback on their acquisition of these new skills on completion – from the group and from the facilitator.

All the elements of this meta-frame provide a helpful framework for teaching supervision skills and, in particular, rapport. For more information on this clinical supervision meta-frame, and this model, the reader can contact the author (Janis) at janis.hostad@hey.nhs.co.uk

Being able to establish a rapport speedily enables the clinician or educationalist to access other useful NLP techniques, such as reframing.

REFRAMING

What is reframing? Just as a picture frame puts borders or boundaries on what you can see in a picture, the frames of reference that you choose as a result of your beliefs about yourself and others, your perceived role in life, your perceived limitations in skills and abilities, can limit what you see as possible. Conversely, the framing you use can open up all sorts of possibilities. You and (if you allow them) others are continually setting timeframes, boundaries, limits, on what you as an individual can and cannot do. This is often without any real thought about the consequences or whether these limitations are real.

Changing the frame of an experience can have a major influence on how you perceive, interpret and react to that experience. Changing the frame of reference is called 'reframing' in NLP. The purpose of reframing is to help a person to experience their thoughts and actions, and the impact of their beliefs, from a different perspective (frame) and potentially to be more resourceful or have more choice in how they react and behave.

When presenting a reframe to another person:

➤ make sure you have rapport and their 'permission' to offer it

➤ understand that while you may believe your reframe is the best ever, it may not work for the other person – simply because they have a different model of the world than you do

➤ explore other possible reframes as well, because according to NLP presupposition, 'there is no failure, only feedback'

➤ be aware that if you present the reframe in the form of a question or a metaphor (story), it will most likely be more fully considered by your client than if you present it as a statement of fact. The best you can do is to ask someone to consider your reframe and then they can choose whether or not it actually reframes their experience.

Example of a student-related reframe

- *'This assignment has got the better of me, I knew I couldn't write at this level, at the beginning, and now I have got so much work done, just to be defeated, I will never get there.'*

  'You haven't got there yet. However, you have achieved a great deal which, at the outset, you thought impossible, so you must be very proud of your endeavours and of proving to yourself that you can work at this level. The end is now much closer than the beginning.'

Example of a patient-related reframe

- *'When my wife visits, she does not bother talking any more. All she ever does is sit there looking at me really sadly, managing an occasional smile, and then she struggles not to cry, but with no success! It hurts!'*

  'It must be very comforting to know that you and your wife are in a mutually special place where you can sit in silence with each other, feeling each other's pain, and know that your love is being expressed through tears and smiles.'

Learning to reframe naturally does take time and those of us who have counselling qualifications and or experience in this field often find it harder to get to grips with reframing, often confusing it with paraphrasing in the first instance. It can be most useful when teaching this skill to illustrate the differences – for example, compare the reframe we have provided above, with the paraphrase below, they both are most useful and effective but each has a different intent and, as a result, a different outcome.

> *'So your wife keeps illustrating how much she cares for you; but is fighting to hide how much of a struggle it is to cover up her emotions, and how, like you, she is affected deeply by your illness.'*

Another exercise which has been most useful in helping students to become more familiar with and experienced in 'reframing' is as follows:

Exercise 4.3 Reframing

The participants are asked to work in triads.
- One person presents a problem and the other two together try to reframe it.
- They make a note of the statement and their reframe to share back in the full group.

This creates much dialogue, particularly about how hard it is to accomplish and the difficulty of ensuring that it is a reframe and not a paraphrase.

WELL-FORMED OUTCOMES

In cancer and palliative care clinical and educational settings, it is crucial that we know what we want to achieve before we set about undertaking the tasks.

In NLP, the term 'well-formed outcome' has been around for over 30 years. However, as with many NLP terms, this name often gets in the way of understanding the simplicity of the model. To put it more simply, what it really means is that you have checked out if this really is the desired outcome by following a process of questioning. If the outcome comes through these processes, it can be deemed well designed or well formed. This process can be used to clarify your own outcomes and can be utilised to assist others in formulating their own well-formed outcome. It is a process that is easily taught and students who go on to use it with patients and carers have reported eliciting positive responses from them. Both authors have achieved similar success with patients, carers, colleagues and students. Although the process of developing a well-formed outcome is relatively simple (*see* Figure 4.5), it does require practice in a safe environment – as indeed does all communications skills training.

It is often difficult in this fast-moving world to stop, re-evaluate and decide what it is you want to achieve, say from a single conversation. Yet if it is an important conversation, it is worth the effort, because it always works better if you have formulated these well-formed outcomes beforehand.

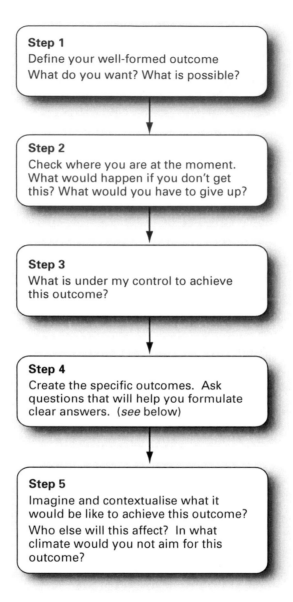

FIGURE 4.5 The well-formed outcome process

Within NLP there are two main models: the Meta model and the Milton model. The Meta model is a useful tool to understand how thoughts are translated into words. It suggests that each sentence spoken can be analysed at two levels: a surface level and also a deeper level. The next section is found within the Meta model. The function of this model is to help us to identify and transform problematic deletions, distortions and generalisations in our thinking and communicating with others and to understand how the language we use can delete, distort and generalise.

DELETIONS, DISTORTION AND GENERALISATIONS

It is important to recognise these concepts because people make judgements based on their own frame of reference, assuming that we all have the same map of the world. When we do successfully recognise deletions, distortion and generalisations, it helps in terms of raising our own self-awareness and in understanding others, therefore improving our overall interpersonal communication.

Deletion

It is impossible for us to take in every stimulus that is around us at any one time; our brains would simply overload. Therefore our brains 'delete' or 'filter out' what is currently unnecessary, thus preventing 'overload' from occurring. In this way, we are continually either 'tuning in' or 'filtering out'.

In a classroom it is easy to illustrate this by playing a DVD – possibly one related to the session – and then seeking feedback on it afterwards. Doing this will help students to understand how much they have deleted.

Exercise 4.4 Recognising deletions

Please watch this excerpt from the DVD (or listen to this track from the CD), observe (or listen out for) as much as you can, and report back on the key points. Also you need to observe and note all the things that you are aware of in the room.

● Write these things down only at the end of the exercise and on your own. Afterwards you can discuss your observations in small groups.
● Notice the differences between what you observed at the time and what other group members observed.
● Think about how these 'deletions' might impact on your communications with other colleagues.
● How might it help you to be aware of similar deletions when talking to patients?

Please nominate a spokesperson to report back, although each individual is encouraged to share their personal comments.

This could then be followed by an exercise which looks at the way individuals 'miss' or 'delete' things from their conversations. Verbs are often used that don't fully explain what is happening and comparisons can be far from clear (Bavister and Vicker 2008). *See* the examples further down.

Distortion

'Distortion' is another commonly used NLP term – it refers to our attaching a certain meaning to things without knowing whether this meaning is valid. For example, we might see that a patient is crying and decide as a result that the patient is not coping. However, it might equally mean that she is coping very well because she is able to openly vent her emotions, which is helping her to manage her problems effectively. If we attach the wrong meaning to such important issues, the distortion can get in the way of helping patients and their families. To reduce the chance of this occurring, we need to find out more accurate detail by asking specific questions in an empathetic manner.

Generalisations

We often use generalisations about ourselves, other people and the world at large. When we make sweeping statements, these are to do with our beliefs – for example, if something happens to us more than just once or twice we might then believe that it always happens, even if it is not true. That is called a limiting belief; it has the effect of stopping us from realising our true potential.

> *'I never get a good mark.'*
>
> *'I always make this mistake.'*
>
> *'I will never be able to give chemotherapy.'*

Due to our assumptions, these beliefs may also negatively affect how we get on with other people.

> *'On that ward, they never answer the phone.'*
>
> *'She is always negative.'*

Giving the student examples like those above means that they can understand the concept. Then they can start to write a list of their own generalisations and discuss them in small groups, looking for similarity and differences and the effect these might have on themselves and others.

So providing the student with examples can be most useful in promoting understanding and in showing how important words can be. However, this aspect of NLP takes some time to learn in all its intricacies; meanwhile exercises need to remain simple and applicable to everyday practice.

Examples of challenging deletion, distortion and generalisation

- Someone might omit an important element of their statement, as in:

  'I am very sad.'

  So the object is to find out about the element that is missing:

  'Very sad about what?'

- Someone claims to know what another person is thinking by saying something like:

  'She thinks I don't like her.'

  So the object is to identify the thinking underlying that assumption.

  'How do you know she is thinking that?'

- Someone makes a broad generalisation:

  'He never thinks of me.'

  So the object is to check for counter examples:

  'Never?' or 'Not even once?'

THE MILTON MODEL

The Milton model was co-created by the two founders of NLP. This approach was modelled on the work of Milton Erikson, the recognised creator of hypnotherapy (Erikson 1983), and it is almost the complete opposite of the Meta model. It is an art form in itself learning to use artificially vague language. This type of language is particularly useful when doing change work with anyone; it encourages a trance-like state by deliberately producing sentences that are open to interpretation, in direct contrast to the Meta model. Questions asked might be as vague as 'And?' or 'So?' or 'Because?. These can be most useful in cancer and palliative care, when dealing with very sensitive topics, because they allow the patients to make their own connections.

METAPHORS AND STORIES

Metaphor and stories are dealt with in great detail in Chapter 3 (by Lorna). However, it would be difficult to write a chapter on NLP and not mention them. Erikson was the master of stories, carefully choosing ones that fitted the needs of the client. In NLP the word 'metaphor' tends to cover all terms such as stories, parables, fables, similes and metaphors. Erikson and others have suggested that metaphors speak directly to the deepest part of the person. When a person starts talking metaphorically, usually they present mctaphors as a way of talking about their problem. A common one with which many of us will be familiar is:

> *'I am feeling out of my depth.'*

You might answer with:

> *'You feel like you might be starting to drown?'*
>
> *'How are you managing to keep your head above the water?'*
>
> *'How deep is it now?'*

All the above responses match and pace the individual, however, if you started to talk about 'no light at the end of the tunnel', you would be failing to stay in rapport. Metaphors are enormously powerful and certainly convey empathy. These will help you to gel with your group if you are teaching and by using them regularly you are acting as an effective role model for the students as they learn to use them too.

An exercise which seems to help participants to feel more confident in using metaphors in practice is detailed below.

Exercise 4.5 Working with metaphors

Ask the participants to sit on their own and come up with metaphors that describe:

- themselves at work
- themselves at home
- themselves in life generally.

Small group work

The participants should then choose one of these metaphors to share in their small group.

In turn, group members share their metaphor, and the rest of the group has to respond using the appropriate language to stay in rapport.

Main group

The small groups feed back in to the main group any metaphors that were particularly difficult, then everyone tries to find an appropriate response.

The facilitator can then join in, providing any other approaches or ideas that the participants have not yet come up with.

Another NLP technique is the use of Anchors, which can be most useful in this field of care.

ANCHORS

'Anchors' are things we all use but not always consciously – for example, how often have you been listening to music on the radio and found yourself smiling because it has connected you to a happy memory? This is an anchor, however, connections could equally anchor to an unhappy memory. It is surprising how a smell or noise or other sensory stimulus can take you back so instantaneously. How is this of benefit in the field of cancer and palliative care? Quite simply, we can change the mood of patients almost instantaneously if they can 'buy into' this approach. By working with patients and finding out their more pleasant experiences, we can help these experiences to be more present, and provide patients with ways of calling these pleasant feelings to mind, when they need them most. They may need a 'trigger' or 'anchor' for doing this, suggesting that when they squeeze their forefinger, the image and positive feeling will reoccur. The exercise will be conducted with the facilitator doing the anchoring and then the patient doing it subsequently. This works in much the same way as Pavlov's dogs, with the repeated signals producing the stimuli to respond in a certain way. A patient could have a picture or photo of some happy event by their bed, which they will be taught to use in this way, as a 'trigger' to transport them into the experience. With all their senses heightened, they can 'associate' into the experience and use it to change their mood and thus help them to cope. Another use for this approach is in helping patients get to sleep by using a simple but very effective 'five finger' exercise in which each finger anchors a special memory; often patients are asleep before they get to the end of it. Both Janis and Lorna have had excellent results using this approach, in different ways, with patients, relatives, staff and students. It can also be very useful as a technique in helping students with exam nerves. So for health professionals and educators alike, this is a most helpful process that is well worth learning. Another approach more familiar to Lorna is phobia cure, used for people with belonephobia.

PHOBIA CURES

Some people have a phobia that impacts significantly on their lives which leads them to take one of several actions, such as avoiding the situation, feeling overwhelmed or becoming highly anxious. Claire Rushworth first taught Lorna this technique over twenty years ago. Lorna has had a significant success rate and many recipients of the NLP phobia techniques have stated that they have achieved a partial or total cure. Belonephobia is an intense fear of needles, pins and other sharp objects. To highlight the usefulness of this phobia cure in the cancer and palliative care clinical setting, the following true scenario is outlined.

A 20-year-old man, John, diagnosed with lymphoma, came to see Lorna in her former role as a Macmillan nurse. The reasons for his visit were varied, but the main one was that he was refusing chemotherapy due to his fear of injections. After discussing this aspect of his care in detail, it became apparent that John had vivid visual memories related to his childhood of being given injections forcibly by the school nurse. Just talking about his childhood experience caused John to become breathless, dizzy and nauseated. He even started to shake and to experience palpitations. He felt he could not go through that again. He vocalised that he would rather die than have the chemotherapy. During the session Lorna explained the NLP phobia treatment, and he agreed to try the technique. The process involves replaying the visual memory of the anxiety-provoking incident but in a completely different way. By replaying the memory in a different way, the loop of seeing a picture (V) and then experiencing unpleasant feelings (k) is broken. This enables the person to process and recode the event to give it new meaning, so that it is no longer a problem or at the very least it is significantly less anxiety provoking. To John's surprise this treatment worked and he went on to receive his six cycles of chemotherapy and to recover from his lymphoma. For those of you who can recall the Jimmys TV series, he played a major role in this with Lorna in a supporting role. He does recount this phobia treatment experience over several episodes. His name has been changed here.

The exact technique is too lengthy to detail here but it is included in the NLP sessions that Lorna teaches. For more information, you can contact the author at lorna@premiermail.co.uk

Lorna has spent many hours teaching on the topic of phobia management and more specifically and has run several workshops at national and European haemophilia nursing conferences. The nurses who attended these conferences have gone on to use this management technique. They have reported back on how effective they have found this technique to be in their clinical areas.

There are many more NLP approaches and techniques which either have not been addressed, or have only been mentioned in passing. Sadly it is beyond the scope of the chapter to do justice to all aspects of NLP, but at least it acts as a 'taster' which 'whets the appetite' of the reader to learn more.

KEY POINTS

■ Practitioners in cancer and palliative care are required to have advanced communications skills and NLP is a largely untapped area from which great advances might be made.
■ This is undoubtedly a fast-growing approach to communications, which with resources spent on research could prove beneficial in this field of care.
■ A number of techniques like phobia cures – for example, belonephobia – have proved themselves to be most effective. Such techniques need to be shared and disseminated to where they can most usefully be introduced for the patients and carers with the greatest needs.
■ 'Associating' and 'dissociating' are very useful techniques in these specialities and there is a need for more staff to learn to use these approaches in order to help distressed patients, relatives, staff and students.
■ Teachers keen to be 'masters' in their own classroom would find NLP awareness-raising workshops (or practitioner courses) most valuable.

CONCLUSION

In this chapter Janis and Lorna have endeavoured to give you a brief overview of this fast-growing model for communications. The four pillars of NLP – namely outcomes, sensory acuity, behavioural flexibility and rapport – have been explored and discussed. They have been applied to education and cancer and palliative care wherever possible. Awareness of the benefits of NLP to education in general is growing. As an educator, you need to be able to build rapport with a group and check their emotional state, and of course use sensory acuity. So much can be achieved with this approach. Within cancer and palliative care, the techniques are enormously beneficial to patients and carers. Clinicians will also benefit from using these NLP techniques. A by-product of this form of learning is that all who do so embark on their own journey of self-discovery in the pursuit of excellence.

Teachers who have mastered many of these techniques and used them in equal measure with their clients, students and colleagues can be likened to the connoisseurs who inhabit the art world. In the NLP context, the connoisseur (teacher) is an individual who brings specific expertise to the evaluation of a given entity (in this case, the student). Expertise in NLP enables the connoisseur to appreciate the subtleties, nuances and complexities in their students. Equipping students to transform themselves from novices to experts in communications skills is like wiping the dust off an old canvas to find underneath a truly authentic human masterpiece.

IMPLICATIONS FOR THE READER'S OWN PRACTICE

1   How will you now integrate NLP techniques into your practice?
2   In what ways will understanding NLP ensure that you become a better teacher in the future?
3   Can you identify which approaches you will now use as part of your daily work?
4   How will you learn more about this in the future?
5   In what way do you think NLP techniques can be audited, and how might some of these different techniques and their usefulness to cancer and palliative care be researched?

REFERENCES

Argylle M (1983) *The Psychology of Interpersonal Behaviour*. London: Penguin Books.

Bavister S, Vicker A (2008) *Teach Yourself NLP*. London: Hodder Education.

Butterworth T (1994) Clinical supervision as an emerging idea in nursing. In: Butterworth T, Faugier J, editors. *Clinical Supervision*. London: Chapman and Hall: 3–17.

Calish A (1994) The metatherapy of supervision using art with transference/countertransference phenomena. *Clinical Supervisor.* **12** (2): 119–27.

Department of Health (1993) *A Vision of the Future: the nursing, midwifery and health visiting contribution to health and healthcare*. London: HMSO.

Dilts R, Grinder J, Bandler R, DeLozier J (1980) *Neuro-linguistic Programming: Volume 1, the study of the structure of subjective experience*. Capitola, CA: Meta Publications.

Einspruch EL, Forman BD (1985) Observations concerning research literature on neuro-linguistic programming. *J Counsel Psychol.* **32** (4): 589–96.

Erikson M (1983) In: Rossi EL, Ryan MO, Sharp FA, editors. *Healing and Hypnosis: the seminars and workshops of Milton H Erikson*. New York: Irving.

Hawkins P, Shohet R (2000) *Supervision in the Helping Professions*. 2nd ed. Milton Keynes: Open University Press.

Johns C (1995) Framing learning through reflection within Carper's fundamental ways of nursing. *J Adv Nurs.* **22**: 226–34.

Jones A (1997) Death, poetry, psychotherapy and clinical supervision (the contribution of psychological psychotherapy to palliative care nursing. *J Adv Nurs.* **25** (2): 238–44.

Kearney M (1996) *Mortally Wounded: stories of soul pain, death, and healing*. New York: Scribner.

Kruijver IP, Kerkstra A, Bensing JM, Van de Wiel HB (2001) Communication skills of nurses during interactions with simulated cancer patients. *J Adv Nurs.* 2001; **34**: 772–9.

Laborde GZ (1998) *Influencing with Integrity*. Camarthen: The Anglo American Book Co.

Mehrabian A, Ferris SR (1967) Inference of attitudes from nonverbal communication in two channels. *J Couns Psychol.* **31** (1): 248–52.

O'Connor J, McDermott I (1996) *An Introduction to NLP*. [CD recording.] Thorsons Element Audio Books.

Rossi EL, Ryan MO, Sharp FA, editors (1983) *Healing and Hypnosis: the seminars and workshops of Milton H Erikson. Vol. 1*. New York: Irving.

Rushworth C (1994) *Making a Difference in Cancer Care*. Guernsey: Guernsey Press.

Sargent P, Thurston M, Kirby K (2004) *Using Neuro-linguistic Programming Techniques to Maximise the Coping Strategies of Carers and Patients Living with Cancer in Ellesmere Port*. Centre for Public Health Research: University College Chester.

Spohrer K (2007) *Teaching NLP in the Classroom*. London: Continuum International Publishing Group.

Timpson J (1998) The NHS as a learning organisation: aspirations beyond the rainbow. *J Nurs Manag.* **6** (5): 261–72.

Turnbull J (1999) Intuition in nursing relationships: the results of 'skills' or 'qualities'? *Br J Nurs.* **8** (5): 302–6.

Walker L (2002) *Consulting with NLP*. Oxford: Radcliffe Medical Press.

Walter J, Bayatt A (2003) Neuro-linguistic programming: the keys to success. *BMJ.* **326**: 165–6.

Walter J, Bayatt A (2003) Neuro-linguistic programming: temperament and character types. *BMJ.* **326**: 133.

Walter J, Bayatt A (2003) Neuro-linguistic programming: verbal communication. *BMJ.* **326**: 583.

Winstanley J, White E (2003) Clinical supervision: models, measures and best practice. *Nurse Res.* **10** (4): 7–38.

Wiseman T (1996) A concept analysis of empathy. *J Adv Nurs.* **23**: 1162–7.

FURTHER READING

Janis and Lorna have chosen two books which give a basic but informative introduction to the topic:

- Millor P (2003) *The Really Good Fun Cartoon Book of NLP.* Carmarthen: Crown House Publishing.

    This is a superb little book which does not cost much but gives the reader a fun and informative account of this approach and its practical application.

    The key principles are enhanced by the cartoon approach which is in keeping with the philosophy of NLP.

    This book is a real favourite of the authors and really 'illuminates' the benefits of NLP. It serves as a basic reminder of all the main techniques and, as such, is a useful addition to the bookshelf.

- Read R, Burton K (2004) *Neuro Linguistc Programming for Dummies Guide*. Chichester: John Wiley and Sons.

    This book is very informative, avoiding the jargon of many other books, and it provides the essentials of this approach. It aims to give you the basic skills with which to think clearly about your own actions and understand the motivations of others.

5

Treasures in jars of clay: working with critical companionship

Angela Brown and Gill Scott

'Self growth is tender; it is holy ground. There's no greater investment.'

Covey 1989: 62

AIM

This chapter seeks to share with the reader the value of critical companionship (Titchen 2001), as discovered by the authors on a journey towards expertise in practice.

LEARNING OUTCOMES

By the end of the chapter, the reader will have:
- gained an introduction to the Royal College of Nursing Institute's Expertise in Practice Project
- shared a process of revealing expertise in practice
- recognised the significance of a helping relationship: critical companionship
- identified the potential of 'digging' for one's own treasures in jars of clay
- considered some approaches for helping others to find their expertise.

INTRODUCTION

This journey will be presented as if it had been an archaeological expedition. This metaphor is used to explain how the treasures of professional expertise are discovered through the relationship between an expert practitioner and a colleague (critical companion). The authors contend it is important to acknowledge that our expertise may be hidden in 'jars of clay' and need to be revealed. This is conveyed by the sharing of some of the reflective journey undertaken as part of the Royal College of Nursing (RCN) Institute's Expertise in Practice Project. This pilot project sought to help practitioners to recognise expertise within their practice through a number of processes. Critical companionship is one of these processes. This account discusses the personal experiences of two participants of the project, Gill Scott as the expert practitioner and Angela Browne as the critical companion.

An archaeological find can be as banal as it is revelatory. Until the investigation is underway, there is an unknown value attached to the potential artefacts found. A degree of investment and commitment to the endeavour is required before this is apparent. The process rather than the outcome of digging is itself, for many volunteers, a personal passion and pleasure. Such features of the archaeological dig are mirrored in the reciprocal critical companionship and expert practitioner relationship. Scarre (2005: 34) tells us that in the study of archaeology, '[t]he multiplicity of views and approaches may sometimes appear confusing, but it is symptomatic of the nature of the enterprise of humans studying themselves', thus acknowledging that the study of archaeology is diverse and interpretable. Searching for the 'treasure' within expertise in practice similarly requires us to study and learn of ourselves. The authors' contention is that within a supportive critical companionship relationship, this extricating process requiring complex interpretations of embedded 'treasure' can bring some sense and reality to the world of clinical practice. This helping professional relationship moves beyond a description of practice to something much more revelatory that reveals not only the 'treasure in jars of clay' but also the treasure of the 'digging' itself.

Through this journey, nursing expertise has been deconstructed and reconstructed to provide insights into clinical expertise. The expert practitioner works within the context of palliative care and the discovery of the treasure at the bottom of the 'jar of clay' led to exploring vulnerability and risk as a paradox in the expert practitioner's expertise. This journey is presented as a narrative of two voices: Angela's reflection of the role of critical companion and Gill's reflections of the impact of critical companionship on her quest to recognise her expertise in practice.

THE ARCHAEOLOGICAL DIG

To assist the reader to follow the process of the 'dig', it is necessary to provide some background and insight into the RCN Expertise in Practice Project.

This project utilised emancipatory action research and fourth-generation evaluation (Guba and Lincoln 1989) as the philosophical framework to test empirically the conceptual framework for expertise developed by Manley and McCormack in 1997 (Manley *et al.* 2005). In May 2000, nursing practitioners were invited to volunteer themselves for inclusion in the project through the production of a self-assessment paper outlining their area of clinical expertise (Hardy *et al.* 2002). Gill's application to participate in the project was successful and the journey began. This journey uses the conceptual framework of critical companionship to explore the experience for Angela as critical companion and the discovery of the 'treasure' in Gill's expertise.

The expert practitioner was required to gather evidence of expertise and to construct a portfolio of evidence. Through observation of practice, 360-degree feedback

(Alimo-Metcalfe 1996) and reflection in and on practice (Schon 1983), the portfolio demonstrated the five attributes and enabling factors for developing expertise as derived from the literature (Manley and McCormack 1997; Titchen 2001; Titchen and Ersser 2001).

Critical companionship is a metaphor for a person-centred helping relationship. The metaphor is conceptual, drawing on critical social theory, human existentialism, spiritualism and phenomenology (Titchen 2000), and in this helping role the critical companion assists another to develop expertise *'by accompanying them on an experiential journey of learning and discovery'* (Manley *et al.* 2005: 12). The critical companionship relationship reflects skilled companionship processes (Titchen 2001), *'the patient-centred helping relationship between practitioner and their patient/client'* (Manley *et al.* 2005). As Manley *et al.* (2005: 12) go on to say, *'critical companions are partners who act as a resource on a journey of discovery – someone who can be trusted, a supporter who had genuine interest in development and growth through providing high challenge and high support'*.

To return to our archaeology analogy, Collis (2001) identifies the vital importance of an archaeological site's management to the project's success. The expertise of the senior archaeologist manages and complements the enthusiasm and sheer availability of the voluntary workforce whose approach to the careful excavation can be coached throughout the shared experience of this one-off and sometimes pressurised exploration. Similarly, critical companionship gave this expert practitioner labels for what she saw in her practice, heightened her awareness of the potential of each moment and also authenticated the expertise she had already developed.

CRITICAL COMPANIONSHIP: AN OVERVIEW

Critical companionship is represented diagrammatically as a *'series of overlapping circles which represent various practical know-how domains'* (Titchen 2003). At the heart of the critical companionship framework lies the relationship between the critical companion and the practitioner. The critical companionship helps the expert to understand their knowledge base – particularly its professional craft knowledge and personal knowledge strands – and it also assists the expert in the integration of these two strands. There is a clear parallel between the skilled companion–patient relationship and the relationship between skilled companionship and critical companionship. However, this will not be explored within the remit of this chapter and the reader is pointed to Titchen (2000) for analysis of such a perspective.

The journey begins

As a fragile artefact is uncovered brushstroke by brushstroke, so it is our intention to reveal the process of companionship.

On first acquaintance with the model, the authors were completely overwhelmed by its sophistication and complexity. Over time, we came to appreciate that that is exactly what successful relationships are, sophisticated and complex.

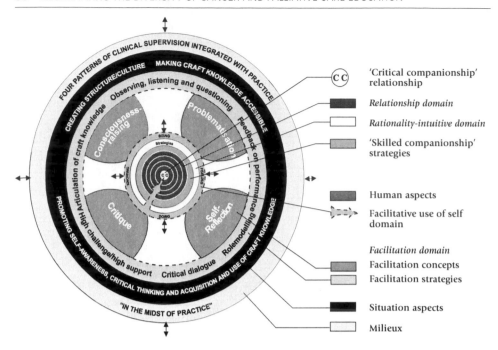

FIGURE 5.1 Critical companionship represented diagrammatically

The relationship domain

You will recall that Gill responded to a national call for volunteers to participate in the Expertise in Practice Project. As a participant, Gill needed to select a critical companion, and Angela was the first respondent to Gill's email to several colleagues.

Mutuality: working with / partnership

Titchen (2001) tells us that *'critical companions build on the practitioner's starting point and tender their knowledge and experience as a resource'*. Within this mutuality Gill and Angela's collegial relationship was defined, carefully negotiated and agreed with a contract. Mutuality is dependent on the other processes within the relationship domain and the critical companion must use and develop these processes. Working together in partnership, the critical companion and the practitioner learn from shared experiences. At the outset of the project we were acquaintances only. At the first meeting we talked nursing, clarified values and beliefs and established what nursing meant to each of us. We shared our goals and aspirations for nursing, the project and ourselves. The critical companion is able through such discussions to individualise the process of facilitation, choosing appropriate interventions and responses after recognising 'where the person is at'.

Particularity: knowing the practitioner

Particularity is about getting to know and understand the uniqueness of the individual practitioner, their details and experiences in the widest possible sense (Titchen 2001). This aspect is seen as the starting point and the basis upon which the facilitation is designed. Gill reflects that at the first meeting, the discussion developed in such a way that she felt comfortable to make the following self-disclosure:

> 'I confessed to my critical companion upon our first meeting when we explored our values about nursing. I said that I had a love–hate relationship with nursing. The fantasy that I always return to when I feel overwhelmed by the constraints and fears of my work are of becoming an art student. I would take a year on a foundation course to experiment with various media and find the expression that suited me. Art was the alternative career option for me when I chose to become a nurse and I have always had a secret regret that it was superseded by what seemed to be a more sensible option at the time.'

Reciprocity: reciprocal closeness, giving and receiving

As time goes by, helpers ask 'what's in it for me?' As a critical companion, Angela felt that spending five hours a month talking nursing with like-minded colleagues was self-indulgent – not often does one have the chance in a busy agenda to enjoy such activities. At the review group meeting, Angela was asked what was in it for her. She responded: 'Working with Gill has been fabulous. I found through these processes that I gained as much as I gave.'

Gill reflects: 'Angela, my chosen critical companion, guided me through the Expert Practitioner Programme.' High support and high challenge (Johns 1997) were the basis of her structured approach to the helping relationship (Titchen 2001). 'What this presented was a refreshing opportunity to luxuriate in exploring and exposing what I demonstrate daily and that would inform the basis of enquiry about the nature of nursing expertise.'

Graceful care: using all aspects of self

Through this process an emotional closeness developed. The hours of discussion, probing, clarifying and defining provided an emotional journey for Gill as the expert practitioner and for Angela as the critical companion. The need to draw upon personal attributes of integrity, compassion and grace was identified. Gill reflects within her portfolio:

> 'This was a rich and mutually beneficial relationship as Angela assisted me in surfacing what I call my "hunches and hang ups" about nursing and being a nurse. I felt valued and respected for my expertise and my personal world view and this gave me the courage to record in-depth reflections with liberty, in a thoroughly new style and with the belief that they had something unique to offer the research enquiry. I was helped by Angela's warmth, acceptance, extraversion and her holistic thinking style.'

Rationality or the intuitive domain

This domain includes three processes: intentionality (acting deliberately), saliency (knowing what matters and acting on it) and temporality (attending to time, timeliness, anticipating and pacing concepts). Titchen (2003) identifies these as prerequisites for the processes within the other two domains: relationship and facilitation. As Angela remembers:

> 'I can recall thinking about these processes as I drove to meet Gill at one of our monthly meetings. Intentionality required me to identify deliberate strategies to support Gill on her journey of discovery. It became obvious that to engage with this facilitation model, the investment of time to think, structure, creativity and resourcefulness would all be necessary attributes. Using these attributes I had to know what was important and focus on the cues (saliency), and time, timing and pacing (temporality) were critical in such a personal and emotional journey of discovery.'

Gill's reluctance to engage with 360-degree feedback is one example of how these attributes and strategies worked. Over several meetings Angela and Gill discussed the process and approach to this element of the project. After each meeting Angela sensed Gill's reluctance to engage with this element: 'I thought about this and at first waited for Gill to feel ready to begin the process. After a while I felt I needed to probe a little more deeply into why there was this reluctance.' Gill was able to recount a very painful experience of receiving feedback in the not-so-distant past and naturally was trying to protect herself from further hurt. The discussion surrounding this brought Gill to a challenging realisation and the surfacing of some of the 'treasure at the bottom of the jar' in the form of vulnerability and risk. Angela recounts: 'We identified a way forward and Gill proceeded to engage with the process of seeking 360-degree feedback.' One of the approaches was to explain the project and the request for participation at an interdisciplinary meeting.

Gill reflects:

> 'When I felt threatened by the need to explain my request for honest feedback from peers about my expertise, Angela was unable to attend the explanatory meeting. She illustrated her companionship by writing a letter to my colleagues adding weight and credibility to the exercise and offering me the support that was required at a crucial time in the project.'

'Interestingly', Gill goes on to say, 'one of my 360-degree peer testimonials stated that I "often go where angels fear to tread"' – an attribute that Zerwekh (2000) identified.

> 'That is because I have faced my own fear, mainly through vicarious but also through some personal experience. As a result, I have a capacity to put myself in the patient's shoes. This also answers the continuing "drive" I feel to improve, develop and expand my sphere of influence.'

Cassidy (1988) wrote eloquently from this same perspective of the vital element of vulnerability in palliative care practitioners. Sometimes, to say, 'I don't know' or 'How can we?' commands respect and trust. Gill further observed: 'Angela would address this too.' As a critical companion, one needs to be able to take risks and also be vulnerable.

Where the clay jar is embedded in the ground, the risk of fracturing it in the attempt to unearth both it and its potentially priceless contents is very prominent in the archaeologist's mind. However, if the risk is not taken and therefore the potential vulnerability not acknowledged, how would we ever find those incredible insights into civilisations, lifestyles and cultures?

The facilitation domain

As the interface between the expert practitioner and the critical companion, this domain involves consciousness-raising, problematisation, critique and self-reflection. 'After a few months, the penny started to drop. We began to internalise the interaction at play', Gill recalls. She continues:

> 'When I first encountered the Titchen model and its description of antennae, I struggled to interpret the practical or operational equivalent of the "antennae" through which expert practitioners sense what is happening within themselves, the relationship and outside within the clinical context. But during one of those defining moments with my critical companion, we recognised something in my daughter's old hand-made painting pinned over my desk. It was [created with] an abstract wheel that threw out paint streaks as the paper had revolved around a turntable. It suddenly epitomised the nature of the patient–expert nurse interaction. Without movement of the turntable, there would still be a painting but of random dots and splashes, though the very same actions had taken place. Movement had created cohesion, patterning and beauty. It reflected Titchen's antennae of the sensitive engagement of the nurse with the patient, the environment and self. This speaks to me of either connected or disconnected nursing, relationship or task orientation, proactive or custodial care and self-giving or self-preservation (because revolving the turntable is far messier). We had entered the facilitation domain! This led us to a bird's-eye view of the conceptual model of critical companionship rather than a slavish interpretation and reductionist approach. We were able to stand back and realise that, like any model, it was there to reflect one's intuitive model against and achieve personal and professional growth in facilitation.'

The archaeologist, too, may have pre-conceived ideas of the outcomes of the 'dig'! How exciting it must be to become aware that despite expectations about the likely era from which the vessel originates, what is revealed may in fact be contradictory or mismatched and lead to new and deeper discoveries.

Facilitation strategies

All of the facilitation strategies were utilised throughout the project: observing, listening and questioning, role modelling, feedback on performance, critical dialogue, articulation of craft knowledge, high challenge and high support. Gill comments:

> 'Careful reflection, discussion and critiquing brought us to the realisation that although the strategies are not new, they are not always obvious to the facilitator or the partner in learning. The labelling of these techniques and approaches and the recognition of them in one's approach to facilitation learning is liberating and productive. Without Angela's

critical companionship, I would have struggled to reconstruct a positive understanding of my practice contribution. I had previously succeeded in seeing the parts of what could be, but never quite synthesised them into a meaningful whole. Like a novice archaeologist I needed the insight and expertise of the site manager to recognise the significance and relationships between the discovered pottery fragments that I had unearthed.'

REVEALING THE TREASURES IN JARS OF CLAY IN PALLIATIVE CARE NURSING

Davies and Oberle (1990), in an attempt to define the aspects of palliative care nursing observed in nurses' descriptions of their work, signal themes of 'valuing' self and others, 'integrity' and 'connecting with' the patient. The core of their argument is that the relational and character-based attributes of the nurse cannot be separated from their behaviours and that any attempt to do so *'led to incomplete conceptualisation of the nurse's role'* (Davies and Oberle: 93). Gill recognised the division of the personal and professional aspects of her practice to be a danger for the Expertise in Practice Project and anticipated that extracting one theme from another could prove impossible, possibly becoming a purely academic exercise. Angela's involvement enabled the exercise to be grounded in reality through her appreciation of Gill's unique contribution.

During the process of research, Gill examined her practice in microscopic detail and analysed it for the attributes of expertise defined by Titchen (2001). For her, the capturing of defined attributes of expertise immediately caused a release of energy and passion about previously unnoticed and potentially insignificant moments. The resultant portfolio was not so much an affirmation of its originating theory as an expression of a personal and unique interpretation of nursing through Gill herself, the agent and creator of these captured moments and responses. It was necessary for her to deconstruct the attributes of expertise in order to recognise them within her own practice. However, it was their reconstruction that led her to the revelation that she was good at what she did. For example, the view that one does not become involved with patients is a long-established one. The protective mechanisms that nurses employ are well documented (Menzies 1960; Benoliel 1982). Yet Gill recognised that her best moments had been at times when she felt helpless, could give no answer or made a choice that had an extremely uncertain outcome. None of these things would have happened if she had simply walked away or socially distanced herself. This quality could be called vulnerability and, as a result of Gill's reflections upon nursing and her own personal practice, she has come to realise that this vulnerability is an attribute underpinning some exciting examples of excellence in nursing.

One of the features of Gill's research participation was being able to present a juxtaposition of experiences, thoughts and evidence within her portfolio. Given this freedom to divulge who she was as a nurse was something unusual to her within her experience of practice and academic life. Aranda (2001) referred to the guilt that nurses felt about an involvement with, or feelings for, patients and noted that they reported an enormous relief in disclosing this. In a similar way, Gill too carried a discomfort about her worldview that is still scantily acknowledged within nursing journals and poorly understood by practitioners – hers is, specifically, a Christian worldview. Functioning within a post-modernist culture that promotes the toleration of eclectic sampling and combinations of various philosophies and belief systems, she had increasingly felt obliged to minimise or conceal her own personal beliefs in the interests of equality and mutual respect. She often felt acutely aware of influences that caused her to subvert her own moral and even spiritual integrity in the name of professionalism where others' expectations or assumptions did not accord with her own worldview. She aligned this very much with Smith's (1992) work on emotional labour. Though her caution was intended to be respectful and often politically correct, it was costly and compromising for her not to be as open as she would like to have been about the way her actions correlated with her beliefs.

One of her favourite Biblical extracts explains this, in 2 Corinthians 4 verses 7–10 (NIV):

> 'But we have this treasure in jars of clay to show that this all-surpassing power is from God and not from us. We are hard-pressed on every side, but not crushed; perplexed, but not in despair; persecuted, but not abandoned; struck down, but not destroyed.'

Paralleling this foundation of her own life with her nursing practice, Gill feels that she has now become more experienced and mature in her practice and insight as she has become increasingly conscious of her own frailty and weakness as a person. This is something she did not set out to develop, but it is a by-product of the self-awareness that once dogged her with thoughts of inadequacy and failure. Now she can live more comfortably with this self-awareness because the very frailty that it reveals is the root of her capacity to identify with and make an impact on people's lives in a significant way. This frailty also helps her to avoid complacency in her personal and professional development or about her achievements.

Angela was very supportive of Gill in articulating these thoughts, excited about their powerful influence in her life and the value of disseminating their principles more widely. Angela's respect for this personal disclosure and its potential was experienced by Gill as liberating – indeed as an emancipatory research experience.

KEY POINTS

- The Expertise in Practice Project provides many exciting prospects. Nursing needs to embrace these concepts and consider how best to implement them in the future.
- The resource implications in implementing this approach on a wider scale will require much thought.
- Critical companionship might with some creativity be incorporated into clinical supervision.
- Health professionals should be encouraged to become involved at a deeper level while being provided with support for sharing their vulnerability.
- Quality vulnerability is a complex phenomenon. Consideration needs to be given as to how this leads to improved care.

CONCLUSION

Gill asks the question at the end of her portfolio *'Is person-centredness or spirituality that which distinguishes the good from the excellent?'* As far as the critical companionship relationship has shown us, nurses that pay attention to their personal ontologies and still engage and connect with their patients' worldviews, tend to be those willing and able to remain person-centred in their care. They can derive treatment pathways for patients that are individualised and not necessarily standardised procedures. Expertise, then, within the context of this discussion, can be seen as a willingness to engage and connect with fellow human beings at the height of their emotional, physical and spiritual existence, to provide a pathway that accompanies that person on their developmental journey.

And so we end this account of our 'dig'. It is our contention that for us this has been a life-changing experience. We commend the processes to the reader; it is a challenging experience but the treasures discovered far outweigh the challenge of the digging.

Readers need to recognise their own jars of clay with undiscovered treasure in relation to expertise and engage with the expertise available in extracting the true value of their contents so that it is discovered and interpreted to this and subsequent generations. We would urge you to use attributes of companionship to nurture and develop others and through these processes to recognise and celebrate expertise with patients and each other.

Readers are directed to *Changing Patients' Worlds through Nursing Practice Expertise* (Manley *et al.* 2005) for a more detailed account of the Expertise in Practice Project. As the Chief Nursing Officer's Bulletin of November 2005 commends:

> '... the RCN's expertise in practice project supports all practising nurses as they implement new developments such as Agenda for Change by offering a practical framework for identifying practice expertise, and in pioneering systems for improved peer review and self-regulation.'

We have considered the risks and vulnerabilities upon both our parts as critical companion and skilled companion within this unique helping relationship. This is akin to that of the archaeological site manager and dedicated archaeologist. As authors, we have continued to experience an exposure to risk and vulnerability by presenting this journey in critical companionship to you, the reader. We challenge you to try to follow this approach and suggest that by raising your awareness, you, too, may fall upon such inner treasures.

IMPLICATIONS FOR THE READER'S OWN PRACTICE

1   What conventions might be constraining the discovery of hidden treasure within your own profession?
2   Through the critical companionship of a 'site manager' you can work with, consider what such exploration of expertise might reveal in its excavation of your unique treasure.
3   Consider the archaeological imagery offered or another preferred analogy to assess

the effectiveness of your own helping skills in developing the impact of learning experiences that you promote.

REFERENCES

Alimo-Metcalfe B (1996) The feedback revolution. *Health Serv J.* 13 June, 26–8.

Aranda S (2001) Silent voices, hidden practices: exploring undiscovered aspects of cancer nursing. *Int J Palliat Nurs.* **7** (4) 178–85.

Benoliel JQ (1982) *Death Education for the Health Professional.* London: McGraw Hill.

The Bible. New International Version (1984) Grand Rapids, MI: Zondervan Publishing House; 2 Corinthians 4: 7–10.

Cassidy S (1988) *Sharing the Darkness.* London: Darton, Longman and Todd.

Chief Nursing Officer (2005) *Bulletin.* London: DoH; Available at: www.dh.gov.uk/cnobulletin

Collis J (2001) *Digging Up the Past.* Thrupp: Sutton Publishing.

Covey SR (1989) *The Seven Habits of Highly Effective People.* London: Simon and Schuster: 62.

Davies B, Oberle K (1990) Dimensions of the supportive role of the nurse in palliative care. *Oncol Nurs Forum.* **17** (1): 87–94.

Guba E, Lincoln Y (1989) *Fourth Generation Evaluation.* Newbury Park, CA: Sage Publications.

Hardy S, Garbett R, Titchen A, Manley K (2002) Exploring nursing expertise: nurses talk nursing. *Nurs Inq.* **9** (3): 196–202.

Johns C (1997) *Becoming an Effective Practitioner Through Guided Reflection* [unpublished PhD thesis]. Luton: University of Luton.

Manley K, McCormack B (1997) *Exploring Expert Practice (NUM65U).* London: Royal College of Nursing.

Manley K *et al.* (2005) *Changing Patients' Worlds Through Nursing Practice Expertise.* London: Royal College of Nursing Institute. Available at: www.rcn.org.uk/publications/pdf/Nursing practiceexpertise.pdf

Menzies IEP (1960) A case study in the functioning of social systems as a defence against anxiety. *Hum Relat.* **13**: 95–121.

Scarre C (2005) *The Human Past.* London: Thames and Hudson: 34.

Schon D (1983) *The Reflective Practitioner: how professionals think in action.* New York: Basic Books.

Smith P (1992) *The Emotional Labour of Nursing.* London: Macmillan.

Titchen A (2000) *Professional Craft Knowledge in Patient Centred Nursing and the Facilitation of Its Development* [D.Phil, University of Oxford, Linacre College].

Titchen A (2001) Critical companionship: a conceptual framework for developing expertise. In: Higgs J, Titchen A, editors. *Practice Knowledge and Expertise in the Health Professions.* Oxford: Butterworth Heinemann: Chapter 10.

Titchen A (2003) Critical companionship: part 1. *Nurs Stand.* **18** (9): 33–40.

Titchen A, Ersser SJ (2001) The nature of professional craft knowledge. In: Higgs J, Titchen A, editors. *Practice Knowledge and Expertise in the Health Professions.* Oxford: Butterworth Heinemann: Chapter 5.

Zerwekh JV (2000) Caring on the ragged edge: nursing persons who are disenfranchised. *Adv Nurs Sci.* **22** (4): 47–61.

6

Reflective practice in cancer and palliative care education

Chris Johns

'In the mirror of reflection, if we gaze earnestly enough, we may see ourselves perhaps for the first time. Such is the revelation we may need another to hold the mirror for us.'

Chris Johns

AIM

This chapter sets out to explore experiential and educational activities that introduce practitioners to reflective practice.

LEARNING OUTCOMES

By the end of this chapter, the reader should be able to:
- identify different perspectives of reflection
- raise self-awareness through reflective practice
- promote effective, high-quality palliative care through reflective practice
- acquire understanding of narrative construction through a series of six dialogical movements
- discuss the use of reflection in palliative care education.

INTRODUCTION

Reflective practice is learning through one's everyday experience to gain insights that change us as practitioners: the way we think, feel, perceive, intuit and respond to situations in practice. In doing so, we intend to become more effective practitioners, more able to live our visions of practice as a reality. Insights are not necessarily conceptualised – 'I have learnt this'. They are more often subliminal, shifting us in subtle ways, like seeds planted in the mind to germinate at appropriate moments, within the complexity of everyday practice (Margolis 1993).

The majority of clinical situations in which practitioners find themselves immersed have no rational solutions. They are messy and indeterminate, or what Schon (1983) refers to as the 'swampy lowlands'. Every situation is unique; it has never happened before. It is not wholly predictable, even though we may have had similar experiences that enable us to predict to some extent the likely outcomes. The difficulty is that we are practitioners of habit, locked into patterns of behaviour that require little thought – 'That's the way we do it'. This leads to complacency and lack of inquiry about other ways of being and responding in practice.

Building on the earlier work of John Dewey (1933), Schon turned the established epistemology of professional practice on its head and staked a claim for an epistemology grounded in the primacy of the practitioner's personal knowing rather than technical rationality, challenging the idea that practitioners can simply apply theoretical solutions to practice situations.

As Schon (1983) notes:

> 'in the varied topography of professional practice there is a high hard ground where practitioners can make effective use of research based theory and technique, and there is a messy lowland where situations are confusing "messes" incapable of technical solution.'

Schon framed the notion of reflection-in-action as a problem-solving approach to situations that caused breakdown. That is where the practitioner's normal smooth performance was interrupted and where their usual pattern of response was inadequate. Schon took his examples from music and architecture, whereby the practitioner could stand back and reframe the situation in order to proceed. Within the immediacy of the clinical moment it is not easy to simply stand back and reframe situations; many situations require immediate response. As such, the idea of reflection-in-action is limited and led me to develop the idea of *reflection-within-the-moment and mindful practice* (Johns 2004: 2).

Reflection has been widely defined (Schon 1983; Boud *et al.* 1983; Boyd and Fales 1983; Mezirow 1981). Mezirow draws on a critical theoretical perspective that grounds reflection as social action towards creating a better state of affairs. As such, reflection has a moral and social agenda towards change that inevitably involves challenging normal patterns of social structures. This idea resonates strongly within nursing, where nurses may not have been able to fulfil their therapeutic potential due to oppressive managerial and professional dominance. I make the point to draw attention to the idea that reflection can merely scratch at the surface of experience but not disturb the normal order of clinical practice, or alternatively it can dig deep into social structures.

This is how I describe reflection:

> *'Reflection is being mindful of self, either within or after experience, as if it is a window through which the practitioner can view and focus self within the context of a particular experience, in order to confront, understand and move toward resolving contradiction between one's vision and their actual practice.*

> *Through the conflict of contradiction, the commitment to realise one's vision, and understanding why things are as they are, the practitioner can gain new insights into self and be empowered to respond more congruently in future situations within a reflexive spiral towards developing practical wisdom and realising one's vision as a lived reality. The practitioner may require guidance to overcome resistance or to be empowered to act on understanding.'* (Johns 2006)

From this description, a number of significant points can be made about reflection.

1 Reflection is always purposeful action towards realising one's vision of desirable practice as a lived reality. As such, it is necessary to have a vision. Through reflection, the practitioner continuously finds meaning in such words as 'suffering' as enshrined within the WHO definition of palliative care and in such ideas as a hospice as a healing sanctuary (Kearney 2000). Vision becomes embodied as something lived, intentional, more realised.

2 Reflective effort is the work undertaken towards resolution of the contradiction between the vision and an understanding of current reality. Factors that constrain the realisation of a vision as a lived reality are identified and understood so that work can be done to shift them. This effort involves not just clinical skills but personal skills such as self-esteem, assertiveness and collaboration.

3 Reflection is a developmental process unfolding over time – the reflective spiral of being and becoming. The idea of reflexivity is one of looking back and seeing how insights have been gained through a series of experiences.

4 Practitioners need to learn how to be reflective. For example, using a model of structured reflection may seem obvious, but the reflective cues within it (*see* Table 6.1) are complex, requiring both experience and guidance to fathom out their learning potential.

5 Reflection spans a spectrum from doing reflection as a technique – for example, using a model of reflection – to being reflective or mindful of self within the clinical moment. The more practitioners reflect and write about experience, the more aware they become of those things they have paid attention to within clinical practice. Hence writing a reflective journal is most significant.

I make no distinction between reflection within and on experience. Both are situations that are happening now yet under different circumstances – one in practice itself and one after practice as a way of looking back at a situation.

A reflective practitioner is someone who reflects within practice itself, not as a problem-solving technique but naturally within each unfolding moment. The reflective practitioner is *mindful* of self – of the way he or she is thinking, feeling and responding within a particular situation – while holding the intent to realise desirable and effective practice, however that may be understood.

As I have suggested, the ability to become mindful is developed through reflection on experience. Writing in a journal or talking through an experience in clinical supervision will enable the practitioner to become more sensitive to the issues spoken or written about in practice. It is like waking up and becoming open and curious about oneself and one's own practice. Indeed these are the prerequisites for reflection (Fay 1987). Nothing is taken for granted. Habitual practice and complacency are swept aside in the commitment to realise one's vision as a lived reality.

6   The significance of commitment is about ensuring that the practitioner really wants to be the most effective practitioner that he or she can be. Without commitment, practitioners turn away from the mirror of reflection. This is where guidance can be most beneficial, to help people face up to their reality. Where practitioner commitment is blunted, then guided reflection can be a gateway to healing.

7   Guidance is vital to realise the learning potential through reflection, especially for novice reflective practitioners.

NARRATIVE CONSTRUCTION AS AN EDUCATIONAL PROCESS

Reflective learning is often presented as a narrative that clearly sets out the insights gained. Narrative can be structured through a series of six dialogical movements:

➤ dialogue with self, written as a 'naïve' or spontaneous story, to produce a story text

➤ dialogue with the story text as an objective and disciplined process, to produce a reflective text

➤ dialogue between the text and other sources of knowing, to frame understandings emerging from the text within the wider community of knowing

➤ dialogue between the text's author and a guide (or guides), to develop and deepen insights

➤ dialogue within the emerging text, to deepen insights and weave the narrative into a coherent and reflective pattern that adequately plots the unfolding journey, to produce a narrative text

➤ dialogue with a wider audience, to trigger social action.

The first dialogical movement: journaling

Journaling is at the core of reflective practice (Street 1995; Holly 1989).

Students new to reflection often find the concepts of reflection difficult to assimilate.

I commence a new reflective class by sharing a story, such as Patricia's story below. This is helpful to role-model what a story might look like. I have been writing my own narrative, as a complementary therapist working with people living with cancer, since 2000. As such, I walk the talk and am prepared to make myself vulnerable, preparing the ground for students' own disclosures and the narrative construction necessary for their assignments through the six dialogical movements.

I then ask the practitioners to write their own story without taking their pen off the paper, paying attention to detail and drawing on all their senses. This taps the spirit of inquiry (Holly 1989). I do not want them to stop and reflect too much, but rather to let the words flow in spontaneous expression. They have twenty minutes.

The class members are always astonished at the result – 'Where do all these words come from and I haven't even focused on what I wanted to say!'

Rich description is vital because it sets up what is reflected on and what can be learned. It is develops the clinical skill of paying attention to detail.

Example: journaling of Patricia's experience

Patricia sits on the edge of her bed leaning on her bed table. She has just vomited her breakfast. She feels her paracetamol triggers the vomiting. I kneel beside her and ask how she is. She says she has vomited continuously since her last chemotherapy cycle for her cancer of the ovary.

She says she knows she is going to die soon and shares her thoughts about her death, what it might be like. She knows the 'curtain will soon come down'. She pauses and I do not fill the silence. She says she has no fear of death. She is not religious, unlike her family, although she has moved closer to religion in the knowledge she is dying. I ask her what she expects after she dies. She says she doesn't know, asks what I think.

I am cautious about imposing my beliefs. I suggest that we have a deeper level of consciousness beyond mind which is revealed when the body and mind fall away at death. I say this consciousness can merge with the light of God when we die.

She likes this image. She thinks it's possible. She talks about Eddie, her husband who died two years ago, about the way they talked about waiting for each other. She feels he's waiting for her. The idea comforts her. She remembers a situation after her son had died. He came and sat on her bed and said everything was okay. He was only 23. She talks about her children and I am mindful of the way people talk through their lives, finding meaning and putting things into perspective.

I tell Pat her green-blue eyes sparkle. 'Really?' she says. She has some eye shadow to enhance the colour. She is pleased I notice, flattered to be admired. Such things are important boosts for people's self-esteem, flattened in the remorseless onslaught of advancing cancer.

She looks wistfully at the garden, 'It must be beautiful in the summer.'

She is astonished that the garden is maintained by volunteers. 'I must come to one of the garden fêtes if I'm still alive next summer.'

We talk of garden smells and she says she loves lavender. She smiles, 'I hope when I die it will be on a nice day.' I bask in this conversation, intrigued to talk with someone contemplating her own death in such an open and curious way.

In talking, I sense the way Patricia tests out and develops her thoughts about her death. She confronts and works through her fears. It is a mutual process as I reflect on my own views and feelings about death.

She gladly accepts my offer of a jacuzzi bath and a foot massage in about half an hour. In the meantime, I fetch her the *Daily Express* to read. She accepts my offer of an aroma stone with lavender so she can smell the garden in her room.

Returning for her bath she informs me that her nausea has ceased. We have struggled to bring this unpleasant symptom under control. I am rather perplexed we have not reviewed her nausea medication since her admission for one week's respite care. Tania laments we no longer keep people long enough in the hospice to respond adequately to symptom management. It is planned for Patricia to go home on Sunday, so how can we adequately adjust her medication?

Pat loves her jacuzzi bath. As she dresses afterwards, she says she used to be 16 stone. Now she is less than 10 stone. The ravages of cancer. She walks back to her room and talks with Tania. In talking, she surfaces and works through her fears. As a therapeutic approach, listening is under-valued and neglected, buried under the symptom gaze and tasks to do.

> 'Sometimes we listen to things, but we never hear them. True listening brings us in touch even with what is unsaid and unsayable. Sometimes the most important thresholds of mystery are places of silence.' (O'Donohue 1997: 99)

As I massage Pat's feet with lavender essential oil mixed in my reflexology base cream, I suggest she close her eyes and relax. I guide her to focus on her breathing – follow her breath in and follow her breath out. To breathe in love and light and to breathe out her fears, simply to flow with her breath. She is very still as I work on her feet and lower legs for about 20 minutes. I hear Tania ask staff to be quiet outside the room as Pat is having a massage. I smile. Tania cares so much it can make her intolerant of what might be construed as carelessness in others. She is passionately loyal to her patients even at the risk of upsetting other staff. Yet they recognise her passion and accommodate her attitude with comment such as 'that's Tania for you'.

Tania has a 'reputation' at the hospital for speaking her mind. My respect for her is grudging because she is fiercely loyal to her patients and her sense of what is right, even at the risk of rubbing staff up the wrong way. She does not play games with misplaced loyalty, although, as I noted with Gus, Tania has a parental trait that can make others feel like naughty children.

Pat is enthused by her massage, 'It was wonderful'. I leave her to enjoy her lunch – fish and chips followed by bread and butter pudding, and no nausea!

At shift report, Mandy, another staff nurse, says it's been quite a week with so many deaths. The chaplain had said yesterday that all the patients he had met the previous week had now died. We spend a few minutes talking about Percy's death. I am informed he died *peacefully* last night. How right we didn't send him back to the treatment hospital for further chemotherapy. The word *peacefully* grates as if it defines the good death.

Yet it feels important that we spend some minutes reflecting on these deaths and releasing our feelings. These people have become part of us and have touched our hearts. We have held them and cried with them, easing them towards as peaceful a death as possible. As we sit, we can honour our patients, their families and ourselves, not in a smug way, but in a way that nurtures and strengthens our purpose and fans our passion. Caring may make us vulnerable, yet it also nourishes and sustains us. A fine balance. I want to say something about *peacefully* but hold my voice. Not a time for surfacing conflict.

Before I leave I say goodbye to Patricia. She smiles and thanks me for my hands and touch. Touch, like genuine listening, is vital to healing. I am reminded of more words from John O'Donohue (1997: 104):

> 'At the highest moments of human intensity, words become silent. Then the language of touch really speaks. When you are lost in the black valley of pain, words grow frail and numb . . . touch offers the deepest clue to the mystery of encounter, awakening and belonging. It is the secret, affective content of every connection and association.'

The second dialogical movement: entering the reflective spiral

Now step back from the story text and gaze at it from a more objective stance. Imagine you are an interested observer. To ask questions of the text in a disciplined way, I can use a model of reflection to guide me. There are many models of reflection to guide the practitioner to reflect in meaningful ways (*see* Further reading). I have developed the model for structured reflection (MSR), as given in Table 6.1. These cues lead us into a dialogue with our text in order to tune into meaning and develop insights.

TABLE 6.1 The model for structured reflection

Reflective cues
Bring the mind home
Focus on a description of an experience that seems significant in some way (story, video etc.)
What particular issues seem significant to pay attention to?
How were others feeling and why did they feel that way? (empathy)
How was I feeling and what made me feel that way? (sympathy)
What was I trying to achieve and did I respond effectively?
What were the consequences of my actions on the patient, others and myself?
What factors influence the way I was/am feeling, thinking and responding to this situation?
What knowledge informed or might have informed me?
To what extent did I act for the best and in tune with my values?
How does this situation connect with previous experiences?
How might I reframe the situation and respond more effectively given this situation again?
What would be the consequences of alternative actions for the patient, others and myself?
What factors might constrain me responding in new ways?
How do I NOW feel about this experience?
Am I more able to support myself and others better as a consequence?
What insights do I draw from this experience?
Am I more able to realise desirable practice? (framing perspectives)

Source: Johns 2009.

The first two cues are not actually reflective cues. The first cue, *Bring the mind home*, is intended to prepare the practitioner for reflection. It has the practical value of teaching the practitioner to centre self using the breath within practice.

As Songyal Rinpoche (1992: 59) says:

> 'We are fragmented into so many different aspects. We don't know who we really are, or what aspects of ourselves we should identify with or believe in. So many contradictory voices, dictates and feelings fight for control over our inner lives that we find ourselves scattered everywhere, in all directions, leaving nobody at home. Meditation [reflection], then, brings the mind home.'

I change the word 'meditation' to 'reflection'. Yet meditation is another way to develop mindfulness. I often spend a few minutes by myself or with groups using meditation to help bring myself and others fully present to ourselves to enhance reflection. As a therapist, I naturally build in relaxation through the breath to prepare patients for 'healing'.

Drawing out significance

What is significant in the journaling may seem obvious, especially as it will be some-thing you have written yourself. On the surface this is probably true. However, to use my example of Patricia's experience, this cue invites me to look deeper, between the lines, or to pull out certain words like *peacefully*. Why do my colleagues say *peacefully* – does it tell something about the staff's need to ensure a good death? I like the text about Patricia's green-blue eyes and the way this flatters her. Recognising her sexuality even as she approaches death seems vital. Talking about her death opens the gate to explore spirituality.

In the process of exploring reflection, you can ask the students: 'What significance do you, the reader, pull out for deeper reflection?' This promotes other poignant and pertinent questions such as 'How was Patricia / how were others feeling?'

It is often our feelings that trigger reflection, especially when we hold powerful negative feelings (Boyd and Fales 1983). It is our feelings that colour perception and the interpretation of situations.

In the text, I realise that I didn't specifically ask Patricia how she was feeling.

As readers, what do you think she would have said? Justify your response. This cue helps the practitioner to develop empathy, by asking how Patricia was really feeling and how I know that.

How was I feeling?

This cue mirrors the previous one – it guides practitioners and students to tune into and know self and to pose a deep, exploratory question of how I was *really* feeling. The cue is vital, given the significance of intimacy and compassion in healing – within a tradition that has encouraged practitioners to be emotionally detached (Menzies-Lyth 1988).

What was I trying to achieve and did I respond effectively?

My therapeutic endeavour is to ease the other's suffering through compassionate and skilled action. My reflective quest!

Yet do I read the pattern of Patricia's suffering well enough? Is my response to her femininity appropriate? Does offering her a jacuzzi exceed my therapist role? Am I compassionate?

What were the consequences?

The more I consider this cue, the more significant it becomes, for without doubt, actions have consequences. Most often people view this in terms of immediate or short-term consequences. What becomes more significant is envisaging the longer-term consequences – not that this is easy to do. Events are not predictable. Yet appreciating consequences in terms of moral endeavour is the core of phronesis or practical wisdom (Delmar and Johns 2008). It is the hallmark of decision-making.

What factors influenced the way I was feeling, thinking and responding?

This is the most difficult cue, simply because it is difficult to see beyond your normative self. Such issues as expectations from others, habitual practice, fear of sanctions, time, resources, emotional entanglement, stress, motivation, lack of skills, negative attitudes – all of these have been encapsulated within a grid of influences to enable the reflective practitioner to systematically check them out (Johns 2006: 45). This cue also reveals the difficulty with unlearning what has become embodied. It is as if our bodies have learned to see and respond to the world in a certain way which may not lead to effective or desirable practice. The inner voices and changing programmed learning are explored in more detail in Chapter 4.

What knowledge informed or might have informed me?

There is a demand for evidence-based practice. All those journals full of *stuff*. It is only through reflection that practitioners can meaningfully assimilate theory and research findings within their practice. The experience is a hook to hang the theory hat on. In the text concerning Patricia's experience, I do not overly engage with theory but I could develop this part of the reflection. For example, nausea management, death and dying talk, sexuality, spirituality, the good death . . . indeed any aspect of the experience can be pulled out to consider its theoretical basis.

To what extent did I act for the best and in tune with my values?

This cue opens the text to ethical review. What would be the best or right course of action? Do I respect the patient's autonomy? Do I intrude into matters that don't concern me, for example talking about God? Is there conflict between myself and colleagues? If so, how can it be ethically resolved?

Indeed all action can be viewed from an ethical perspective. To do so requires me to appreciate the situation from each person's perspective and then to consider ethical principles. Is there conflict? If so, how best can it be resolved considering issues of authority and tradition. I call this 'ethical mapping' (Johns 2009).

Now reader, how many dilemmas can you spot in my story of Patricia?

How does this situation connect with previous experience?

I have worked with many patients like Patricia who have influenced my practice. Writing a narrative over six years has enabled me to draw connections between my experiences. For example, topics like spirituality have been a constant focus while others, such as sexuality, have taken less focus. I am aware of my natural tendency to avoid difficult issues like noise and attitudes to the good death. Through reflection, I strive to develop a more informed and assertive voice and view conflict as a positive aspect of the learning organisation. Some things, within ourselves and within organisational culture, have to be carefully chipped away rather than swept away.

The forward-looking cues

I haven't addressed these cues in my reflection on being with Patricia.

Readers, can you consider if you were in this situation how you might respond? What options do you have? Challenge yourself to think outside your normal patterns and comfort zones. What would be the consequences? What might stop you from responding in the way you would choose? It is all very well to say 'given the situation again, I would respond like this', but could you? What skills would you need to develop?

What insights have I gained? / Am I more able to realise desirable practice?

Commentators have questioned the value of reflection in terms of leading to patient outcomes (Burton 2000; Mackintosh 1998). Yet through reflective narratives, beneficial outcomes for patients are evident, although readers may question the authenticity of such accounts (*see* Johns 2002).

To frame insights, I have developed the framing perspective tool (*see* Table 6.2).

TABLE 6.2 Framing perspectives and their application

Framing perspective	How has this experience enabled me to ...
Philosophical framing	confront and clarify my beliefs and values that constitute desirable practice?
Role framing	clarify my role boundaries and authority within my role, and my power relationships with others?
Theoretical framing	access, critique and meaningfully assimilate relevant theory / research findings with my personal knowing?
Reality perspective framing	understand the barrier of reality while helping me to become empowered to act in more congruent ways?
Problem framing	focus problem identification and resolution within the experience?
Temporal framing	draw patterns with past experiences while anticipating how I might respond in similar situations in new ways?
Parallel process framing	make connections between learning processes within my supervision process and my clinical practice?
Developmental framing	frame my realising of desirable practice within appropriate theoretical frameworks?

An example of developmental framing is found in the 'Being available' template, as discussed below. The vision of the hospice where I practised is based on holistic values. So how might my development of effective holistic practice be known? In response to this challenge, I developed the 'Being available' template based on the core holistic therapeutic – namely that of the practitioner being available to enable the patient to find meaning in their experience and to make best decisions about their healthcare, and to assist the patient to meet their health needs.

Being available template

The extent to which the practitioner can be available is influenced by six inter-related dynamics:

- the extent to which the practitioner intends a valid vision for practice
- the extent to which the practitioner is concerned for the patient and family
- the extent to which the practitioner knows the patient and family
- the extent to which the practitioner can make effective clinical judgement and respond with skilled ethical action to meet patient and family need
- the extent to which the practitioner knows and manages self within the relationship with equanimity
- the extent to which the practitioner can create and sustain an environment where being available is possible.

Source: adapted from Johns (2004).

The reader can apply this template over my text of being with Patricia and with subsequent accounts.

Other frameworks may be helpful in looking at more discrete aspects of practitioner performance. For example:

➤ expertise using the Dreyfus and Dreyfus model for skill acquisition (Dreyfus and Dreyfus 1996)

➤ the Thomas and Kilmann conflict management grid (Cavanagh 1991)

➤ the assertiveness ladder (Johns 2006).

Indeed, any theory can be converted into a map to enable the practitioner to position self within.

The third dialogical movement: the dance with Sophia

In the third dialogical movement, I engage in a dialogue between my emerging insights and the wider community of knowledge, informing and deepening my insights. My reflection on the experience with Patricia helped me to realise that I knew very little about sexuality and palliative care. I undertook a literature search using BNI and CINAHL search engines, yet found that they revealed nothing of any significance. However, there is an informative chapter on *teaching* sexuality relating to palliative care by Hostad (2007) in the previous book in this series.

Eventually I unearthed a paper by Kralik *et al.* (2001) entitled 'Constructions of sexuality for midlife women living with chronic illness'.

They quote:

> *'Women wrote of the discomfort shown by health professionals when talking about sex and sexuality. Such discomfort was not conducive to women disclosing their experiences and in some instances effectively closed off any further communication about sex.'* (185)

This made me reflect on my own discomfort in addressing sexuality, caused by not wanting to embarrass either myself or patients. Without doubt, sexuality is a taboo topic and yet its being taboo closes down what may be a vital therapeutic space for patients. Subsequently a more recent paper by Lemieux *et al.* (2004) has been inform-ative (Johns 2006).

The fourth dialogical movement: co-creating insights

I shared the experience I have in my peer clinical supervision with two of the hos-pice sisters. Clinical supervision is a formal process whereby I can be guided to learn through reflection to develop and sustain expertise, and to take responsibility for ensuring that my practice is effective. There are many reasons why reflection may need guidance (Johns 2006), not the least being that it can help the practitioner to develop the skill of holding creative tension and opening up possibilities to see other ways of being within the situation.

Only one sister was present. She asked me what I felt was significant about the experience. I picked out the contextual issues – staff noise, nausea management, the value of massage in terms of Patricia's well-being, her being visited by her son and the way such ideas are ridiculed by some staff. I emphasised the significance of sexuality based on the paper by Kralik *et al.* (2001).

Maud, the sister, felt challenged by my revelations in terms of her own practice, confessing that she was unaware of these issues, and sharing two experiences of her own. Confession under conditions of trust is a powerful factor in creating team learn-ing (Senge 1990), although it might also be seen negatively as a new form of social surveillance and control (Gilbert 2001; Cotton 2001).

As noted earlier, team learning is learning together through dialogue. As such, group guided reflection opens a *potential* learning space for the multi-professional team to grow rather than act out its multi-professional rhetoric.

A key role for the teacher or reflective practice enabler is to provide expertise and guidance in these learning spaces.

I say *potential* because practitioners, in my experience, need expert guidance to achieve it. This is a key role for the teacher or reflective guide. Aspects of this teacher's or guide's work will include the following:

➤ Rekindling commitment that practice matters to practitioners, at a time when they may be feeling burnt out. Clearly, burnt-out nurses are not available to their patients and colleagues. If practitioners have lost commitment, then this must be the point where guidance commences. There is no other place, simply because burnt-out people avoid the mirror. Linked to this point is nurturing compassion as the most significant therapeutic use of self. Arthur Frank (2002) writes of the demoralisation working in an environment where he is not valued or cared for adequately – hence guidance is a form of care to re-moralise the practitioner, for only if practitioners feel valued and cared for can they value and care for their patients. It is a simple equation, but does anyone listen? (*see* Johns 2006).
➤ Getting practitioners to face up to and harness anxiety when the natural inclination is to defend self against anxiety. People often say to me, 'don't we all

reflect?' That is true to some extent, but I argue that people reflect to rationalise anxiety not to learn from it.

➤ Getting practitioners to effectively use the MSR cues – otherwise people get stuck on the surface of these cues and wonder why reflection doesn't lead to meaningful learning. I might also add that a purpose of guidance is to nag practitioners to keep a journal. It may sound easy, but many practitioners are unable to find time to dedicate to journaling.

➤ Unearthing contradiction and understanding those factors or hindrances that constrain realising desirable practice. People usually view themselves as normal, and so it is actually quite difficult to persuade them to include self in problems. People often project their own inadequacy into the environment rather than accepting responsibility for self.

➤ Helping the practitioner to get up when they stumble and fall against the hard face of reality. Reflection can be tough, and those engaged in it need a compassionate yet firm hand to make it across often rocky ground.

➤ Infusing the practitioner with courage to act on insights. Kieffer (1984) noted that an external enabler was the single most important factor that empowered people to act. Perhaps that is the sense of not being alone? It is also why group guided reflection is so invaluable – creating as it does some peer pressure to act. Practitioners must learn to be assertive – this is always an underlying theme of reflective practice.

➤ Shifting ways of thinking so that practitioners are willing to contemplate new ways of responding to situations. Practitioners often struggle to generate new options, as they have become stuck in one, limiting way of thinking. Guidance helps to open them up to new possibilities, and illuminates practice from new vistas, creating lateral thinking and freeing the mind to follow paths of imagination and creativity. It is a form of play.

➤ Linking practice with theory in meaningful ways. I am always astonished that practitioners cannot name the theories or research they use. In an attempt to rectify this, I offer a mine of theory and research information which can be introduced into guidance when the practitioner is best positioned to assimilate it into practice. Without doubt, an effective practitioner is an informed practitioner.

➤ Summarising the insights and learning gained. Guidance enables the practitioner to look back and see progress, affirming the value of guided reflection within the reflective spiral of being and becoming.

The fifth dialogical movement: weaving the narrative

I now weave the four dialogical strands into a coherent and reflective narrative form that adequately plots my journey of realising desirable practice. I plot this journey by applying appropriate markers, as discussed earlier in the chapter. Writing the narrative releases the artist within to present a narrative that both enchants and challenges the reader. Okri (1997) urges the writer to transgress normative boundaries, challenging the normal order of things. An in-depth exploration of coherence and reflexivity are beyond the scope of this chapter. However, I have alluded to the significance of reflexivity as a looking back and a plotting of the emergence of one's effectiveness through a series of unfolding experiences. The point is worth reiterating, in that reflection is a learning process that unfolds over time rather than being instantly realised. It takes time and commitment to journal and discover the depth and subtlety of each reflective cue. It takes time to dwell within the stories and find insight. It takes time to be guided and write narratives. As such, reflection must be the core of the curriculum.

The sixth dialogical movement: dialogue with others

While writing the narrative has intrinsic value for the writer, it also has value for the interested reader. Reading my narrative will stir the reader's imagination. Some readers may take offence at what I have written, drawing out their own prejudices. I use my narratives as the basis for teaching palliative care to stimulate the students' own stories. I call this 'camp-fire teaching' (Johns 2004). I prefer it to teaching abstract theory, simply because story sets the scene within which relevant theory can be contextualised. Specific aspects of palliative care can be pulled out and foregrounded against the holistic palliative care background.

KEY POINTS

- Reflection can be viewed as a spectrum of activity from a technique to something lived as a way of being in practice.
- Reflection is a developmental reflexive process unfolding over time.
- Reflection needs to be guided to enhance its learning potential.
- Reflection is the art of holding and working towards resolving creative tension.
- Reflection must be at the core of the curriculum.
- Reflection is the hook to hang the theory hat on.
- Reflection is always challenging habitual ways of practice.
- Being a reflective practitioner is something lived in practice itself, requiring a reflective culture and systems to reinforce and sustain it.

CONCLUSION

In this chapter I have outlined reflection as a learning process through six dialogical movements. I have not explored reflection as a way of structuring clinical practice through the Burford Nursing Development Unit: Caring in Practice model. However, I do want briefly to draw the reader's attention to the significance of creating reflective learning environments within practice itself – through the way we appreciate the life pattern of our patients and families; through the way we communicate both verbally and orally; through the developmental systems we establish; and through the way we monitor quality and generally create the organisational culture.

I make these points simply to emphasise that being a reflective practitioner is something that is lived moment to moment in practice, not something done in educational programmes (Johns 2009).

IMPLICATIONS FOR THE READER'S OWN PRACTICE

1   What models of reflection do you use and how effective are they?
2   How often do you use reflection in your teaching practice?
3   How might you utilise similar narratives to teach reflective practice in your area?
4   How might your development of holistic practice become transparent?

REFERENCES

Boyd E, Fales A (1983) Reflective learning: key to learning from experience. *J Hum Psychol.* **23** (2): 99–117.

Boud D, Keogh R, Walker D, editors (1985) *Reflection: turning experience into learning.* London: Kogan Page.

Burton A (2000) Reflection: nursing's practice and education panacea? *J Adv Nurs.* **31** (5): 1009–17.

Cavanagh S (1991) The management style of staff nurses and nurse managers. *J Adv Nurs.* **16**: 1254–60.

Cotton A (2001) Private thoughts in public spheres: issues in reflection and reflective practice in nursing. *J Adv Nurs.* **36** (4): 512–19.

Cowling R (2000) Healing as appreciating wholeness. *Adv Nurs Sci.* **22** (3): 16–32.

Delmar C, Johns C (2008) *The Good, the Wise and the Right Clinical Nursing Practice.* Aalborg: Aalborg Hospital and Aarhus University Hospital Press.

Dewey J (1933) *How We Think.* Boston, MA: JC Heath.

Dreyfus H, Dreyfus S (1996) The relationship of theory and practice and the acquisition of skill. In: Benner P, Tanner C, Chesla C, editors. *Expertise in Nursing Practice.* New York: Springer.

Fay B (1987) *Critical Social Science.* Cambridge: Polity Press.

Frank A (2002) Relations of caring: demoralization and remoralization in the clinic. *Int J Hum Car.* **6** (2): 13–19.

Gilbert T (2001) Reflective practice and clinical supervision: meticulous rituals of the confessional. *J Adv Nurs.* **36** (2): 199–205.

Goldstein J (2002) *One Dharma: the emerging Western Buddhism.* London: Rider.

Holly M (1989) Reflective writing and the spirit of inquiry. *Camb J Educ.* **19** (1): 71–80.

Hostad J (2007) 'Let's talk about it, we never do', sexual health in cancer and palliative care: an educational dilemma. In: Foyle L, Hostad J, editors. *Innovations in Cancer and Palliative Care Education.* Oxford: Radcliffe Publishing.

Johns C (2002) *Guided Reflection: advancing practice.* Oxford: Blackwell Publishing.

Johns C (2004) *Becoming a Reflective Practitioner.* 2nd ed. Oxford: Blackwell Publishing.

Johns C (2006) *Engaging Reflection in Everyday Practice: a narrative approach.* Oxford: Blackwell Publishing.

Johns C (2009) *Becoming a Reflective Practitioner.* 3rd ed. Oxford: Wiley-Blackwell.

Jones B, Jones G (1996) *Earth Dance Drum: a celebration of life.* Salt Lake City, UT: Commune-A-Key.

Kearney M (2000) *A Place of Healing: working with suffering in living and dying.* Oxford: Oxford University Press.

Kieffer C (1984) Citizen empowerment: a developmental perspective. *Prev Hum Serv.* **84** (3): 9–36.

Kralik D, Koch T, Telford K (2001) Constructions of sexuality for midlife women living with chronic illness. *J Adv Nurs*. **35** (2): 180–7.

Lemieux L, Kaiser S, Pererra J, Meadows L (2004) Sexuality in palliative care: patients perspectives. *Palliat Med*. **18**: 630–7.

Mackintosh C (1998) Reflection: a flawed strategy for the nursing profession. *Nurse Educ Today*. **18**: 553–7.

Margolis H (1993) *Paradigm and Barriers: how habits of mind govern scientific beliefs*. Chicago, IL: University of Chicago Press.

Menzies-Lyth I (1988) A case study in the functioning of social systems as a defence against anxiety. In: Menzies-Lyth I. *Containing Anxiety in Institutions: selected essays*. London: Free Association Books.

Mezirow J (1981) A critical theory of adult learning and education. *Adult Educ*. **32** (1): 3–24.

O'Donohue J (1997) *Anam Cara*. New York: Bantam Books.

Okri B (1997) *A Way of Being Free*. London: Phoenix House.

Rinpoche S (1992) *The Tibetan Book of Living and Dying*. London: Rider.

Schon D (1983) *The Reflective Practitioner*. Aldershot: Avebury.

Senge P (1990) *The Fifth Discipline: the art and practice of the learning organisation*. London: Century Business.

Street A (1995) *Nursing Replay: researching nursing culture together*. Melbourne: Churchill Livngstone.

FURTHER READING

- Besides the referenced texts, a number of others may be helpful:
- Bulman C, Shutz S (2005) *Reflective Practice in Nursing: the growth of the professional practitioner*. 3rd ed. Oxford: Blackwell Publishing.
- Ghaye T (2005) *Developing the Reflective Healthcare Team*. Oxford: Blackwell Publishing.
- Johns C (2004) *Being Mindful, Easing Suffering: reflections on palliative care*. London: Jessica Kingsley Publishing.
- Johns C, Freshwater D (2005) *Transforming Nursing through Reflective Practice*. 2nd ed. Oxford: Blackwell Publishing.
- Rolfe G, Freshwater D, Jasper M (2001) *Critical Reflection for Nursing and the Helping Professions*. Basingstoke: Palgrave.
- Taylor B (2000) *Reflective Practice: a guide for nurses and midwives*. St Leonards, NSW: Allen & Unwin.

7

Learning and teaching critical thinking skills

Janet Holt

'It is the mark of an educated mind to be able to entertain a thought without accepting it.'

Aristotle

AIM

The aim of this chapter is to demonstrate how critical thinking skills can be useful in cancer and palliative care education and practice.

LEARNING OUTCOMES

By the end of this chapter, the reader should be able to:
- explore the reasons for teaching critical thinking in cancer and palliative care education
- discuss philosophical method as a strategy for learning and teaching critical thinking
- present examples of learning and teaching strategies for developing critical thinking skills.

INTRODUCTION

Critical thinking is a useful skill to develop in professional life and essential for academic study. We all engage in some form of critical thinking in everyday life, but developing these skills to use in a more systematic way can be beneficial to health professionals in practice. Proficiency in critical thinking skills is an expectation of graduates, and necessary for healthcare practitioners working in highly complex clinical environments where they need to consider, analyse, synthesise and evaluate evidence to make choices about treatment and care. In cancer and palliative care, health professionals are often faced with complex ethical dilemmas such as withdrawing treatment or evaluating the potential futility of treatment. In these situations, empirical evidence will not necessarily be present to evaluate, and practitioners will need skills in reason and argument to make moral judgements based on analysis and evaluation of the arguments advanced by others and their own personal views.

This chapter will explore the concept of critical thinking and investigate why developing critical thinking skills is important for health professionals. Ways of introducing critical thinking skills into the curriculum will be examined and the chapter will conclude with some examples of learning and teaching strategies for this.

DEFINING CRITICAL THINKING

In the healthcare literature, there are a number of definitions of critical thinking. Glen (1995) for example defines critical thinking as both a philosophical orientation to thinking and a cognitive process allowing judgement. Other authors describe it as a composition of knowledge, attitudes and the application of skills (Staib 2003); as having the ability to identify problems, to reason and make decisions (Yuan *et al.* 2007); and as a cognitive activity of critically analytical and evaluative thinking (Cottrell 2005). The definitions emphasise the importance of judgement, reason and cognition, which is summarised in a more lengthy definition from the American Philosophical Association (APA). For the APA, critical thinking means:

> 'purposeful, self regulatory judgement which results in interpretation, analysis evaluation and inference, as well as explanation of the evidential, conceptual, methodological, criteriological or contextual considerations on which the judgement is based.' (American Philosophical Association 1990: 3)

Critical thinkers therefore are inquisitive, well informed, open minded, flexible and able to make judgements; they have an ability to think in a reasoned ordered and diligent fashion, and reflect sceptically (American Philosophical Association 1990; Cottrell 2005).

WHY TEACH CRITICAL THINKING?

As can be seen in the definitions above, developing skills in critical thinking is useful for everyday life, but having the ability to analyse, reason and evaluate is essential for practitioners in contemporary healthcare with all its complexities. Education for healthcare practitioners has changed considerably over the past 20 years, particularly with the move into higher education for programmes of study that had previously utilised an apprentice style of training. The importance of theoretical knowledge for practice-based disciplines is now an expectation, and practitioners begin their professional careers with a minimum of diploma level qualifications and many are graduates. Experienced practitioners also return to higher education for further study, both at undergraduate and postgraduate levels. Analytical skills are recognised as important in higher education and the need to practise from an evidence base is an essential requirement of contemporary practice. Programmes of study are designed to develop analytical skills in health practitioners to enable them to *'think, examine assumptions and provide reasoned argument to support ideas and judgements'* (Holt and Clarke 2002: 77). Consequently, there is an expectation that practitioners will have a deeper understanding of concepts rather than just of their practical application. But it cannot be assumed that students will develop critical thinking skills simply because of being registered in programmes of higher education.

Critical thinking can make a significant contribution to knowledge development in healthcare and is essential for:

➤ finding ways to help students to move from black and white (dualistic) thinking, to being able to work through complex problems and explain their reasoning and conclusions
➤ developing skills in clinical judgement and clinical decision-making
➤ evidence-based practice
➤ stimulating and continuing debate about the nature of healthcare and its knowledge and practice base
➤ giving account for our actions to the public and to the profession.

MEASURING CRITICAL THINKING SKILLS

There are a number of published studies, particularly in the North American literature, where the critical thinking abilities of students have been investigated and measured and a review of these methods can be found in Daly (2001) and Mundy and Denham (2008). There are a number of standardised measures that can be used to measure critical thinking, but the two most popular are the Watson–Glaser Critical Thinking Appraisal (Watson and Glaser 1991) and the California Critical Thinking Skills Test (Facione 1990), both of which are broad spectrum measures of critical thinking attributes. Generally speaking, the tests can be used as before and after measures either of a programme overall or of a specific intervention. However, even in North America where it is common to routinely test critical thinking, students have differing levels of ability on entry to programmes, making it difficult to obtain baseline data. Furthermore, there are problems associated with the assessment tools, most notably that they are not discipline specific and may not adequately capture critical thinking skills that emanate from practice situations (Mundy and Denham 2008). The tools can also be problematic when used in countries other that the United States, as they are culturally contextual and there is the possibility that critical thinking characteristics may differ between cultural groups (Tiwari *et al.* 2003).

Further evidence of the confusing picture of the efficacy of the assessment tools can be seen in an investigation into the impact of philosophy on students' ability to think critically. In this study using the Watson–Glaser Critical Thinking Appraisal, the researchers found that while a one-term course in logic had an impact on the students' ability to think critically, the results were less conclusive for students who took other philosophy courses (Annis and Annis 1979). Given that the foundation of philosophy is critical thinking, it is not unreasonable to believe that taking a course in philosophy would by definition improve and develop critical thinking skills, so these results are surprising. However, the researchers acknowledge that the participants had only studied the subjects for one term, which was a very short time for critical thinking skills to develop to such an extent as to show a statistically significant difference in a pre- and post-test design.

Developing critical thinking skills in students continues to be a goal of higher education programmes, and there appear to be sound arguments to support this for pre- and post-registration healthcare students. But the findings from research in this area are inconsistent, raising concerns about the ability of the standard instruments to measure critical thinking. This is particularly the case for healthcare students, and Mundy and Denham (2008) propose the development of a discipline-specific instrument and for more research specifically focused on how healthcare students think about their diverse roles and the way the critical thought is translated into practice in clinical settings.

LEARNING TO THINK CRITICALLY

The key issue in critical thinking is the development of skills in reason and argument and this has a threefold purpose:

➤ to enable us to critically evaluate our own beliefs
➤ to enable us to present these verbally and in written format to others
➤ to enable us to evaluate and analyse the arguments presented to us by other people.

Much of the foundation for critical thinking can be found in the academic discipline of philosophy, and according to Warburton:

> 'Philosophy is an activity: it is a way of thinking about certain sorts of questions. Its most distinctive feature is the use of logical argument. Philosophers typically deal in arguments: they either invent them, criticise other people or do both. They also analyse and clarify concepts.' (Warburton 1999: 1–2)

Despite the findings in Annis and Annis's (1979) study, by definition critical thinking skills can be developed using philosophical enquiry to explore and analyse concepts, arguments and claims (Clarke and Holt 2001). It should be noted that in order to do this, it is not necessary to study philosophy as a subject *per se*, but to introduce students to methods of philosophical enquiry to explore fundamental questions in healthcare.

Whether critical thinking can be taught or not has been a matter of debate. However, it is unclear how students are to acquire skills in critical thinking if this is not directly addressed in the curriculum. Maudsley and Strivens (2000) examine the evidence for and against teaching critical thinking and conclude that it can be taught as long as the learning and teaching strategies are directed towards techniques to develop thinking skills. It is important to distinguish between learning about a subject and learning to think, as thinking skills are not necessarily developed simply as a consequence of subject knowledge. For example, healthcare practitioners in cancer and palliative care are expected to respect the dignity of service users and this is the focus of a recent campaign of the Royal College of Nursing (RCN). The importance of respecting dignity is often stated explicitly in professional codes of practice and/ or ethics, such as in The Code for Nurses and Midwives: '*You must treat people as individuals and respect their dignity*' (Nursing and Midwifery Council 2008: 2). But what does it mean exactly to say that we respect someone's dignity? The emphasis on respecting dignity in The Code implies that nurses have a duty or are obliged to do this, particularly as The Code is the document by which nurses are held to account for their actions. Therefore, it is plausible that respecting dignity is included within the healthcare curriculum. One learning strategy to approach this subject could be to give examples of how a person's dignity can be respected and how it can be violated. For example, a common understanding of maintaining dignity in healthcare is ensuring that service users are not exposed during clinical procedures. Hence, the student will learn about how to respect a person's dignity, but while learning the practicalities of maintaining dignity are arguably essential for nurses, this approach will not enhance their understanding of the concept of dignity.

Is knowledge of the practicalities of respecting dignity enough or is there an expectation that highly educated professionals are able to demonstrate not only how to treat people with dignity, but also that they have a broader and deeper knowledge base of the subject as a whole? To achieve greater understanding, the concept of dignity can be examined in the published literature. For example, a paper by Ann Gallagher explores not only the concept of dignity but also that of respect for dignity (Gallagher 2004). The paper is a very good example of a philosophical analysis of the concepts, and someone reading this paper would gain a much broader and deeper knowledge of dignity rather than simply understanding the practicalities of maintaining dignity. Edwards (2001) indicates that a typical characteristic of philosophy is its concern with second-order questions. While first-order enquiry involves acquiring *knowledge* of the subject, second-order or philosophical enquiry involves examining the *meaning* of the subject. In the example of dignity, first-order questions could include those that might be answered empirically, such as 'How do nurses respect dignity?', or 'What are service users' experiences of respect for dignity?' Second-order enquiry would focus on what is meant by dignity, such as examining definitions of dignity or asking what it means to say that dignity must be respected. Nevertheless, understanding a paper such as the one cited by Gallagher (2004) presupposes a capacity to recognise, evaluate and make judgements of the arguments presented, in other words, an ability to demonstrate use of critical thinking skills.

INTRODUCING CRITICAL THINKING SKILLS INTO THE CURRICULUM

If students are to be encouraged to develop critical thinking skills, then time will need to be found in the curriculum for this and facilitators will need to be identified. Learning and teaching strategies and resources will also need to be developed. Different methods and approaches can be used, for example, Toofany (2008) proposes concept mapping as a useful technique, while Maudsley and Strivens (2000) recommend problem-based learning. There is also the issue of who should teach and facilitate the development of critical thinking skills. Mundy and Denham (2008) suggest that it should not be assumed that members of academic staff, no matter how highly educated, are proficient in critical thinking abilities. Furthermore, even if the member of staff does have clearly refined critical thinking abilities, they may not necessarily be able to communicate this to help others to develop their skills. Therefore critical thinking skills teaching is no different to that in any other aspect of healthcare and those who have the necessary skills, knowledge and aptitude to do so should teach it (Holt 2007).

As considered above, Maudsley and Strivens (2000) also discuss the need to separate subject knowledge from strategies specifically directed to develop critical thinking skills, and this can be particularly useful for pre-registration students at the beginning of a programme of study. Two good resources for this are Anne Thompson's *Critical Reasoning* (1996) and Stella Cottrell's *Critical Thinking Skills* (2005). Both contain a number of exercises that can be used for classroom activities, but Cottrell's book has a much broader scope and the advantage of being written specifically for students. Hence it can be used both for classroom teaching and by the students to study independently.

For more senior students in health-related courses and particularly for post-registration students, the need to separate subject learning from learning skills in critical thinking is less obvious. Earlier in this chapter, the example of respecting dignity was presented to illustrate the process of philosophical enquiry. Students in the preliminary stages of healthcare courses are introduced to a range of theoretical subjects to prepare them for experiential learning in practice settings. Hence, it is crucially important that they understand the practicalities of respecting a service user's dignity and, arguably, it is less important for them to explore dignity as a concept at this stage in a programme of study. However, for students who have had exposure to the realities of the practice setting, a deeper exploration of concepts such as dignity, holism or evidence-based practice is valuable. This is of particular importance for post-registration students who might not see the relevance of being given general exercises designed to help them to identify arguments made by others and to improve their own reasoning skills. Therefore, for students who are already aware of the importance of fundamental concepts such as respecting dignity, it can be particularly helpful to embed the development of critical thinking skills in contextually specific examples.

Members of staff in the School of Healthcare at the University of Leeds have successfully used this approach for a number of years in two modules in post-registration nursing degrees (Clarke and Holt 2001; Holt and Clarke 2002). The learning and teaching strategies include lecturer-led sessions and student-led tutorials as well as private study time. The students are introduced to skills in philosophical analysis, but in a nursing context. So for example, an early session in the module explores the use of language and meaning, and students are given a simple statement to discuss:

> *'Is the train standing here in the station at platform 1 the same train your sister took to London yesterday?'*

Typically the discussions centre around the physical attributes of the train or whether the timetable is the important factor. What is important in this example is that the students explore the meaning of the word 'same' and this exercise allows them to do this. In turn, it allows them to realise that what is at issue here is a verbal disagreement (Hospers 1997), not what the train actually looks like, how many carriages it has or what time it left and subsequently arrived at the destination. The aim of the exercise is therefore for students to appreciate and understand that different interpretations of the word 'same' are being used. Once this key issue is grasped, the exercise is then immediately followed by a nursing-related example, such as:

> 'Is Tom the same person that he was since he suffered a head injury and exhibits different behaviours to those prior to his injury?'

Other exercises centre on defining and accompanying characteristics. Again using an example from Hospers (1997), the students look at the defining and accompanying characteristics of objects such as a triangle, horse, dog and cat. The aim here is to identify what are essential characteristics – that is, characteristics that it is necessary for the object to have – and then separating these from accompanying characteristics, namely, those that are not defining, such as colour or the number of legs. One of the defining characteristics of a triangle is that it has three sides, and should one or more sides be removed, then the object would cease to be a triangle. However, any other characteristics such as colour or size could be altered without substantially affecting the definition. Similar to the previous example, it is crucial to move swiftly to a clinical illustration of the point, such as 'How do we define nursing?', 'What are the defining characteristics of nursing that are essential to the meaning of nursing?', 'What are the less important (accompanying) characteristics?' or 'What do we mean by branches or specialities of nursing?' Specific cancer and palliative care examples can be substituted instead of the head injury example, and for exercises to explore definitions, examples could be 'What is palliative care?' or 'How do we define death?' In our experience, we have found the students need little prompting to move from the more general to the clinical examples, and in the majority of cases they provide their own examples from practice to illustrate the points made. This has been found to be a good stimulus for discussion, however, it does require skilful facilitation to keep focus.

For tutorials, we have selected articles and chapters from the nursing literature that explore particular concepts. The journals *Nursing Philosophy* and the *Journal of Advanced Nursing* are useful resources for this, as are position statements produced by professional bodies, such as the RCN's definition of nursing (Royal College of Nursing 2003). It is important that the students are given the resources and a short series of questions to act as prompts at the beginning of the module, to ensure that they have sufficient time to locate the material, read and reflect on the content. Some papers may be long or complex, an example of this being John Paley's interesting and comprehensive paper, 'An archaeology of caring knowledge' (Paley 2001). To overcome this, either the students can be split into groups to look at different sections of the paper, or specific arguments or sections can be identified for analysis. To keep the students' interest in the subject, it is advisable to choose papers that are directly related to their clinical experience, but this can still include exploration of broader concepts such as caring, or dignity. Even if the papers are not specific to cancer and/or palliative care, extrapolation of the theories, concepts and arguments from the papers and debating them in the context of cancer and palliative care is particularly helpful in further developing critical thinking skills.

As noted above, there is concern about the lack of evidence to support the efficacy of critical thinking skills learning and teaching, but assessment of this can still be made through formal evaluation and assessment of the strategies used. Methods of assessment directed towards making a judgement of the students' critical thinking skills will at least show evidence of the achievements of specific students and allow for some appraisal of the approaches to learning and teaching. In our experience, the selective use of philosophical methods of enquiry can be beneficial to help students acquire skills in critical analysis and to encourage them to think about, analyse, evaluate and be sceptical about concepts important to practice. Subsequently, this approach can make a positive contribution to the development of knowledge (Holt and Clarke 2002).

KEY POINTS

■ Critical thinkers are inquisitive, well informed, open minded, flexible and able to make judgements, have an ability to think in a reasoned, ordered and diligent fashion, and reflect sceptically (American Philosophical Association 1990; Cottrell 2005).
■ Cancer and palliative care education provides opportunities to develop critical thinking.
■ Critical thinking should be an essential part of the curriculum.
■ Examples to demonstrate the benefits of critical thinking abound in cancer and palliative care.

CONCLUSION

There is general agreement that critical thinking skills are necessary for practitioners practising in complex setting such as cancer and palliative care. Pre- and post-registration programmes of study for health professionals aim to develop critical thinking skills, but it cannot be assumed that students will develop such skills simply as a result of their exposure to higher education. This is further complicated by inconsistencies in research in this area and doubt about the limitation of using the standardised measures with healthcare students. If it is important to help students become independent critical thinkers, then the curriculum must directly address this issue and methods of learning, teaching and assessment of critical thinking made explicit in programmes of study. There are a number of resources currently available to help facilitators to prepare material for classroom study and for students to use independently. However, some of the better examples of this material are directed to learning to think critically in general and are not contextually specific.

As has been shown in this chapter, these resources can be used as a foundation for learning and as a basis to develop specific exercises related to cancer and palliative care. It is important that links to practice are explicit, as students, particularly those who already have some knowledge, are less likely to appreciate the value of learning that does not seem to be directly relevant or meaningful or to resonate with their experiences. Even without evidence from systematic investigation, local assessment of learning, teaching and assessment strategies together with student evaluation of the experience will indicate where improvements need to be made and show areas of good practice contributing to knowledge development.

IMPLICATIONS FOR THE READER'S OWN PRACTICE

1 How will you develop and measure the critical thinking of your students in the future?
2 What exercises could you use in the classroom that promote critical thinking in practice?
3 How would you improve first-order and second-order techniques?
4 What examples specific to cancer and palliative care can you think of to explore critical thinking?

REFERENCES

American Philosophical Association (1990) *Critical Thinking: a statement of expert consensus for purposes of educational assessment and instrument.* The Delphi Report: research findings and recommendations prepared for the committee on pre-college philosophy. Newark, NJ: APA.

Annis LF, Annis DB (1979) The impact of philosophy on students' critical thinking ability. Contemp Educ Psychol. **4**: 219–26.

Clarke DJ, Holt J (2001) Philosophy: a door to open the door to critical thinking. *Nurse Educ Today.* **21**: 71–8.

Cottrell S (2005) *Critical Thinking Skills.* Basingstoke: Palgrave Macmillan.

Daly WM (2001) The development of an alternative method of assessment of critical thinking as an outcome of nursing education. *J Adv Nurs.* **36** (1): 120–30.

Edwards SD (2001) *Philosophy of Nursing.* Basingstoke: Palgrave.

Facione PA (1990) *The California Critical Thinking Skills Test: form A and form B.* Millbrae, CA: California Academic Press.

Gallagher A (2004) Dignity and respect for dignity – two key health professional values: implications for nursing practice. *Nurs Ethics.* **11** (6): 587–99.

Glen S (1995) Developing critical thinking in higher education. *Nurse Educ Today.* **13** (2): 170–6.

Holt J (2007) Teaching ethics in cancer and palliative care. In: Foyle L, Hostad J, editors. *Innovations in Cancer and Palliative Care Education.* Oxford: Radcliffe Publishing.

Holt J, Clarke D (2002) Philosophy and nursing: a useful transferable skill. *Nurs Philos.* **1** (1): 76–9.

Hospers J (1997) *An Introduction to Philosophical Analysis.* 4th ed. London: Routledge.

Maudsley G, Strivens J (2000) Promoting professional knowledge, experiential learning and critical thinking for medical students. *Med Educ.* **34**: 535–44.

Mundy K, Denham SA (2008) Nurse educators: still challenged by critical thinking. *Teach Learn Nurs.* **3**: 94–9.

Nursing and Midwifery Council (2008) *The Code: standards of conduct, performance and ethics for nurses and midwives.* London: NMC.

Palcy J (2001) An archaeology of caring knowledge. *J Adv Nurs.* **36** (2): 188–98.

Royal College of Nursing (2003) *Defining Nursing.* London: RCN.

Staib S (2003) Teaching and measuring critical thinking. *J Nurs Educ.* **42** (11): 121–5.

Thompson A (1996) *Critical Reasoning.* London: Routledge.

Tiwari A, Avery A, Lai P (2003) Critical thinking: disposition of Hong Kong Chinese and Australian nursing students. *J Adv Nurs.* **44** (3): 298–307.

Toofany S (2008) Critical thinking among nurses. *Nurs Manag.* **14** (9): 28–31.

Warburton N (1999) *Philosophy: the basics.* 3rd ed. London: Routledge.

Watson G, Glaser EM (1991) *Critical Thinking Appraisal Manual.* Kent: Harcourt Brace.

Yuan H, Williams B, Fan L (2007) A systematic review of selected evidence on developing nursing students' critical thinking through problem based learning. *Nurse Educ Today.* **28**: 657–63.

8

Advanced nursing practice: the potential sword of Damocles in education?

Martin Towers

'Change does not necessarily assure progress, but progress implacably requires
change. Education is essential to change, for education creates new wants and the
ability to satisfy them.'

Henry Steele Commager

AIM

This chapter is intended to give a brief overview of the development of
advanced practice in nursing and the implications this brings for practitioners and those who educate them, particularly in relation to the professional
and legal accountability of the nurse. There is necessarily some outline
given of what might be considered the 'nuts and bolts' of the legal and
professional issues and it is to be hoped that this may form a basis of discussion and debate for those undertaking education in this area.

LEARNING OUTCOMES
By the end of this chapter, the reader should be able to:
- discuss the changing boundaries in relation to advanced nursing
  practice
- define and discuss legal and professional issues in relation to
  advanced nursing practice
- explore the educational responsibilities in raising awareness of
  employers' attitudes and liabilities in the NHS and voluntary sector
- identify the challenges in cancer and palliative care education in
  advanced nursing practice.

INTRODUCTION

Nursing in general has undergone some major shifts over the last ten to fifteen years or so, not only in terms of educational preparation (the move into higher education being a good example) and opportunities for further professional development but also in terms of the boundaries of practice. Areas such as prescribing and diagnosis that were once considered to be the sole preserve of medical practitioners have been opened up and nurses are now working in areas and developing skills that would have been considered impossible even twenty years ago. Palliative care has been affected by these changes as much as any other area of nursing and the potential scope for developing the role of palliative care nurses both as individuals and as part of a team must be seen as considerable.

The pace of change and reform of how healthcare is delivered has also had a major impact. The government can be seen to have pushed professional boundaries further as a result of initiatives such as 'Liberating the talents' (DoH 2002) and it could be argued that the professions, education and other stakeholders have been left to play 'catch-up' in dealing with the consequences of the changes brought about by government policy. It is also very important to note that the government does not seem to have been discriminating about the areas where this advanced practice could be developed. Therefore it is quite difficult to entirely focus on cancer and palliative care, as the direction that the development of advanced practitioners is moving in is still not, at this stage, entirely clear.

The growth of the autonomous practitioners may, however, have brought problems in its wake relating to issues of legal and professional accountability. It is the aim of this chapter to highlight some of these issues from both a practice and educational perspective. Because of the possible nature and scope of developments in clinical practice, partly due to the lack of precision in the definition and perceived scope of advanced practice (Nursing and Midwifery Council 2005), some of what may follow is necessarily speculative and general in nature, but this chapter may also offer insights into current as well as future practice and the subsequent training of practitioners.

CHANGING PROFESSIONAL BOUNDARIES

There has always been a tendency for nurses to have extended their practice, for example prior to World War II nurses did not perform blood pressure readings and many of the dressings to patients wounds were carried out by junior medical staff (Baly 1995). In the final quarter of the twentieth century, this trend appears to have accelerated. The new roles that nurses undertook (for example, administration of intravenous additives, and ear syringing) could be seen as extended roles that quite easily 'fitted in' with what was taken as the basic nurse's role (Dimond 2008; Mackay 1993). They were largely uncontroversial, as the roles (or tasks) were ones that the medical profession largely considered to be routine and the time thus saved could be put to a better use. From an organisational point of view, it also appeared to be advantageous given the seemingly relentless pressure on medical staff time and resources as well as budget (Mackay 1993). Such roles were carefully controlled by employers and were generally limited in scope and relied on the nurse's following a set of clearly defined protocols.

As an example, readers who qualified after the late 1970s may recall the training that was given to undertake the administration of intravenous medications.

In 1992 the United Kingdom Central Council (UKCC) produced the Third Edition of the Code of Professional Conduct (UKCC 1992) and supported this with a number of supplementary documents, one of which was titled 'Exercising accountability' (UKCC 1992a). This document removed the concept of the 'extended' role of the nurse and replaced it with the concept of 'expanded' practice. The same year also saw the passage of the Medicinal Products (Prescribing by Nurses) Act 1992 that followed on from the first Crown report (DoH 1989) that recommended that some nurses be allowed to prescribe from a limited formulary. It is against this background that an expansion of the areas of nursing practice developed and a whole range of new roles were created that, while being firmly rooted in the matrix and culture of nursing practice, have led to the creation of new areas of practice that require the use of skills usually associated with the medical profession, such as diagnosis and prescribing. This trend has also been encouraged by initiatives from the UK Government, such as the NHS Plan (Department of Health 2000), and the changes to general practitioner contracts. From an educational perspective, that has led to the development of a whole range of new courses being offered at higher academic levels.

Therefore, we have now reached the stage where there are a number of nurses who have a range of roles and are considered to be practising at what can be termed an advanced level. As well as such issues as the blurring of professional boundaries, there may be challenges in the shape of how advanced practitioners are to be held accountable for their practice. This is something that those engaged in preparing nurses for advanced practice need to consider, as an advanced practitioner may be exposed to a higher level of risk than has been the case for nurses. To help those being prepared for advanced practice and those involved in their preparation, the next section will look at the concept of accountability, especially from a legal perspective.

ACCOUNTABILITY

Dimond (2008) uses the phrase 'arenas of accountability' when defining how nurses can be held accountable for their practice. She identifies four areas: accountability to the employer, to the profession, to the patient and to the public. It is with accountability to the patient and the profession that we are going to be primarily concerned here.

The individual legal accountability of a nurse for their practice appears to be a concept that has taken a while to take hold. This is probably a reflection of the status that nurses have held within healthcare organisations. In *Gold v. Essex CC* (1942), Lord Goddard could comment that

> *'It is part of the nurses' duty, as servants of the hospital, to attend the surgeons and physicians and carry out their orders. If the surgeon gives a direction to the nurse which she carries out, she is not guilty of negligence even if the direction is improper.'*

While today that would not be considered good law, it does raise the question of how nurses (and indeed, other healthcare professionals) are held to be legally liable for their actions.

In civil law terms, if a patient is injured as a result of an alleged act of negligence by a professionally qualified practitioner, then they may be entitled to compensation. This is the only effective mechanism available to patients where they have been injured seriously and may require long-term care. To obtain compensation, the following steps are necessary.

1   A patient (claimant) has to establish that a practitioner (defendant) owed the claimant a duty of care, i.e. that the relationship between defendant and claimant was sufficiently close to impose a duty on the defendant not to injure (by action or omission) the claimant. 'Relationship' in this context means that the defendant could reasonably foresee that their professional actions could have an effect on others. This has been interpreted quite strictly by the courts (*see* Herring 2008).

2   Once duty of care has been established (and in practical terms, this is not a problem in relation to the NHS), the claimant then has to show that the defendant has breached the duty of care. This is done by reference to what is termed the Bolam test, named after the case of *Bolam v. Friern HMC* (1957). In outline, professionals' actions are judged against a 'responsible body of clinical opinion' and could therefore be considered as essentially a professional rather than a legal test, although the courts assert that they make the decision on breach of duty. There are a number of modifications to the concept in *Bolam* (which are concisely and clearly discussed by Greene 2005) and it should be noted that the concept in *Bolam* is not without its critics (Greene 2005; Mason and Laurie 2006; Brazier and Miola 2000).

3   As a direct result of the breach of duty by the defendant, there has to be injury suffered by the claimant. The injury must be reasonably foreseeable, i.e. it has to be an injury that can only have resulted from the defendant's action and which would have not occurred but for the actions of the defendant (Mason and Laurie 2006).

It can be seen that this process requires the claimant to establish fault on the part of the defendant and that no recovery can be made if the injury arose accidentally. Under our current system, accidental injury is not compensated outside of an injured person's personal insurance (Pattinson 2006). Other jurisdictions, most notably New Zealand, have introduced the concept of 'no fault' liability with apparently mixed results (de Cruz 2003). To try to stem the large sums of money (£633.3 million in 2007–08, NHSLA 2008) that are spent on settling claims within the NHS, the UK Government has introduced a new system of enforceable mediation and settlement without the need for litigation. This is contained in the NHS Redress Act 2006 that came into force in October 2008. This legislation applies to claims where the damages will be less than £20 000 and where there has been negligence by a healthcare professional. The Act is not beyond criticism and a useful, if somewhat critical, analysis is offered by Farell and Devaney (2007). It will be interesting as to how well it will work in the future to satisfy the demands of injured patients for compensation and to encourage healthcare providers to be more proactive in dealing with errors and incidents.

Irrespective of the mechanism of gaining (i.e. legislation or litigation), compensation so received as a result of a successful action is paid in the form of monetary damages and here it is important to note that, unlike the USA, damages in the UK are purely compensatory in nature and do not contain a punitive element. Damages are also decided by the trial judge according to a strict formula and guidelines which are designed to place the claimant in the position they would have been had they not suffered the injury (Ingham 2008).

The basic concept of legal liability outlined above applies across the whole spectrum of practice irrespective of the type of role nurses were undertaking. However, some issues around breach of duty in respect of advanced practice could be important and are briefly discussed below.

In fact, it would be unlikely that a nurse would be sued as an individual (Dimond 2008). This is because most nurses are employed by another party and that employer – whether the NHS, a GP practice or a charity – would be vicariously liable for the actions of the nurse. Vicarious liability is a legal doctrine whereby an employer, even if not at fault themselves, becomes legally liable for the negligent actions of their employee, provided that the employee was acting within the scope and course of their employment. In the NHS this is dealt with under the terms of NHS Indemnity (NHS Executive 1996). Nurses employed by GPs and charities should be covered by the indemnity insurance that their employers should have (Greene 2005).

For nurses working as advanced practitioners, there are a number of issues for consideration. These are:
➤ the standard of care that nurses would be expected to adhere to
➤ recognition by employers and educators of the importance of the novel risks faced by nurses undertaking advanced roles
➤ recognition by practitioners of their own legal accountability.

Standard of care

One of the difficulties in looking at any issue involving potential litigation lies in the record of cases. Most books dealing with negligence in healthcare (often rather revealing having the word 'medical' rather than healthcare in the title) have to rely on the case law. Any review of this case law (and collected examples can be found in Stauch *et al.* 2006; Jackson 2006) will reveal that the cases are overwhelmingly related to medical rather than nursing or any other section of the healthcare professions. Even in the titles aimed at nurses (e.g. Dimond 2008; McHale and Tingle 2007; Fletcher and Holt 1995), most of the cases cited involve doctors as the professional under scrutiny.

Given that most of the professional staff employed in healthcare are nurses and that they will be responsible for a large proportion of healthcare interventions, this may seem surprising. The question could be asked whether nurses are less negligent than doctors; logically the answer should be 'no', but it seems that statistics giving any impression as who is being negligent do not exist (Montgomery 2003). The answer may be that traditionally doctors have been more exposed to risk from litigation as they have been carrying out activities that may be seen as potentially harmful to patients. After all, it could be argued that while major surgery or the use of potent medicines in oncology may carry a high risk of injury or mortality, a patient would be very unlikely (not to say unlucky) to die of a bed bath. Of course, as nurses increasingly undertake roles that can be seen as carrying an increased level of risk, this may be well alter.

Cultural issues may also have played a part. It could be argued that traditionally the essential relationship between the nurse and the patient was of quite a different nature from that between the doctor and the patient. In the past, as authors such as Salvage (1985) and Hart (1994) have commented, public perceptions of nurses have not always been terribly accurate, but it would appear that notwithstanding cases such as those involving Beverly Allitt, Barbara Salisbury and Colin Norris, the public have generally been well disposed to the nursing profession. Reports like the Allitt Inquiry (1994) reflect society's unwillingness to accept the idea that members of a 'caring' profession would wish to cause harm to patients and this may have been translated into a reluctance to blame individual nurses rather than an organisation. Financial issues may also have played a part. It was only in 1995 that the NHS took full responsibility for settling negligence cases involving doctors; prior to that date the medical defence bodies (e.g. Medical Defence Union and Medical Protection Society) acted on behalf of doctors and were very active in defending claims, as indeed they still are with respect to general practitioners and others not directly employed by the NHS. The NHS Litigation Authority is keen to resolve cases through mediation (NHSLA 2009), which, apart from savings in time, is considerably cheaper than going to court. This means that only quite difficult cases are fully litigated (about 2% according to the NHSLA 2009).

However, in the future it may be the nurses who, through advanced and autonomous practice, create the difficult legal problems. Over the years the law has established its tests to decide how a standard of care may be met by reference to practitioner standards. This has largely taken place in the context of medical practice. With a whole range of new practice areas opening for nurses (and other health professionals), how confident can we be as to how we define standards of care with respect to advanced practice? At first, there may be reliance on applying the standards expected of medical practitioners, but at some stage the courts, or whoever is charged with deciding how liability is apportioned, are going to have to decide on how they deal with a profession that operates in a very different manner to medicine. Those involved in education may have to make practitioners much more aware that their practice carries risks, which can have serious consequences, not only in terms of patient safety but also in terms of accounting for their practice, as can be seen below.

Recognition of risk

Professionally, nurses, perhaps much more than doctors, have been subject to tight control by their employers and the professional regulators (Montgomery 2003). Most nurses will be familiar with the use of a whole range of procedures and protocols that govern their practice and there seems to be an expectation that they will abide by these. This is also reflected in the hierarchical structure of nursing and the concepts of obedience, even to the point of litigation (*see Hefferon v. UKCC* 1988 and Hart 1994). At the same time there has been a growing awareness within the NHS organisations that the level of settlements for negligence needs to be controlled.[1] One of the ways this can be done is through the use of various risk management initiatives that NHS bodies have put in place. For those who are not directly employed by the NHS (i.e. nurses who are employed by charities or general practices), the same issues still apply as there will be pressures from the organisation's insurers to reduce their exposure to risk as well as to meet performance targets that will form part of any contracts. However, it must be remembered that the advanced practice that employees may be undertaking requires the application of skills and knowledge that are not always amenable to a process of protocol and policy. Examples would be in relation to nurse practitioners who may be involved in using diagnostic skills to assess and offer treatment for patients and those who act as independent prescribers. These groups quite clearly may offer novel challenges to the organisations they work for, as they will not fit closely into the classic mould of protocol-led practice. Although these nurses will work to quite closely agreed guidelines, there is going to be a margin of uncertainty to some of their work. This can be demonstrated by considering what could happen. If a nurse acting as an advanced practitioner makes a decision based on their autonomous diagnosis of a patient's or service user's condition that turns out to be incorrect, and if as a result the patient or service user is injured in some way, then there is potential liability. It would be quite straightforward, providing that adequate procedures were in place, to demonstrate whether the nurse had been acting as they should have been in terms of following agreed guidelines. However, the problem then arises of trying to evaluate if the decision made by the nurse was the right decision and protocols and policies may offer only limited help. The fact that this margin is precisely in the area of work where one of the major problems surrounding litigation often occurs is something that employers and educators have to be aware of, if they are going to adequately support not only their employees or students, but also their patients or service users.

The importance that is placed on the development of decision-making skills as part of the preparation for advanced practice, as well as on ensuring that it is supported by an adequate knowledge base, is quite clearly an investment that potentially will pay rich dividends in terms of producing practitioners who may be less likely to make errors of judgement and who will recognise the limitations of their practice.

Awareness by practitioners of their own knowledge and limitations

As well as employers and educators having a clear concept of the types of risks that advanced practitioners may be open to, the individual also has a responsibility. Nurses are familiar with the concept of personal accountability – the Code of Conduct (NMC 2008) is very clear on this point and any of the legal ethical texts aimed at nurses give clear accounts of the nurse's accountability to the law (Dimond 2008; McHale and Tingle 2001). Added to this, the professional guidelines that have been issued in respect of some areas of advanced practice also reinforce the point. As an example, when pre-scribing by nurses was introduced as a result of the Crown reports and the subsequent Medicinal Products (Prescribing by Nurses) Act 1992, the UKCC issued quite detailed guidance for nurses undertaking courses of preparation as extended and independent prescribers. The guidance specifically highlighted the need for practitioners to be aware of their accountability in this particular area of practice as well as defining some of the issues to be considered in relation to their accountability (UKCC 2001). In terms of education, this will have had obvious implications for providers to design courses that highlight concepts and issues of personal accountability.

Nurses who act as advanced practitioners and those who educate them have a clear duty to themselves and their patients to ensure that they are familiar with the possible consequences of their actions and the processes by which they may be held to account for those actions.

This seems particularly relevant at present considering the claims that are made in respect of a possible 'compensation culture' and concerns that have been expressed about 'defensive practice'. While this is an interesting area in itself, there is insufficient space to discuss this issue within the confines of this chapter. Readers are directed to Herring (2008), Mason and Laurie (2006) and the report by the House of Commons Constitution Affairs Committee (House of Commons 2006).

PROFESSIONAL REGULATION

Professional regulation is another area where there may well be challenges to advanced practice in the future, especially in areas where nurses could be perceived to be at special risk because of the nature of the practice that they undertake and the risk of causing harm. Advanced practice, by its very nature, may be leading nurses into areas where the profession as a whole has little experience of dealing with both ethical and legal issues, and it may become difficult for those who have to give advice to practitioners (for example, the nursing unions, managers, even possibly the regulatory body). In the field of palliative care, as a result of changes in legislation, advanced practitioners are now able to prescribe controlled drugs, including opiates (DoH 2009).

This represents a major expansion of nursing practice into areas previously considered to be firmly within the scope of medical practice and is an area not without potential problems, as evidenced by the discussion over prescribing as a result of the Harold Shipman case and subsequent inquiry (Shipman Inquiry 2004).

It is interesting to note that the whole area of prescribing opiates is potentially one of some concern and it could be argued that the problems that practitioners appear to face in the USA with regard to opiate prescribing – with practitioners being under investigation from local law enforcement agencies when they appear to have prescribed 'too many' opiates' (Pain and the Law 2009) – may serve as a warning to practitioners in the UK. In view of the current interest in issues surrounding the end of life, especially against the background of the debate over assisted suicide and the recent media interest in this area, practitioners may feel apprehensive over dealing with this area of practice (Brazier and Cave 2007).

All nurses will be aware of the statement in the Code of Conduct (NMC 2008):

> 'As a professional, you are personally accountable for actions and omissions in your practice and must always be able to justify your decisions.'

In terms of advanced practice, this takes on special importance as some of the decisions taken by practitioners could clearly injure or have other adverse effects on their patients in a way that is novel in terms of nursing practice. For example, if a palliative care practitioner prescribes a particular medication to a patient and it is given by another nursing practitioner, then in the event of injury both practitioners could be held accountable to the regulatory body. One nurse (the prescriber) could be acting as an autonomous practitioner as an independent prescriber. The NMC would then have to decide if there had been misconduct and arrive at appropriate penalties for both practitioners based on their level of culpability. This may or may not be a relatively straightforward task, although there seems to be scope for discussion in terms of the expectations placed upon the practitioners. It seems, too, that the professional relationship between the nurses would be essentially different from that so far encountered in terms of medication errors where the issues have centred on the relationship and expectations between two (or more) different groups of professionals. The Code (NMC 2008) seems to set high standards of conduct expected from nurses. In the previous edition of the Code (NMC 2004), paragraph 8.5 expected nurses to intervene in emergency situations both inside and outside of the workplace situation. While it is easily imagined that nurses would intervene in emergency situations within the workplace, the imposition of such a duty outside of the workplace implied a higher standard of conduct than that imposed by the current law of negligence and, unlike some other jurisdictions, England has no 'Good Samaritan' legislation (Mason and Laurie 2006). Whether this would be the case under the 2008 Code is unclear, as it is not explicitly mentioned.

A far more potentially worrying issue from a regulation perspective lies within the nature of advanced practice. Nurses who are working at this level will often be using skills that are much more akin to those of doctors, as in the use of diagnostic and prescribing skills. They could be, from a lay point of view at least, considered to be much nearer to doctors than nurses in the way that they work. Even though they will have been educated as nurses and may still have aspects of what can be considered to be nursing culture as part of their background, they may be working in ways that are quite different from older and more accepted ways of nursing practice. When it is considered that these roles evolved at quite a rapid rate, it would be interesting to consider how the NMC will deal with practitioners who are seen as having transgressed.

It would seem that there are a number of difficulties for the NMC. Neither the NMC nor their predecessors (the UKCC) appear to have adequately addressed the issue of advanced practice in a concrete form, despite a number of years spent discussing proposals. The rapid pace of change that government policy has created has almost certainly made it difficult for the NMC to respond to changes to professional practice, but the move towards higher levels of practice has been underway for some years now. Also, in fairness to the NMC, it seems to be that definitions of advanced practice are difficult to agree on. The NMC issued a consultation document in early 2005 (NMC 2005) and published the results in May 2005 and it was expected that what the NMC considers to constitute an advanced practitioner and their preparation for practice would have been known before the end of 2006 (NMC 2008). However, this process appears to be stalled while further discussion takes place over wider issues of regulation for the healthcare professions and there is now some doubt as to the commitment of government to ensure that advanced practice is subject to statutory regulation (Health Republic 2009). The rapid rate of development of practice means that any future advice could soon become outdated. How the NMC would deal with cases in relation to advanced practice remains to be seen.

It could also be seen that this lack of guidance makes it very difficult for both the practitioner and the educationalist to determine what are the acceptable limits of advanced practice and how the professional body intends to deal with such cases. Even when the appropriate guidance is issued by the NMC, there could probably be issues over the future shape and direction of the regulation of advanced practice, given the current consultations over the shape of future healthcare professional regulation (Secretary of State for Health 2007).

IMPLICATIONS FOR EDUCATORS

Quite clearly, the challenges of changing practices in the NHS and the expansion in the scope and range of nursing practice to encompass new areas have implications for educators. There has already been examination of the clear need for nurses undertaking advanced practice of any description to ensure that they are fully aware of the scope of their professional and legal accountability for practice and the implications of that accountability. This also imposes a duty on educators who are involved in preparing practitioners to undertake those roles: they must themselves be adequately aware of the implications of new roles and able to make those practitioners aware of the issues of accountability as well.

Another potential issue arises from the nature of higher education itself. In recent years, the relationship between students and the higher education institutions where they study has been seen in a more commercial light and there has been discussion that this may take the form of a quasi contract. This would mean that in certain circumstances the student would have a right of action against the institution if it could be shown that the institution had failed in its duty to provide appropriate teaching.

For example, Birtwistle (2002) examines the possible extent to which educational providers could be held liable in negligence if they fail to properly provide appropriate information to their students that adversely affected that student's competence. Obviously, this could have implications in nursing, as there is a complex relationship between preparation for practice, the clinical area, the practitioner and the professional regulator. It could be argued that the professional has a duty to maintain their own competence (and this could reasonably include the awareness of issues around accountability), but how far does the educator have a duty to ensure competence in all relevant areas and how far is that duty enforceable?

KEY POINTS

- In preparing practitioners to undertake roles that significantly extend their former roles and include elements that could be considered to be higher risk, educators need to be aware themselves of the implications for accountability of the practitioner.
- Practitioners need themselves to be fully aware of their own accountability in a number of different arenas.
- In preparing practitioners, educators should consider if there are particular elements of practice that could carry a greater degree of risk. Examples could be in areas of practice that already appear to attract high levels of complaint or litigation (obstetrics, neo-natal care).
- Educators should also consider the nature of the intended practice. For example,

if the role involves diagnosis, then this may carry higher risks of potential harm compared to many of the roles that nurses have carried out in the past.

■ Practitioners and those who educate them need to be aware of the attitudes of actual and potential employers. For example in the NHS, the issues of vicarious liability are relatively straightforward, but issues around insurance, especially in the voluntary sector, may need to be explored.

■ It is important to consider that as more nurses take on advanced practice and develop their skills, there will be greater confidence and familiarity with the risks. In the future, any concerns about the level of accountability for advanced practice will probably be easier to contemplate as there will be a greater level of experience to rely on.

CONCLUSION

The delivery of healthcare and the nurse's part in that delivery has seen rapid and profound change within a relatively short period of time. This has been mirrored by major changes in the educational preparation of healthcare practitioners at both pre- and post-registration level. As in any periods of change, there are uncertainties and there is some confusion. This can be in relation to the directions that change may take and also to what the nature of the eventual outcomes will be.

This is surely true of the development of the advanced practitioner's role, as in other areas, as can be seen by the difficulty that the regulatory body has had in defining the nature of advanced practice and role of the advanced practitioner. However, this role is clearly not about to disappear. As this role matures, then the challenges that loom for practitioners – and those who educate, regulate and employ such practitioners – must and will be faced and resolved.

IMPLICATIONS FOR THE READER'S OWN PRACTICE

1 How current is your knowledge in relation to forthcoming changes in advanced nursing practice?

2 In what ways will you channel this knowledge into educational activities to raise student awareness?

3 How will you increase your knowledge of legal and professional issues in order to become a better educator?

4 Which other professionals' help can you enrol in order to illuminate your teaching?

5 What activities could you create to use in the classroom to engage with the importance and serious nature of accountability?

NOTE

1 According to the National Health Service Litigation Authority, in 2007–08 it made payments of £633 325 299. This can be compared to 1997–98 when £49 460 000 was paid out (NHSLA 2008).

REFERENCES

The Allitt Inquiry (1994) *Independent Inquiry Relating to Deaths and Injuries on the Children's Ward at Grantham and Kesteven General Hospital During the Period February to April 1991.* London: HMSO.

Baly M (1995) *Nursing and Social Change.* 3rd ed. London: Routledge.

Birtwistle T (2002) Liability for 'educational malpractice'. *Educ Law J.* **2**: 95–9.

Bolam v. Friern Hospital Management Committee [1957] 1WLR 582.

Brazier M, Cave E (2007) *Medicine, Patients and the Law.* 4th ed. London: Penguin.

Brazier M, Miola J (2000) Bye-bye Bolam, a medical litigation revolution? *Med Law Rev.* **8**: 85–114.

De Cruz P (2001) *Comparative Healthcare Law.* London: Cavendish.

Department of Health (1989) *Review of Prescribing, Supply and Administration of Medicines.* (Crown report.) London: DoH.

Department of Health (1999) *Review of Prescribing, Supply and Administration of Medicines.* Final Report. (Crown report.) London: DoH.

Department of Health (2000) *The NHS Plan: a plan for investment, a plan for reform.* Cm 4818. London: HMSO.

Department of Health (2002) *Liberating the Talents.* Available at: www.dh.gov.uk/en/ Publicationsandstatistics/Publications/PublicationsPolicyAndGuidance/DH_4007473 (accessed 3 September 2008).

Department of Health (2006) *A Prescription for Patient Satisfaction.* Available at: www.dh.gov. uk/en/Publicationsandstatistics/Pressreleases/DH_4134390

Department of Health (2009) *Nurse Independent Prescribing.* Available at: www.dh.gov.uk/en/ Healthcare/Medicinespharmacyandindustry/Prescriptions/TheNon-MedicalPrescribing Programme/Nurseprescribing/index.htm

Dimond B (2008) *Legal Aspects of Nursing.* 5th ed. London: Longman.

Farell AM, Devaney S (2007) Making amends or making things worse? Clinical negligence reform and patient redress in England. *Leg Stud.* **27**: 630–48.

Fletcher N, Holt J (1995) *Ethics, Law and Nursing.* Manchester: Manchester University Press.

Gold v. Essex CC [1942] 2 All ER 237.

Greene B (2005) *Understanding Medical Law.* London: Routledge Cavendish.

Hart C (1994) *Behind the Mask.* London: Baillière Tindall.

Health Republic (2009) DoH 'may regret' regulating advanced nurses on the cheap. Available at: www.healthcarerepublic.com/news/Nurse/890623/DoH-may-regret-regulating-advanced-nurses-cheap/

Hefferon v. UKCC [1988] 10 BMLR 1.

Herring J (2008) *Medical Law and Ethics.* 2nd ed. Oxford: Oxford University Press.

House of Commons Constitutional Affairs Committee (2006) *Compensation Culture.* London: HMSO.

Ingham T (2008) *The English Legal Process.* Oxford: Oxford University Press.

Jackson E (2006) *Medical Law Texts, Cases and Materials.* Oxford: Oxford University Press.

Mackay L (1993) *Conflicts in Care.* London: Chapman and Hall.

Mason JK, Laurie GT (2006) *Mason and McCall Smiths Law and Medical Ethics.* 7th ed. Oxford: Oxford University Press.

McHale J, Tingle J (2001) *Law and Nursing.* 2nd ed. Oxford: Butterworth Heinemann.

McHale J, Tingle J (2007) *Law and Nursing.* 7th ed. Oxford: Butterworth Heinemann.

Medicinal Products: Prescription by Nurses etc. Act 1992. Elizabeth II, Chapter 28. London: HMSO.

Montgomery J (2003) *Healthcare Law.* 2nd ed. Oxford: Oxford University Press.

National Health Service Executive (1996) *Arrangements for Handling Clinical Negligence Claims against NHS Staff.* HSG(96)48 NHS Indemnity.

National Health Service Litigation Authority (2008) *Report and Accounts.* London: HMSO.

National Health Service Litigation Authority (2009) *Claims.* Available at: www.nhsla.com/Claims/

NHS Redress Act 2006. Elizabeth II, Chapter 44. London: HMSO.

Nursing and Midwifery Council (2004) *The NMC Code of Professional Conduct: standards for conduct, performance and ethics.* London: NMC.

Nursing and Midwifery Council (2005) *NMC Consultation on a Proposed Framework for the Standard for Post-registration Nursing.* London: NMC.

Nursing and Midwifery Council (2006) Advanced nursing practice update. Available at: www.nmc-uk.org/aArticle.aspx?ArticleID=2038

Nursing and Midwifery Council (2008) *The Code: standards of conduct, performance and ethics for nurses and midwives.* London: NMC.

Pain and the Law (2009) Available at: www.painandthelaw.org/

Pattinson S (2006) *Medical Law and Ethics.* London: Thomson, Sweet and Maxwell.

Salvage J (1985) *The Politics of Nursing.* London: Heinemann Nursing.

Secretary of State for Health (2007) *Trust, Assurance and Safety: the regulation of health professionals in the twenty-first century.* Cm 7013. London: HMSO.

The Shipman Inquiry (2004) *Fourth Report: the regulation of controlled drugs in the community.* Cm 6249. London: HMSO.

Stauch M, Wheat B, Tingle J (2006) *Text Cases and Material on Medical Law.* 3rd ed. London: Cavendish.

United Kingdom Central Council (1992) *Code of Professional Conduct.* 3rd ed. London: UKCC.

United Kingdom Central Council (1992a) *Exercising Accountability.* London: UKCC.

United Kingdom Central Council (2001) *Code of Professional Conduct.* 5th ed. London: UKCC.

9

Integrating knowledge, skills and compassion to reconfigure a cancer service: a managerial perspective

Sarah Bates and Wendy Page

The Blind Men and the Elephant

It was six men of Indostan
To learning much inclined,
Who went to see the Elephant
(Though all off them were blind)
That each by observation
Might satisfy his mind

The First approached the Elephant
And happening to fall
Against his broad and sturdy side
At once began to brawl:
'God bless me but the Elephant
is very like a wall'

The Second, feeling of the tusk,
Cried 'Ho what have we here
So very round and smooth and sharp?
To me 'tis clear mighty clear
This wonder of an Elephant
Is very like a spear!'
The Third approached the animal,
And happening to take
The squirming trunk within his hands,
Thus boldly up and spake:
'I see' quoth he, 'The Elephant
Is very like a snake'

The Fourth reached out an eager hand
And felt around the knee,
'What most this wondrous beast is like
Is mighty plain' quoth he:
''Tis clear enough the Elephant
Is very like a tree'

The Fifth who chanced to the ear,
Said 'E'en the blindest man
Can tell what this resembles most;
Deny the fact who can,
This marvel of an Elephent
Is very like a fan'

The Sixth no sooner had begun
About the beast to grope,
Than, seizing on the swinging tail
That fell within his scope,
'I see', quoth he, 'the Elephant
Is very like a rope!'

And so these men of Indostan
Disputed loud and long
Each of his own opinion
Exceeding stiff and strong,
Though each was partly in the right,
All were in the wrong!

Moral
So oft in theological wars,
The disputants, I ween,
Rail on in utter ignorance
Of what each other mean,
And prate on about an Elephant
Not one of them has seen!!!

John Godfrey Saxe (1816–87)

AIM

The aim of this chapter is to explore the learning that occurred when reconfiguring a cancer centre. It will also evaluate some of the relevant theories and structures required to redesign cancer care, and how this information could be utilised to educate others.

LEARNING OUTCOMES

By the end of this chapter, the reader should be able to:
- identify the learning that has contributed to re-engineer the centre
- evaluate the relevance of theories in the process of changing and improving quality of care
- reflect on the impact of the process on healthcare professionals and staff
- discuss the educational processes required to implement the changes
- reflect on how managerial and educational theory dovetail together
- reflect on ways that this experience might help others and how it might be used as a teaching tool.

INTRODUCTION AND BACKGROUND

Mintzberg *et al.* (2009) propose that when it comes to strategy formation, we are the people who are blind and strategy is the elephant. No one has the perception of the beast as a whole, so each therefore has his or her own interpretation of the phenomenon. Mintzberg *et al.* (2009) note that like the elephant, strategy is more than the sum of its parts, and yet to comprehend strategy as whole we do need to understand the individual elements that contribute to it.

It was with this in mind that we set about our plans for the redesign of a cancer service: a new £70 million build on the horizon, a massive undertaking and much to plan. It was important to try to break down such a huge and daunting task, both to better understand it and also to be able to plan and implement it successfully.

This chapter seeks to discuss the key theories regarding strategy development and implementation. It will then critically analyse these in relation to the strategic development of cancer services within the Hull and East Yorkshire Hospitals NHS Trust. As well, we shall explore the extent to which people involved with developing and implementing the strategy actually understood the process they were engaged in.

First we need to describe something of the political climate that has influenced the development of the Cancer Centre strategy within the Hull and East Yorkshire Hospitals NHS Trust. This is a large acute Trust comprising a Specialist/Tertiary Centre, Trauma Centre and Cancer Centre; it is also a teaching hospital and the major NHS partner in the Hull York Medical School. Hull and East Yorkshire Hospitals NHS Trust was established in October 1999 through the merger of the former Royal Hull Hospitals and East Yorkshire Hospitals Trusts. The Trust employs approximately 7000 staff and has an annual turnover in the region of £400 million (2008/09).

The Trust's secondary care service portfolio is comprehensive, covering most of the major medical and surgical specialities, routine and specialist diagnostic services and other clinical support services. These services are primarily provided to a catchment population in the region of 0.5 million, but the Trust also provides a number of specialist services to a catchment population of between 1.05 and 1.25 million (varying by service) in a broader geographical area extending from Scarborough in the north to Grimsby and Scunthorpe in the south. The Trust is the accredited Cancer Centre for the Humber and Yorkshire Coast area; it is this aspect of strategic development and implementation that will be discussed within this chapter. It is hoped that readers who work in cancer and palliative care will be interested to see the amount and type of strategising and planning that goes into preparing for a change of this magnitude. Similarly, it is hoped that educationalists will find it useful to see how underpinning theories are also interwoven in the work of managers. For those who teach healthcare policy in cancer and palliative care, this might be incorporated into useful teaching exercises. It may also be useful to those planning significant changes in their working practice to consider the 'positives and pitfalls' of the authors' endeavours.

THE NEED FOR CHANGE

The authors are senior nurses within the Cancer and Clinical Support business unit of the Hull and East Yorkshire Hospitals NHS Trust; Sarah is the Head of Nursing and Wendy is the Matron for the Cancer Centre. We were two individuals ideally placed and with a vested interest in getting the strategy right for the benefit of patients and staff alike.

Between 2001 and 2009 the strategic direction of the organisation and the business units within it has been focused towards achieving the modernisation agenda set out by the Department of Health (DoH) in the NHS's *A Plan for Investment, a Plan for Reform* (DoH 2000). The plan is both radical and ambitious in what it sets out to achieve in its core principles, but also fundamental to its success is the key strategy of devolving power away from Strategic Health Authorities (SHA) and into individual organisations (Foundation Trusts) and of these organisations in turn devolving that power further to individual business units responsible for the delivery of patient services. During this period, the strategy for the development of the Cancer Centre was being formulated and it needed to reflect and integrate national and local strategy while simultaneously re-designing the way in which patients were cared for in this speciality.

The *NHS Human Resources Strategy* (DoH 2000) which was developed in conjunction with the *NHS Plan* (2000) clearly states that for a Trust to achieve its strategy, it has to invest in the organisational culture promoting staff involvement and partnership working (DoH 2000). Trusts are required to demonstrate a clear commitment through effective leadership, education, training and policy development and through evidence of staff engagement in the evaluation and redesign of services at both an operational and strategic level. The *NHS Plan* (DoH 2000) stresses the requirement for employees to be given the freedom to be innovative, creative and essentially to solve old problems in new ways. This was seen as being essential in planning the approach and strategy for the new Cancer Centre; engaging staff and service users was seen to be pivotal in the success of the strategy and therefore the success of the massive change ahead and the delivery of our services.

Achieving these objectives required the Trust and its staff to understand the environment in which it has to operate, especially when the NHS both nationally and locally is a going through a period of radical change. Talbot-Smith and Pollock (2007) state that the NHS has changed from a tax-funded, centrally planned, publicly owned accountable service to operating within a market in which patients are free to choose where and who provides their healthcare and, as a result, organisations have to compete for business. This is a new concept and somewhat shocking to many, with marketing being viewed as abhorrent to the ethos on which the NHS was established (Thorpe 2008). The introduction of the competitive market has been seen by some to be undermining the spirit of collaboration on which the foundations of the NHS lay (Unison 2007). However, with the advent of 'Payment by Results' (DoH 2000) and 'Any Willing Provider' (DoH 2000), essentially patients are free to commission their own healthcare and obviously the quality of that healthcare will be high on their agenda. The competitiveness of the marketplace therefore must ensure that organisations are driven to provide and deliver high-quality and evidence-based care. This can only be to the advantage of the patients in terms of quality service delivery.

Within such a challenging and diverse climate, it has been paramount for the Trust to articulate its strategy, a summary of which can be seen in Table 9.1. The document sets out the Vision, Values and Strategic direction for Hull and East Yorkshire Hospitals NHS Trust over the next five years. These five years will see continuing change in the way health services are provided and as an organisation it is essential that we develop a strategy that prepares us for these challenges as well as taking into account national and local policy and the needs of the population we serve. In the redesign of the cancer services, it was important to reflect the Trust's vision and strategic objectives and these are as follows:

TABLE 9.1 The Trust's strategic objectives

Hull and East Yorkshire Hospitals NHS Trust
Strategic Objectives
• to continue to be the major provider of secondary and tertiary healthcare services to patients in Hull, the East Riding of Yorkshire and surrounding districts
• to improve clinical outcomes and quality of care
• to improve the patient experience
• to plan, develop and deliver services in partnership with the Primary Care Trusts, neighbouring Trusts and other organisations
• to continue to provide, in partnership with other organisations, a comprehensive range of clinical teaching
• to expand programmes of research and development in priority areas
• to achieve and sustain financial viability
• to ensure our workforce is fit for purpose and can deliver the Trust agenda effectively and efficiently.

The NHS is continually exposed to external influences which often enforce changes to its services (Mannion *et al.* 2005). For any senior manager within the Trust it is a valuable skill, and in some ways imperative, to have the ability to internalise change quickly and reflect on what has been learnt previously. Hooper and Potter (2000) deem it as a failure not to adapt to change sufficiently quickly and this sits within the remit of senior managers within an organisation. This is supported by Kolb *et al.* (1994, as cited in Mullins 2005) who state that '*a key function of strategic management development*

. . . is to provide managers with access to knowledge and relationship networks that can help them become lifelong learners and cope with the issues on their continually changing agendas'.

Speaking with other senior managers and some of the Trust directors about how the Trust developed its strategy, it is very much perceived as a 'top-down approach' and seems to lend itself to the 'positioning' school of thought (Mintzberg *et al.* 2009). The strategy developed through the Chief Executive's office utilising a small project team with the aim of fulfilling the requirements of becoming a Foundation Trust and meeting government targets. The strategy's development was neither inclusive of nor considered the views, thoughts and opinions of all staff members at varying levels throughout the organisation. Approaching the formulation of strategy in this manner can lead to some key players becoming disenfranchised (Johnson and Scholes 2002). Understanding the 'new' NHS is already confusing for the general public and also for staff who work in a healthcare arena, with many no longer understanding the organisation they are employed by (Talbot-Smith and Pollock 2007). Abrahamsson (1977, cited in Beardwell and Clayton 2007) describes this process as 'indirect mechanisms of participation' which can be viewed as a political process that contributes to high-level decision-making. Such a process contrasts with direct participation, which may take longer but views employees as valuable assets to be nurtured as they become potentially a source of competitive edge with their commitment, adaptability and skills (Legge 2005, cited in Beardwell and Clayton 2007). This brings us back to the *NHS Plan* (DoH 2000) and the key to succeeding, with the desired strategy being staff participation and engagement. This was felt to be absolutely crucial in the redesign and planning for the successful opening of the new Cancer Centre. Our staff are our biggest asset; we were moving to a wonderful, purpose-built unit but recognised that without the engagement and participation of our staff teams, this challenge would be an unsuccessful one. This carried with it risk and had huge connotations for our staff but also for our patients and service users.

REDESIGN OF CANCER SERVICES

With regard to the redesign of the cancer services in Hull and East Yorkshire NHS Trust, specifically the move to a purpose-built oncology and haematology unit, staff engagement was seen to be essential from the very beginning. The process began long before the first bricks and mortar were laid. The principles of care required for this specialist group of patients and the specific needs of patients were explored and analysed. Patients themselves were used to influence the planning for the new centre; patient representatives were involved during the commissioning of the new building and their views, along with those of many current service users, were sought. A plan was then formulated as to how they could be cared for, based on the mapping of their individual and specific needs and taking their views and ideas into consideration. One of the main issues to be elicited from patient groups was that they wanted to be cared for in the right place, not be 'lodged' on a non-oncology/haematology ward where staff were unsure how to care for them. They also expressed the need for easy access to inpatient beds and services as they were needed.

This list represents the core of their wants and needs.

➤ 'We'd like comfortable waiting areas but not too large that we feel insignificant or forgotten about.'

➤ 'It would be good to have easy access to inpatient beds as and when we need them, rather than have to go through Accident and Emergency.'

➤ 'It would make such a difference if every staff member could care for any diagnosis, no matter which ward we were on.'

➤ 'We need to be cared for by knowledgeable and skilled staff with expertise in our particular cancer.'

➤ 'We want to feel cared for, as individuals.'

All of their needs were considered and as much as possible the plans adapted to accommodate these requests. For example, this strategy was developed using creativity and innovation, moving away from the traditions of nursing in this area where the norm would have been for separate speciality wards – a chemotherapy ward, a radiotherapy ward, a haematology ward and many more. The transfer involved moving a haematology ward from one hospital site and two oncology wards from a different site across the city. In addition, two brand new wards were being created within the new Cancer Centre. It was decided that on transfer to the new Centre, the wards would all care for both oncology and haematology patients, offering a full range of treatments from diagnosis through to palliation and end-of-life care. The criteria for where the patient received care would be based on their clinical needs and level of dependency. The concept of a palliative care ward, medium and high-dependency wards was created. In order to achieve this, the staff groups were carefully assessed; their experience, knowledge, skills and competencies were measured; and from the three original inpatient ward teams, five new teams of staff were reconfigured to facilitate the transfer to the new Centre. This was a major change for the service and also within the Trust; our reason for undertaking this was to improve the standard of care delivered to our patient groups, as well as to ensure that patients had the right care, in the right place, at the right time. It was also recognised and acknowledged that this would fit with our philosophy of staff development – the aim being to create a team of Cancer Centre staff with the knowledge and skills to care for any cancer patient at every stage of their illness. This value was seen as being very important both to patient and staff groups.

In order to support this, many 'time-outs', information briefings, educational sessions and social events were planned in the years and months prior to the move. The time-outs were joint educational and managerial events, which *all* staff of all grades were expected to attend. The dual approach, as well as ensuring that the outcomes were met, was designed to illustrate the commitment, care and support which was being offered. These events were full days and had a formal programme in order that all groups were given the same information. However, it was planned that the sessions be in keeping with the holistic, individualised care which is synonymous with cancer and palliative care. Therefore each session was experiential in nature, including a questions and answers section, to ensure that everyone's needs were met. The days also encompassed information on change management, how it might affect them and how they might find ways to cope. These days were run by the managers (ourselves) and our educationalist.

We have also developed a new programme of rotation in order that all nursing staff of all grades will have placements on the five wards and, in doing so, complete an underpinning learning programme and competency framework. The competency framework is detailed and extensive, covering many aspects of care for oncology, haematology and palliative care patients. Each individual embarking on this rotation will have an achievement log to complete. This again involved the dual 'managerial and educational' approach, which we believe leads to maximum learning and the highest level of competency as well as the ability to measure our success. Another bonus of this approach is that, because of the way the achievement log has been written – with specific competencies and an underpinning learning taxonomy – and following the negotiations between our educationalist and the local universities, it is anticipated it will be accredited. Completing the achievement log during placement is compulsory whereas the academic route requires some extra work. In the long term, this will produce skilled and knowledgeable nurses who are able to care for any cancer patient, oncology or haematology, at any stage of their illness from diagnosis to death.

TABLE 9.2 The strategy of cancer care

The strategy of cancer care within the new Centre includes:
• a flexible workforce that should be able to meet the challenges of the diverse patient group and allow the service to respond to changing agendas
• a specialised workforce which can adapt to the needs of the cancer patient and not be restricted around a patient's diagnosis
• core competencies for all staff
• patient involvement as paramount in this process and the patient experience being reflected within this strategy
• stronger working relationships between patients and staff
• the highest standards of patient care.

The strategy for care delivery was developed over a long period of time, approximately three years. To understand the process of the strategy development, the key theories pertaining to strategy development and implementation in relation to developing cancer services will be further explored.

KEY THEORIES OF STRATEGY DEVELOPMENT AND IMPLEMENTATION

What is strategy? The concept was born out of the history of the military: from ancient times, much has been said about the greatness of the military commanders and the strategies they developed. The word 'strategic' comes from the Greek word *stratego* which literally means a military general. The ideas of military strategy seem to have been transposed into business strategy within the second half of the twentieth century; it was developed throughout the 1950s and thrived in 1960s, 1970s and 1980s. Like military strategy, business strategy has not stood still but instead has kept on evolving (Shimizu *et al.* 2006).

TABLE 9.3 SWOT analysis

STRENGTHS	WEAKNESSES
Committed individuals	Services on three sites
Patient focused	Old building
Highly skilled	Working in silos
Excited to develop services	Little opportunity for integration
Dedicated to high-quality care	Segregated working that limits knowledge
Low turnover of staff	Different ways of delivering the same thing
	New ideas not always listened to
	Don't like 'top down' approach
	Some areas hard to find recruits for
OPPORTUNITIES	**THREATS**
Development of new cancer service	New teams
Blank canvas/ripe for development	Not being listened to
All working on the same site	Don't want to change
Able to learn from one another	People who sabotage development
Diagnostics on site	Not enough staff to do things properly
Chance to be listened to	
Ability to do something different	
Ability to be flexible	
Ability to integrate better	

The literature review of strategic management is vast. The word 'strategy', now used both liberally and lovingly by managers, is most influential; managers are judged by their greatness if they appear to have developed and successfully implemented planned strategies (Mintzberg *et al.* 2009). However, strategies must be specific to the organisation and its intent; Johnson and Scholes (2002) state that 'strategy is the direction and scope of an organisation over the long-term: which achieves advantage for the organisation through its configuration of resources within a changing environment, to meet the needs of markets and to fulfil stakeholder expectations'. Leuke (2005) notes that a good strategy combined with outstanding implementation is every company's best guarantee for success. He goes on to say that 'strategy creation is about doing the rights' whereas 'implementation is about doing things right'.

Mintzberg *et al.* (2009) maintain that the complexity of strategy requires that it has a number of definitions and they developed their work around 10 'schools' of thought for determining strategy. These included: design, planning, positioning, entrepreneurial, cognitive, learning, power, culture, environmental and configuration. It is important to stress that although there are different explanations as to how strategy is developed and implemented, it is unlikely that any one of these works in isolation and offers 'the' answer; success is more likely with a mix of approaches (Johnson and Scholes 2002). This is certainly what was seen and experienced within the development of our strategy for cancer services. Mintzberg *et al.* (2009) speak about the strategy-formation process which, without a doubt, is one of the most influential aspects of a project. Many of its principles underpin several tools used today, such as the SWOT (Strengths, Weaknesses, Opportunity and Threats) analysis, and this was one of the tools used to progress the strategic development within cancer services in Hull. At the earliest opportunity for staff involvement in the development of a strategy for cancer services, professionals met through facilitated groups and undertook a SWOT analysis. The salient points of this work became the foundations upon which we based our strategy design.

The design school origins can be traced back to the work of Selznicks (1957) and Chandler (1962). However, Mintzberg *et al.* (2009) and Porter (1980) critique this school, suggesting that a great deal of the core strategic management comes from assumptions and although perfectly plausible they can sometimes be misleading. When critiquing this in relation to the SWOT analysis undertaken, we assumed that the opportunities that were suggested by the professionals were a good thing and these assumptions did form the basis of the planning of the new service. This view is also shared by Kenny (2006), which he describes as strategy shortfall, alluding to the fact that these assumptions may not take into consideration other external factors that influence strategic development. Mintzberg *et al.* (2009) imply that the design school is the best place for strategy formation if there is to be a major shift for an organisation, or when it is coming out of a change process into a period of relative stability.

Mintzberg *et al.* (2009) broke down the steps of strategic planning into the following and these were tools used throughout the stages of planning for the Cancer Centre. The examples given below relate to workforce development within nursing at each of Mintzberg's stages.

TABLE 9.4 Mintzberg's stages

The objective-setting stage	The need to develop a flexible workforce equipped with core competencies to be able to care for cancer patients.
The external audit stage	What are the core competencies that other Cancer Centres had designed for their nursing workforce?
The internal audit stage	What were our skills deficits? The need to develop an up-to-date database of competencies held by the current nursing workforce.
The strategy-evaluation stage	The need to develop a competency document and teaching package to address these needs.
The strategy operational stage	Implementation. All nurses currently are working to the core competency document.

In much of the theory relating to strategic planning there seems to be a sense that planning and control are unquestionably linked. Hamel (1996) argues that strategic planning has little to do with strategy, which he believes is a much more radical and innovative process. He deems that strategic planning is much more about maintaining control within an organisation. This is supported by Goold and Campbell (1987), who wrote about strategic control and one of its key elements being strategic planning and another being financial control.

We certainly used strategic planning tools to take control of our strategy – with such a large-scale task, we had to ensure that our strategy was going to be successfully implemented, so we had to have detailed operational plans in place. Johnson and Scholes (2002) suggest that this does not need to be seen in a negative context, that a benefit of strategic planning is that it offers a high level of control and co-ordination which the organisation is able to apply over a strategy. This was important and integral to the change for cancer services, as control was seen to be a vital part for all the key team members in order to transfer to the new build smoothly and efficiently, and with a minimum of disruption for the staff and most importantly for our service users. This was viewed by the patients as being critical. These patients were already in the midst of a distressing journey of cancer care and treatment, so the move and transfer to the new service had to be smooth, controlled and well organised in order to reduce the impact on them as individuals and on their treatment/care pathway.

Reviewing the literature, it would be a reasonable assessment that although planning doesn't guarantee strategic success, it certainly has a place within strategic development. Certainly within the changes in the NHS there has to be a conscious move away from using strategic planning as an annual, calendar-driven ritual (Hamel 1996) and instead to use it as robust tool for strategic business success (Talbot-Smith and Pollock 2007).

We would suggest that health professionals both pre- and post-qualification need to be taught not only about policy drivers but also about strategic planning. It is only with good teaching – providing the theories, research and encouraging not just the 'know about' but 'the 'know how' – that they can become involved in the wider strategic decision-making process, as they grow in ability and confidence. If this happens, then as health professionals qualify, they can become immediately involved with strategic development on a micro scale, but understand the wider macro approach. This approach will lead to bridging the gap between managers and those working by the bedside, thus working towards a more compassionate caring reciprocal arrangement. Unfortunately, many health professionals see strategy as something imposed on them, rather than something in which they ought to be involved.

While not educationalists, we suggest the following exercises to facilitate learning about strategy.

Exercise 9.1
- Provide the students with some of the theoretical concepts of strategy, for example Mintzberg's stages/schools of thought.
- Ask them to plan to reconfigure a cancer service which is expanding and moving to a new building. This has to be achieved by integrating knowledge, skills and compassion in to their chosen approach.
- Ask students to consider the following:
- What policy drivers must influence your approach?

- Which theory do you think will be most appropriate to this type of change and why? (You could use one of the approaches provided or find another which you might prefer.)
- Describe how you would go about this process with actions and time limits?
- What do you see as being the biggest challenges and opportunities which you might face?
- How do you think all staff might be involved?
- What will they use to measure their success?
- What else do they need to consider?

This activity would need the theory to be taught first (useful references are given in the References section of our chapter). This chapter could be useful to the facilitator to provide ideas, and might be useful to the student to read as homework to compare their work to ours.

Exercise 9.2

At a subsequent session, learners could report back on:
- What were the similarities and differences of methods of their approach to the Hull project?
- What did they forget that was important?
- What did the Queens Centre in Hull not do which might have helped?
- How useful are the theories in practice?
- What other learning did they glean from reading about this experience?

NB: Alternatively they could do a SWOT analysis to reflect on these different approaches.

The understanding of clinicians about strategy formation has the potential to engage them proactively in the process. The outcome of motivating the workforce will propel specific projects forward to achieving their aims and objectives.

Strategic development has accrued a number of models and perspectives. The positioning school saw strategy formation as a means of establishing a strong position within the marketplace so that it was able to withstand competition. The criticism of this school of thought is that is far too rigid and does not allow for creativity, therefore the strategy formation may be thwarted. Mintzberg *et al.* (2009) suggest that this approach to planning lends itself to traditional big businesses and has a 'top down' approach which potentially does not engage with those lower down the hierarchy who may also have a valuable contribution to make. This line of thought is reinforced by Hamel (1997), who suggests that innovative strategies do not occur through sterile analysis but through experience and creativity. The positioning school lends itself to what was described in the introduction regarding the formulation of the overall Trust strategy. If a Trust or service line (in this case, cancer) is to be successful within the healthcare arena, it must establish a robust market position and be able to compete. In addition, in order to contribute to the success of the strategy and gain engagement and commitment from its workforce, staff too should be involved in its design, evolution, implementation and subsequent evaluation.

Within the development of the Cancer Centre strategy all these factors had to be addressed but the ethos of the strategy was always for staff engagement and not a 'top down' approach. We endeavoured to do this by involving all grades of staff in time-out sessions, facilitating team meetings, circulating regular information about the new build and ensuring that all managers were heavily involved in the project and so were equipped to answer staff queries and address their information needs. We believe this is vital and were driven by a passion and desire to make this right both for our staff and our service users. We are both compassionate individuals and care deeply about our patients, always putting them first, at the centre of everything we do. Every initiative and project we have developed has been for the benefit of our patients, to make our service better for them. However, we feel equally passionate about our staff and recognise that they are our most valuable resource and are key to the delivery of a caring and compassionate service to our patients. We also acknowledge that working in this speciality is hard, emotionally exhausting at times, and one of our key outcomes was that staff felt cared for and valued.

While we had ideas and a vision for the future, this remained fluid and was adapted with input from others as the strategy development progressed. The 'entrepreneurship' school (strategy as a visionary process), as signalled by Mintzberg *et al.* (2009), moves away from the prescriptive schools into the realms of the descriptive, seeking to understand strategy as it starts to unfold. It focuses on strategy development being led totally by an individual with vision, judgement, wisdom and experience. It is solely down to this individual to create or at least articulate the strategy and for others to follow. Shimizu *et al.* (2006) describe this as being the process of creative intuition, giving the visionary leader the ability to create and implement strategy successfully. Activities associated with strategic leadership often include making strategic decisions and being able to communicate the vision for the future (Boal and Hooijberg 2001). We tried to communicate 'the vision' by the previously mentioned time-out days and by ensuring that ward managers were fully aware of the vision so they could disseminate it to all their teams.

The obvious weakness of this school of thought is its reliance on one individual, therefore the key decisions regarding strategy are centralised to that one person's focus and vision and may not reflect any others' viewpoints or contributions. However, it is recognised that strategy does rely on a vision of the future and the ability to turn this into reality; without this, there would be no strategy.

As a result of this weakness, although we considered this model and used some relevant elements, we considered it not to be so useful in the context of the strategic planning for the Cancer Centre. Certainly in the redesign of the cancer services there were ideas and visions of the future (those of the senior managers), however, these were challenged, changed and further developed by the engagement and involvement of others. It was deemed essential to effective implementation that all staff have an opportunity to be involved, engaged and perceive that there was a contribution for them to make. To assist with this, 'blue sky thinking' events were held with many groups of staff and patients to canvass their visions for the future, and many of these visions contributed to the final strategy.

The 'learning' school discusses strategy as an emergent process that can develop in parallel with other processes (Shimizu *et al.* 2006). This is an incremental view of strategy development and this was demonstrated within the design of the Cancer Centre strategy. There was clearly a vision of how staff and patients wanted to see the design of the new services, with specific outcomes which had to be delivered and achieved – for example, the cost implications of delivering the service within the financial envelope and within the time scale. However, the practicalities and detail of service design and operational strategy remained flexible, being changed and adapted during the consultation and emergent process.

THE DESIGN TEAM

The design team had never been involved in developing a strategy of such a scale and therefore the business unit commissioned the formulation of small project groups to look at the different aspects of the overall service strategy. As a group, through a process of service mapping, they highlighted issues of concern with regard to the current service provision and identified possible solutions. The overall direction was led by core members of the project team, comprising of managers and individuals with a transformational leadership style and excellent communication skills that were used to engage the wider team in the strategy design. Their backgrounds were diverse and included personnel, administration, educational, senior nursing, operational management and senior medical staff.

During the development of the new oncology and haematology departments, the inpatient unit has increased from three to five wards, as previously discussed. The aim was to change the way patient care was managed and to review the flow of patients through the inpatient unit. There were many initial thoughts as to how this could be done, from disease specific to treatment specific, and the initial strategy included this. However, as the strategy evolved it became clear this was going against our desire to allow for as much flexibility as possible, and the final strategy was to integrate oncology and haematology patients on all wards and to nurse them according to clinical dependency. Another reason for undertaking this was to create and manage capacity of patients. We knew through the preparatory work undertaken that we would rapidly exceed the capacity of inpatient beds and therefore needed to create a way of dealing with patient flow and demand as effectively and flexibly as possible. This way of nursing also allows the teams to have a more strategic overview and, more so than would have done five individual wards, helps the teams to think and work together to create increased efficiencies and effectiveness. Furthermore, this was felt to be an effective way of overcoming the 'working in silos' ethos which had been identified as a weakness by team members themselves during the SWOT analysis.

The implementation began long before the planned move in August 2008; in fact, discussion and planning began at least two years prior to this. Work included discussing and planning ideas with senior nursing staff initially and ensuring their engagement and involvement in the process. The time-out and study days for staff took place in 2007 and into 2008, as already mentioned, providing all staff with the opportunity to be involved and become engaged in the change process and this allowed us to listen to their ideas, concerns and feedback. As a result of this feedback, the ideas around the original concept were changed and adapted accordingly, with new strategy developing. Staff were obviously uncomfortable and anxious about the process, the management and the transition of such a huge change. Their thoughts, concerns and opinions were all listened to and taken into account at every stage of the pathway. The changes made as the strategy emerged were reported back to the staff groups, ensuring acknowledgement of their ideas and contributions. We hoped that through all this, they heard our message that we truly care for them, and were doing our utmost to respond to their requests and make the change as enjoyable and stress free as possible.

The development of the Cancer Centre strategy started with a clear vision of the required outcome; however the realised strategy is one that emerged through the engagement and involvement of many team members, harnessing learning throughout the process. This resulted in the production of a detailed and well planned strategy that was then implemented within the new Cancer Centre.

ASSESSMENT OF UNDERSTANDING

In order to assess individuals' understanding of the concept of strategy development within the Cancer Centre, two focus groups involving nurses took place. Each group consisted of between five and seven nursing staff and was facilitated by a senior manager.

A focus group was chosen as the preferred tool, as it is particularly suited for obtaining several perspectives about the same topic and gaining insight into people's shared understanding of everyday situations and the way in which individuals are influenced by others and group situations (Morgan 1997). The focus group is also useful to draw on respondents' attitudes and beliefs (Morgan and Kreuger, cited in Morgan 1993), as can be seen from Table 9.5.

TABLE 9.5 Key focus group questions

Key open questions asked of the group:
• Can you describe key aspects within the strategy for service delivery within the Cancer Centre?
• How did the Cancer Centre strategy develop?
• Do you feel that you contributed to the strategy development?

The data from the focus groups were analysed and collated, with key concepts being identified. All the focus group participants found it hard to articulate an answer to the question regarding key aspects of the strategy. Many were silent initially, until the facilitator prompted them by exploring what their understanding of strategy is. A few staff said that the Cancer Centre didn't have a strategy, with several other nurses expressing that strategy and a vision for a service were the same.

The word 'vision' was key; once used, other staff members relayed to us the key aspects of the strategy. It seemed to be the term 'strategy' that confused most people, with one nurse expressing that nurses were not familiar with the term 'strategy' but were more able to discuss in terms of a vision for service delivery. However, most nurses, when asked if they knew what outcomes were being attempted with the new Cancer Centre, could discuss the advantages of flexible working and of nurses having core competencies to deliver safe, high quality care to all cancer patients.

Some staff in the focus groups had been part of the project groups and clearly recalled SWOT analysis, 'blue sky thinking' sessions and time-outs which resulted in the strategy formation. To others, these concepts remained clearly alien despite their own attendance at these seminal events! Some described how strategy is something developed by the management and given to them to achieve. Others expressed and questioned why there was a need to change how services were delivered and still could not see how the strategy might successfully be implemented. Some acknowledged they had been sceptical of the strategy and its advantages for staff and patients but were now beginning to see the benefits for both. Some staff were exceptionally positive, and were honest in admitting how sceptical they had been prior to the move but asserted that now they were happy in their work area and could see real and tangible benefits to this new way of working, both for themselves and their patients.

In terms of the strategy development and the participants' contributions, there was a real mix of those who felt engaged in the process and had actively participated and those who felt that they had not been consulted and had had no opportunity to contribute. This was interesting, as although not all staff had been on the project groups, every staff member had attended time-outs where the strategy had been discussed and their contributions and ideas had been actively sought. Some believed this was too late in the design process, perceiving the outline strategy to be the final version, which was not the case. Conversely, others believed that their contributions had influenced the final strategy and were proud of their input.

From the analysis of the data generated from the focus groups, it was clear that the key to staff perceiving and understanding their involvement in the strategy development process was through effective communication. Some felt that they had had appropriate information throughout the process of service redesign and had an active involvement in the decision-making process. Others clearly felt that communication had only been at high level and had not filtered through the hierarchical ranks. It was this group of staff who felt disengaged from the process. For those staff who felt disengaged, further workshops and meetings were set up to ensure that staff had more opportunities to become involved and contribute to the implementation of the strategy. Ward managers also held team meetings and ensured communication with all staff on a daily basis.

WHAT DID WE LEARN?

The key to the survival and growth of an organisation is strategy, being aware of changes and adapting to them continually.

Anyone else contemplating a similar change in their working practice or that of others might find the following checklist useful as a guideline.

➤ When planning a massive change, remember that the devil is in the detail!
➤ Involve staff at every step of the process and ensure that they disseminate information to their teams.
➤ Communication is essential and should take place in many different forms. You cannot do too much of this.
➤ Ensure that there are frequent opportunities for staff to ask questions and to seek further information.
➤ Ensure that all disciplines of staff are involved as such a major change affects many staff groups.
➤ Listen to the ideas and suggestions of others and, where possible, feed them into the planning process.
➤ Listen to patients and service users, because their input and experiences, too, should be influential in such a process.

As managers, we had anticipated and expected the mixed feedback and understood the theory of change and its implications for the wider teams. However, as individuals who had committed so much time and energy to the process – little short of the proverbial blood, sweat and tears – it was sometimes disappointing to us and very difficult to cope with. The knowledge of theory and research did not serve to protect our feelings at all times. The work involved in the management and 'driving' of this massive challenge must not be underestimated and has certainly taken its toll on the key staff in this undertaking. Our survival has depended on effective working together, excellent communication skills and an ability to think quickly, adapting to any given situation. We have shared tears as well as joy, have grown emotionally and professionally, and have learned a great deal about the redesign of a cancer service and its leadership. We have drawn strength from those who have been supportive, hard working and enthusiastic in their efforts, of whom there were many. We have also drawn strength from our patients and their feedback prior to the opening of the Centre, as well as after we moved in; this valuable input has been essential in further developing our strategy and ways of working.

In relation to the Cancer Centre strategy, the strategic direction was created with stakeholders and was subsequently implemented. This process was clearly a process of emergent strategy, although aspects were planned and analysed throughout the commissioning period.

This strategy, although not yet formally reviewed and evaluated, is appearing to have benefits in terms of quality of patient care and efficiency within the service line. It was clear from evaluating the focus group data that there was a mix between those who felt that they had been fully engaged in the strategy development and implementation and those who had felt disengaged from this process. The significant key difference in the staff groups was between those who felt that they had received communication throughout the process and those who believed that strategy had been developed at a higher level and imposed upon them. Despite the deliberate actions undertaken to achieve the engagement of all staff, it was still perceived by some to be a historical 'top down' approach and true engagement at all levels was therefore not achieved.

The lack of true engagement was disappointing for us on a personal and a professional level, as a huge amount of work and emotional effort had been invested in this vision and strategy. However, it is important to balance this with the positive feedback received from others, including different staff groups, some of whom had little preparatory work. It is recognised that it will always be notoriously difficult to achieve full staff engagement with large and diverse teams (Mintzberg *et al.* 2009). In terms of organisational learning throughout this process, many good and successful approaches have been explored and used, and the benefits are evident. The communication aspects have been recognised as a major factor in the success of the strategy process in some areas; some negativity still exists in staff who feel that they were not given the opportunity to participate or in those areas where the communication process is less advanced. It would be interesting to undertake further research in the future comparing effective teams with less effective teams, investigating the levels of ownership of strategy and whether this can be directly improved through the use of different, diverse and repeated communication techniques.

Prior to the move

We organised 'drop in' days to help familiarise the staff with their new working environment; these were very well attended. Our educator (supported by the planning team) ran induction days for three months leading up to the day of the move, which every member of staff attended. This induction was interdisciplinary in nature, with specific sessions on such topics as building a team and staff support. A member of the planning team came at the end of every day to answer questions. Each group was given the opportunity to share their anxieties, ideas and queries, which the educator fed back to the team. In turn these queries were dealt with and information provided as appropriate, the induction days were given excellent feedback. They also gave opportunity for staff to become more familiar with their new surroundings. This was aided by a specially developed induction handbook.

The day of the move

On the day, we know we got it right; everything went smoothly and without any hitches. It was a very happy day, the strategising really paid off; all that planning provided a very organised, efficient and patient-friendly move. On arrival, patients were heard to say that the Centre was like a hotel and they were impressed with its airy and welcoming feel. They were also pleased with their actual transfer from other hospital sites to this one; it was a smooth and well-organised move, even down to knowing which patients were on their way from the transferring wards and what wards and bed numbers they were going into within the new Centre. Staff, too, seemed happy and commented that they were proud to be a part of such a successful day. There was a real excited, anticipatory atmosphere and much team camaraderie. Everything went well on the day of the move, from transferring the patients, to the multidisciplinary teams on all three sites working together to ensure a successful outcome. The photographs illustrate a 'snapshot' of all the enthusiasm, hard work and effort by all of our staff involved in making 23 August 2008 such a special and significant day for the patients, their loved ones and the staff (*see* Figures 9.1–9.3).

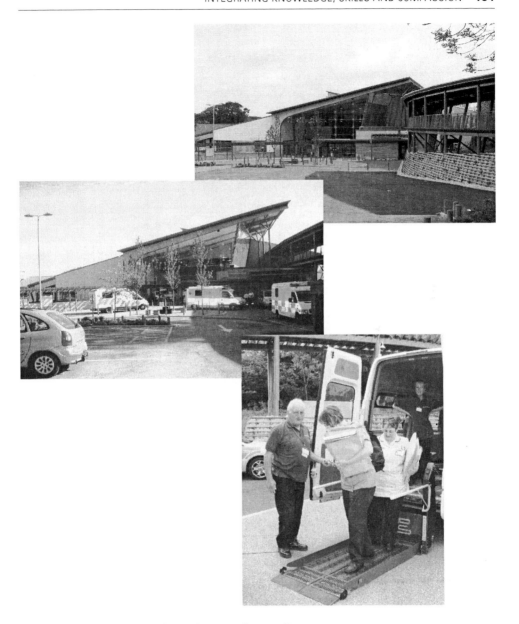

FIGURES 9.1–9.3 Moving in to the new Cancer Centre

The transition to the new Cancer Centre continues, however, eight months into the new build and staff, on the whole, appear very positive. The new teams on each of the wards are settling well and becoming efficient and cohesive, each at a slightly differing stage of the change process (Tuckman 1965). The staff are beginning to think and work much more as a whole team of five wards, rather than as a singular ward; they are keen to support and help each other, sharing knowledge, skills and experience. We are very proud and humbled to be part of this compassionate and caring team.

The Centre has recently been officially opened by Her Majesty The Queen and HRH Prince Phillip – a fantastic day and a real celebration for every staff member involved in the Centre. This has been a real mark of achievement and one of which each person must feel very proud for the part they played in making it happen.

We have received some excellent feedback from patients and their families –about the building, its state-of-the art appearance and artistic features, but also and even more significantly about the systems of care we have implemented and developed. Some of our patients wept on moving into the building and were overwhelmed by their surroundings, with some articulating that they didn't deserve to be cared for in such a wonderful environment! However, we are not perfect and like any other NHS organisation face problems and challenges on a daily basis. Yet our aim remains to have a fantastic service delivered in this wonderful building and so to provide our patients and their families with an outstanding, second-to-none service.

KEY POINTS

- Senior managers can influence workforce participation in strategic management.
- Strategic management is underpinned by a range of perspectives and theories.
- Education is pivotal to facilitate smooth transition in service developments.
- All stakeholders value consultation in strategic development and this must always be completed when any venture of this type is being planned.
- Senior managers not only focus on delivering a high standard of care but also on care for their staff – although this is not always recognised and acknowledged by the workforce.

CONCLUSION

In terms of learning with regard to the process, it must be remembered that strategy development is extremely complex and diverse; it is a continuous journey which must be undertaken in partnership. We have tried to illustrate the different elements of thought around strategic development. It is also hoped that this chapter might be useful as a teaching tool for health professionals and students to learn about planning strategic developments and change. Perhaps learning from our mistakes and successes? These should not be seen in isolation and attention must be given to the whole process, as well as acknowledgement that successful strategy formation combines many elements. Integrating knowledge, skills and compassion to reconfigure a cancer service was most certainly not easy but it was definitely worth all the hard work, emotional soul-searching and effort. Opportunities for being involved in strategic development often present themselves; we hope this chapter has motivated others to become engaged in similar processes.

Returning to the analogy of the elephant, we must see strategy as the whole beast and not simply the sum of its parts.

> *'It was the gang from strategy*
> *To action much inclined,*
> *Who went to find their cagy beast*
> *As they left the schools behind.*
> *Cried they, 'Having rode on the safari*
> *Can we be no longer be so blind?'*

(Mintzberg *et al.* 2009)

Then we, the managers, educators and bedside nursing staff might embrace change; continuing to work together compassionately and in harmony, to provide the highest quality of care to all our patients.

IMPLICATIONS FOR THE READER'S OWN PRACTICE

1 What would you need to learn to develop your knowledge and understanding of strategic management theories and practice?
2 How have you been involved in strategic management in the past, and how might you increase your involvement in the future?
3 What sort of creative activities can you devise to teach about strategic management?
4 How can you evaluate the impact of teaching about strategic management to the relevant stakeholders?

REFERENCES

Beardwell J, Clayton T (2007) *Human Resource Management: a contemporary approach.* 5th ed. London: Prentice Hall.

Boal KB, Hooijberg R (2001) Strategic leadership research: moving on. *Leader Q.* **11** (4): 515–49.

Chandler AD Jr (1962) *Strategy and Structure: chapters in the history of the industrial enterprise.* Cambridge, MA: MIT Press.

Department of Health (2000) *The NHS Plan: a plan for investment, a plan for reform.* London: DoH.

Department of Health (2000) *The NHS HR Strategy.* London: DoH.

Goold M, Campbell A (1987) *Designing Effective Organisations.* San Francisco, CA: Jossey-Bass/ Wiley.

Hamel G (1996) Strategy as a revolution. *Harvard Business Review.* July/August.

Hooper A, Potter J (2000) *Intelligent Leadership.* London: Random House.

Johnson G, Scholes K (2002) *Exploring Corporate Strategy.* 6th ed. Financial Times Series. London: Prentice Hall.

Kenny J (2006) Strategy and the learning organization: a maturity model for formation of strategy. *Learning Organ.* **13** (4): 353–68.

Leuke R (2005) *Strategy: create and implement the best strategy for your business.* Harvard Business Essentials. Cambridge, MA: Harvard Business School Press.

Mannion R, Davies HTO, Marshall MN (2005) *Cultures for Performance in Health Care.* Maidenhead: Open University Press.

Mintzberg H, Ahlstrand B, Lampel J (2009) *Strategy Safari: the complete guide through the wilds of strategic management.* Financial Times Series. London: Prentice Hall.

Morgan DL (1993) *Successful Focus Groups.* London: Sage.

Morgan DL (1997) *Focus Groups as Qualitative Research.* 2nd ed. London: Sage.

Mullins LJ (2005) *Management and Organisational Behaviour.* 7th ed. London: Prentice Hall.

Porter ME (1980) *Competitive Strategy: techniques for analysing industries and competitors.* New York: Free Press.

Selznicks P (1957) *Leadership in Administration: a sociological interpretation.* Evanson, IL: Row Peterson.

Shimizu T, Caravalho MM, Laurindo FJB (2006) *Strategic Alignment Process and Decision Support Systems: theory and case studies.* Hershey, PA: Idea Group Publishing.

Talbot-Smith A, Pollock A (2007) *The New NHS: a guide.* London: Routledge Publications.

Thorpe D (2008) *The Real NHS: the benefits of a marketing approach.* London: The Chartered Institute of Marketing.

Tuckman BW (1965) Development sequence in small groups. *Psychol Bull.* **63**: 384–99.

Unison (2007) *Unison response to DH consultation document 'Code of Practice on the Promotion of NHS Services'.* London: Unison Policy Unit.

10

Issues in research teaching and learning: what should we focus on?

David Clarke

'In the culture I grew up in you did your work and you did not put your arm around
it to stop other people from looking . . . you took the earliest possible opportunity
to make knowledge available.'

James Black (1995)

AIM

The aim of this chapter is to explore the factors influencing teaching and
learning about research in the context of developing skilled and knowledgeable practitioners within cancer and palliative care services.

LEARNING OUTCOMES

By the end of this chapter, the reader should be able to:
- consider the recent shift in attitudes regarding the importance of
  research and evidence in healthcare practice
- examine the concept of information literacy and consider its
  importance in research education and research utilisation
- explore the ways in which cancer and palliative care professionals can
  develop skills in locating, understanding and appraising research
- consider how research evidence can be utilised in education and
  clinical practice.

INTRODUCTION

In the quotation above, James Black was talking about the future of modern medicine;
more than fourteen years on, his comments remain very relevant in terms of developing and providing effective cancer and palliative care services. The concept of making

new knowledge and research evidence available to practitioners as soon as possible is now firmly embedded within the culture of most health services across the world (Muir-Gray 2001; Pearson *et al.* 2007). The contribution of research in the development and provision of effective services for patients with cancer has long been established (Doll and Peto 1981; DoH 1995, 2000b). The growth of research in relation to palliative care provision is rather more recent, but its importance is recognised by policymakers, health professionals and users of these services (DoH 2004; Pilgrim Projects 2007). There has been a positive shift in the attitudes of healthcare professionals towards learning about and understanding research in the last five to ten years. This shift should result in real benefits for the provision of cancer and palliative care services in the short to medium term. However, the shift has also challenged educators to find effective ways of helping healthcare professionals to locate and understand the range of information and research evidence now available, and to use these resources appropriately in their practice. This chapter will explore some of those challenges, and suggest ways in which educators and cancer and palliative care practitioners can develop essential skills and knowledge in relation to research.

CONTEXTUAL FACTORS IMPACTING ON ATTITUDES TOWARDS RESEARCH TEACHING AND LEARNING

Over the last 30 years there have been many calls for nursing and the allied health professions to base their practice on research (Committee on Nursing 1972; UKCC 1986; DoH 1993; Trinder and Reynolds 2000). However, it is perhaps only in the last ten years that significant progress has been made towards ensuring that health professional practice is based on firm evidence of its effectiveness (DoH 1996; Muir-Gray 2001; Pearson *et al.* 2007). Educators have long been exhorted to include research in their teaching and to teach health professionals about research methods in order that these professionals may participate in research activity related to their discipline. A number of factors made these requirements challenging until relatively recently; these included the availability of research evidence, the educational preparation of lecturers, the location of health professional education and the relative presence or absence of a research-oriented culture within health services.

Medical research relating to cancer treatment is well established; however, its primary focus has been on demonstrating the effectiveness of surgery, chemotherapy and radiotherapy (Corner and Bailey 2001; DoH 2007). Randomised controlled trials (RCTs) have understandably dominated the medical research agenda. The complexity of many of the interventions trialled has meant that for many non-medical healthcare professionals, their only engagement with this kind of research has been with the implementation of findings. This had two consequences. First, the role of educators was perceived as primarily being to identify and then convey the results of (primarily) medical research to practitioners. Second, this kind of educator and practitioner engagement with research implied that the design and conduct of research was a kind of specialised scientific endeavour sometimes far removed from day-to-day healthcare practice. As a result, many healthcare professionals perceived research to be an abstract and theoretical subject. One consequence of this was that attitudes towards understanding research methods and developing skills for critical appraisal of research were often negative. It proved difficult for some healthcare professionals to see the relevance of research for their day-to-day clinical practice. More recently, there has been a significant increase in the availability and quality of non-medical research in cancer and palliative care. However, changing attitudes towards understanding and using research has remained a challenge for many educators.

An important factor in developing more positive attitudes towards research teaching and learning was the transfer of health professional education into higher education, a process that was complete by the mid-1990s in the UK. This encouraged educators to undertake research degrees and also exposed them to an educational culture where research activity and teaching had a very high profile (DoH 2006; UKCRC 2006). This had a direct impact on development of new programmes for health professionals, as research teaching was required at all academic levels. The content of these programmes began to reflect contemporary research agendas evident in clinical practice and also the research interests of educators and their colleagues within faculties of health and medicine (Fallowfield *et al.* 2002; Shilling *et al.* 2003; Hopkinson *et al.* 2005). A continuing dilemma for educators, however, was to decide where to focus research teaching and learning; essentially this dilemma relates to making decisions about whether to focus on developing health professionals' research skills, or to focus on developing their skills as consumers of research. This important issue will be addressed in more detail later in the chapter.

Perhaps the most significant factor affecting attitudes towards research teaching and learning has been the growth in interest in the concept of evidence-based practice, and the impact of this in healthcare practice settings. Most authors acknowledge the important contribution made by the physician Archie Cochrane in the late 1970s in raising awareness of the importance of clinical and cost effectiveness in the provision of health services (Trinder and Reynolds 2000; Muir-Gray 2001; Pearson *et al.* 2007). However in the UK, the growth of interest in evidence-based practice among healthcare providers and service managers coincided largely with the publication of *Promoting Clinical Effectiveness: a framework for action in and through the NHS* (DoH 1996) and the post-1997 focus on modernising and improving health services through identification key standards for healthcare organisation and delivery. The introduction of the *NHS Plan* (DoH 2000a), National Service Frameworks (DoH 2000c, 2000b, 2001a) and the establishment of the National Institute for Health and Clinical Excellence (DoH 1999a) were hugely significant in that, perhaps for the first time in many instances, evidence-based clinical standards were clearly identified and achievement of those standards would be the subject of regular monitoring. While not all of these standards were based on high-quality research evidence, their introduction and the identification of the evidence on which they were based meant that healthcare professionals at all levels (rather than just researchers) were required to consider the effectiveness of their practice and the evidence on which that practice was based.

DEFINING EVIDENCE-BASED PRACTICE

These terms are now in common use but may not always be clearly defined or understood in the context of their relationship to the kinds of evidence and research identified within documents outlining national clinical standards. One of the most commonly cited definitions was provided by Sackett *et al.* (1996: 71):

> '*Evidence based medicine is the conscientious, explicit and judicious use of current best evidence in making decisions about the care of individual patients. The practice of evidence based medicine means integrating individual clinical expertise with the best available external clinical evidence from systematic research.*'

Although Sackett *et al.* (1996) were talking about evidence-based medicine, the above definition translates quite easily into the broader areas of evidence-based nursing and evidence-based practice in general. Similarly, Cullum *et al.* (1998: 38) highlighted three key elements of evidence-based practice which were transferable to all disciplines:

> '*Evidence based healthcare integrates the best evidence from research with clinical expertise, patient preferences and existing resources into decision making about the healthcare of individual patients.*'

Cullum *et al.* (1998) provided an important reminder that evidence alone is not sufficient to improve the effectiveness of health services. The central importance of balancing patient preference with available resources is a key factor in ensuring that the available evidence is used judiciously to inform and support decision-making. This focus on patients' views and experiences as central to the organisation and delivery of health services has recently been given further prominence in the review of the NHS conducted by Lord Darzi which culminated in the *High Quality Care for All: NHS next stage review report* (DoH 2008). In cancer and palliative care, the *Cancer Plan* (DoH 2000b), the *Improving Outcomes* Guidance (DoH 1999b), the *Manual of Cancer Services Standards* (DoH 2001b) and *Building on the Best* (DoH 2004) provided a detailed and evidence-based framework designed to help configure services, select effective drugs and technologies and make patient-orientated decisions which result in consistent delivery of high-quality care. In part, making such decisions depends on the level and strength of the evidence underpinning national clinical standards; levels and hierarchies of evidence will be explored in the later section on systematic reviews and meta-analysis.

So from a position of perhaps limited research evidence and some negative attitudes towards research, most educators are now working with health professionals who recognise the contribution of research evidence in providing effective cancer and palliative care services. These professionals are now more actively seeking education in evidence-based practice and research. Equally importantly, these practitioners are now working in health services where the requirement to meet or exceed national standards has impacted on the culture of those services (Healthcare Commission 2007). Where once research may have been seen as an enterprise sometimes peripheral to mainstream care delivery, it is now recognised as a fundamental part of health service policy and practice (Hamer and Collinson 2005; DoH 2006; UKCRC 2006). In shifting the policy emphasis from continually restating the importance of research to a focus on the evidence of clinical effectiveness, policymakers may have inadvertently removed some barriers to health professionals engaging with research evidence.

CONTEMPORARY RESEARCH TEACHING AND LEARNING: WHERE SHOULD THE FOCUS BE?

There seems to be little doubt that to improve the standard of healthcare provision, health professionals in all fields should develop research knowledge and skills. There is, however, some debate in higher education institutions and some areas of practice as to how such knowledge and skills should be developed. In essence, there are two positions within this debate. The first argues that the most appropriate way to develop research knowledge and skills is to ensure that undergraduates participate in small-scale research activities in all three years of their programmes of study; ideally these activities should be directly related to research projects being undertaken by academic and professional researchers in their field of study. Students work in small groups as well as individually, they design and conduct small-scale projects and evaluate data generated in these projects. The primary (educational) purpose is to focus on learning *through* research, in order to develop students' knowledge of and participation in research related to their discipline. In some settings, students supported by experienced researchers can contribute directly to the generation of new knowledge in their chosen field (Council on Undergraduate Research 2007). This approach, which is somewhat more common in the USA, is championed by Jenkins and Healey (2007) and Huggins *et al.* (2007). This is also the focus of the Research Based Learning-Centre for Excellence in Teaching and Learning (CETL) project at the University of Warwick. These authors maintain that development of students' research skills is a fundamental requirement for universities if students are to usefully contribute to their professions, the economy and to the development of society as a whole. Such an approach anticipates that involving all students in the research process increases knowledge and understanding of the importance of research inquiry and should increase the number of undergraduate students who will consider careers in research. The success of learning through participation in research activities depends in large part on two related issues. First, there needs to be a critical mass of research-active staff in university departments. Second, research-active staff must be willing to participate in educational programmes committed to developing learning through participation in educationally orientated small-scale research projects and also ongoing staff research projects. While there have been significant developments in terms of increasing the research capacity in nursing, midwifery and the allied health professionals, there is only limited evidence that the learning through research model identified above could be successfully adopted at present (Johnson 2006; UKCRC 2006).

The second position in the debate surrounding research teaching and learning within health professions therefore adopts a more pragmatic stance and focuses on developing students' awareness and utilisation of research evidence in developing high-quality healthcare provision. In this approach, developing knowledge and skills

TABLE 10.1 An approach to research teaching and learning: progression from basic to advanced competence in information retrieval, critical appraisal and research skills

Foundation knowledge and skills	Intermediate knowledge and skills		Application and utilisation	Advanced knowledge and skills
Information literacy	Research processes and methods: consumer	Critical appraisal and systematic review	Application in practice settings	Research processes and methods: researcher
Recognising information needs	Understanding the need for systematic and rigorous methods of enquiry	Understanding the nature and purpose of critical appraisal	Interpreting and using clinical guidelines, and National Service Framework standards	Developing focused research questions Reviewing the existing knowledge base – advanced literature searching
Understanding and utilising relevant resources • NHS Evidence • Electronic Databases • The Internet	Differentiating between audit and research	Differentiating between traditional literature reviews and systematic reviews and meta-analysis	Working collaboratively and across networks to develop evidence-based policies and protocols • using journal clubs • developing research utilisation programmes	Seeking research funding Developing appropriate research designs Working with NRES Applying for ethical (LREC) and research governance approval
Developing skills in searching and retrieval • search strategies • saving and retrieving searches	Developing knowledge of common research methods in healthcare	Selecting appropriate tools for appraisal: • the Critical Appraisal Skills Programme • Consort Guidelines	Working collaboratively in considering the recommendations of systematic reviews and improving outcomes guidance	Understanding, planning and managing sampling strategies Reviewing, deciding on and using data collection methods/tools
Developing the skills required to judge the quality of online information • using RDN Virtual Training	Research approaches • experimental • survey • ethnographic	Using relevant resources • Cochrane Library • Centre for Reviews and Dissemination	Sharing examples of evidence-based practice through teaching others, presenting at conferences and publications	Planning, understanding and managing data analysis Writing research reports Disseminating research findings
Introduction to literature reviewing	Reading research publications			
Understanding the concept of evidence-based practice	Recognising the importance of clinical guidelines			

is a progressive undertaking, moving from basic to more advanced competencies in information retrieval, and critical appraisal of research evidence. These are regarded as foundation skills for the progression to development of the skills required to design, conduct and evaluate research. It is significant that recent reports, making recommendations regarding the development of the research capacity of healthcare professionals, place most emphasis (in the short-term) on postgraduate or qualifying training in research (DoH 2006; Johnson 2006; UKCRC 2008). However, these policy documents also recognise the importance of developing educational and practice cultures where scholarship and research are considered core elements of health professional activity. Implicit in this approach is recognition of the need for progression from research awareness, through research appraisal and utilisation, towards research participation. The ways in which such an approach can be developed are outlined in Table 10.1.

DEVELOPING INFORMATION LITERACY

It has been argued that we live in an 'information age' and that it is essential that universities contribute to and develop the 'knowledge economy' (Romer 1990; Castells 1996). Few would dispute that as a result of the increased availability of research evidence, in part due to the growth of the Internet, it has never been more important that health professionals develop the knowledge and skills required to locate and discriminate between poor and high-quality healthcare information. The term 'information literacy' is now commonly used to describe this process; this is defined as follows:

> *'Information literacy is knowing when and why you need information, where to find it, and how to evaluate, use and communicate it in an ethical manner.'* (Society of College, National and University Libraries (SCONUL) 1999)

Information literacy is now internationally regarded as a core element of undergraduate preparation and as a significant contributor to developing the skills of lifelong learning in professional groups (American Library Association 1989; SCONUL 1999; Bundy 2004). The Seven Pillars Model for information literacy developed by SCONUL (1999) (*see* Figure 10.1) provides a framework which can be utilised to design appropriate learning and teaching activities. These activities can be progressed through a variety of academic levels or can be designed specifically around the needs of health professionals on short courses at different points in their careers. The following section identifies the ways in which health professionals in general, and those working in cancer and palliative care practice specifically can benefit from developing information literacy skills.

At various stages in their professional careers, practitioners are likely to *recognise information needs* – for example, in relation to understanding the nature and progression of site-specific cancers; developing knowledge of effective treatment interventions; and understanding the range of specialist care and management strategies required to meet the needs of patients being treated for cancer and/or requiring palliative care. Given the huge amounts of information now available to practitioners, *distinguishing ways to address gaps* in knowledge and understanding is an area where educators can

SCONUL Seven Pillars Model for Information Literacy
© Society of College, National and University Libraries

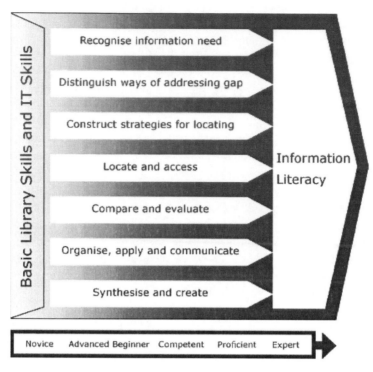

FIGURE 10.1 SCONUL Seven Pillars model for information literacy

help practitioners to *construct strategies for locating* and also to *locate and access* high-quality healthcare information and research findings (SCONUL 1999). An information box nearby identifies a key – but at present under-utilised – information source which can be used in a targeted way by health professionals to meet information needs.

NHS Evidence

(Formerly the National Library for Health)

Acts as a web-based port and an information gateway.
Using the simple search screen, users can access high-quality and up-to-date information including:
● Guidelines from the National Institute for Health and Clinical Excellence

The Cancer Collection includes:
● Evidence summaries and links to Health Technology Assessments, Systematic Reviews and ongoing trials, and the 'grey' (unpublished) literature. There is also a section on medicines and devices where information on individual cancer drugs can be accessed.

Searches can be filtered to pursue specific areas of interest, such as those above, via:
- links to policy documents, e.g. the *NHS Cancer Plan, Improving Outcomes* Guidance and *Building on the Best: end of life care* initiative, from the Department of Health
- see also the Behind the Headlines from NHS Choices archive, where media reports on contemporary research are evaluated, e.g. in relation to funding cancer drugs such as Herceptin. Over 170 cancer-related articles were reviewed by mid-2009. This can be accessed by searching NHS Evidence or more directly at: www.nhs.uk/News/Pages/NewsIndex.aspx
- NHS Evidence can be found at: www.evidence.nhs.uk/

The NHS Evidence Health Information Resources website (which has some content previously seen on the National Library for Health site) will continue to run in parallel to the NHS Evidence website. At the time of publication, this can be accessed at: www.library.nhs.uk

A similar resource is provided by INTUTE, where high-quality peer-reviewed educational and research resources are grouped by subject speciality, including health and life sciences (INTUTE can be accessed at: http://intute.ac.uk). Information gateways such as the NHS Evidence, and INTUTE are currently under-utilised by health professionals in general but represent important consolidated resources for busy practitioners seeking to find specific research or information related to particular areas of professional practice. Two additional areas are important in terms of developing basic information literacy skills; these are namely understanding and using electronic databases, and discriminating between good and poor quality information available on the Internet. In most higher education institutions, subject-specific librarians and educators are working collaboratively to ensure that students understand: first, the range of electronic databases related to their professional interests, and second, how to develop effective search strategies to locate specific research information within these databases. An information box nearby lists some key electronic databases for health professionals working in cancer and palliative care services.

Healthcare-related electronic databases
- CINAHL
- MEDLINE
- Science Direct
- PsychInfo
- AIDS and Cancer research abstracts
- AMED
- EMBASE
- Web of Science
- The Cochrane Library

While subject-specific electronic databases should be the first port of call for health professionals, it is recognised that the ubiquitous nature of the Internet means that guidance is also needed on recognising the strengths and weaknesses of information which can be found there. Health professional education programmes, including the INTUTE Virtual Training Suite tutorials on using the Internet effectively, provide an opportunity for students to develop knowledge and skills related to judging the quality of online health and research-related information. Providing targeted activities for health professionals to develop the skills outlined above ensures that the foundation knowledge and skills required for undertaking a literature review can be developed or revisited where appropriate. The term 'foundation' is important here, in that these skills are sometimes regarded as basic and yet the ability to design and conduct an effective search strategy and literature review is a fundamental requirement for both novice and experienced researchers. The importance of developing these skills should not be underestimated. An effective way to consolidate these skills is to engage practitioners or students in conducting a small-scale literature review as part of an investigation into a particular treatment or care intervention, or to support the new evidence-based care pathway or protocol, either in practice settings or as part of a programme of study. Using the resources available via NHS Evidence should also encourage practitioners to follow Black's (1995) example and share information and research evidence, as opposed to working in isolation and repeating work which may already have been undertaken elsewhere. Cancer and palliative care networks, too, seek to foster dissemination and sharing of research evidence and practice development (DoH 2007). Explicitly linking these educational processes to contemporary agendas for networks increases practitioners' understanding of the relevance of skills development and stimulates interest in developing competencies in these areas.

UNDERSTANDING RESEARCH METHODS AND SKILLS IN CRITICAL APPRAISAL

While learning how to locate high-quality research evidence is essential, it is imperative that health professionals can progress in terms of information literacy and develop the knowledge and skills to *compare and evaluate*, that is, to critically appraise research and other forms of evidence identified. Critical appraisal is a higher-order skill which is unlikely to be understood and used effectively unless it is developed alongside, or following exposure to, an overview of the research process and examination of research methods. Defining and locating research in the context of current issues in clinical practice is an effective way of engaging health professionals with the debates surrounding the relative strengths and weaknesses of different research methodologies in answering questions arising from cancer and palliative care practice (Pearson *et al.* 2007).

In developing understanding of research methods it is also important that the process of clinical audit is examined so that health professionals understand the similarities and differences between audit and research (Cheater and Closs 1998). Garland (2005: 136) suggested that *'research is used to define good practice, whereas audit measures the extent to which good practice is implemented on a daily basis'*. We could add to this straightforward definition that the primary purpose of research activity is to generate new knowledge or to investigate the effectiveness of new or existing interventions. In contrast, audit examines whether existing practice in a given clinical area is consistent with identified standards, such as those identified in the *Improving Outcomes* Guidance (DoH 1999b) and National Service Frameworks (DoH 2000b). Both audit and research contribute to improving the effectiveness of healthcare, and both require careful critical appraisal before their recommendations are accepted.

It is also important to establish the necessity for systematic and rigorous approaches to developing and examining clinical practice questions as these are hallmarks of the quality of research (Long and Godfrey 2004). The research process can be seen as analogous to the way in which most health professionals assess and manage the needs of patients in their care. In both situations, health professionals begin with a clinical problem or question and need to gather specific data using recognised tools or techniques. These data must be analysed rigorously and objectively; the conclusions drawn should derive from the data and provide a plausible explanation on which future actions can be based. If assessment of need is not systematic, then interpretation and analysis of data and subsequent diagnosis may be inaccurate and planned treatments may prove ineffective. The same criteria can be applied to research. If research or audit questions are poorly defined, if sampling is inappropriate and if data collection methods are not valid and applied systematically, then it is likely that data generated and the subsequent data analysis will be of limited value in providing new knowledge or in determining whether interventions are effective (Bowling and Ebrahim 2005). Encouraging health professionals to explore the similarities in these two processes can help to demystify research and develop an understanding that particular research approaches provide frameworks which practitioners and researchers can use in the exploration of particular clinical issues. The same frameworks can also provide the basis for external appraisal of the quality of research (Burns and Grove 2005).

However, an appreciation of the research process alone is not sufficient. Health professionals will not develop the capacity to critically appraise published research unless they have had the opportunity (previously or concurrently) to develop understanding of common research approaches, that is, experimental, survey and ethnographic approaches. It is beyond the scope of this chapter to review the strengths and weaknesses of these approaches; the texts by Bowling and Ebrahim (2005), Holloway and Wheeler (2002) and Polit and Beck (2006) provide excellent summaries for readers unfamiliar with these approaches. The volume and availability of published research in healthcare is both a help and a hindrance. Finding research relevant to the practice of cancer and palliative care professionals is not difficult; the problem is that it is also not difficult to be overwhelmed by the volume of available literature. For example a search using the terms 'cancer and fatigue' using the CINAHL and MEDLINE databases produced 1207 and 3448 hits respectively. The almost impossible number of published research papers which healthcare professionals would have to read in order to stay abreast of developments within their field is recognised by most healthcare professions (Davidoff *et al.* 1995; Nail-Chiwetalu and Ratner 2006; Ratner 2006; Malone 2007). The next two sections will briefly examine ways to make learning about and use of research relevant for health professionals, and comment on the important contribution of systematic reviews and meta-analyses as a means to manage the problems caused by the sheer volume of research now published.

USING NATIONAL SERVICE FRAMEWORK OR CANCER STANDARDS AS EXEMPLARS

If teaching about research methods is not to be perceived as an abstract theoretical exercise, then it is necessary to find ways to capture health professionals' interest in research methods and help them to develop the skills to determine the quality of research evidence. Health professionals are increasingly familiar with national clinical standards and targets for service improvement (DoH 2000a, 2001b, 2004). The majority of these standards are based on research evidence. Developing short programmes or practice-led exercises where health professionals locate, read and then compare and evaluate the research in small groups provides a means to use contemporary practice standards to develop understanding of research methods, review the available litera-ture and develop skills in critical appraisal. Table 10.2 illustrates the kind of activities which can be used.

TABLE 10.2 Developing understanding of research methods and applying this in critical appraisal of research

Locate the evidence	Select a topic area	Identify research to read and review	Discuss the research methods used	Use the Critical Appraisal Skills Programme (CASP) (PHRU 2006) tool for RCTs
Access the NICE guidelines via NHS Evidence ⟶ DoH DoH publications	Improving outcomes in colorectal cancers Use the PDF 'Research Evidence for the Manual Update'	Focus on anal cancer treatments (p. 249) identifies 3 studies examining primary non-surgical treatment of anal cancer • Bartelink (EORTC) (1997) • Flam (RTOG) (1996) • UKCCCR (1996)	RCTs • inclusion and exclusion criteria • sample sizes • data collection and outcome measures • data analysis • findings and recommendations	Working with a facilitator • use the CASP questions to appraise each element of the research • discuss the appraisal process • identify further learning needs

The Critical Appraisal Skills Programme Resource (CASP) developed by the Public Health Resources Unit (PHRU 2006) provides a set of high-quality appraisal tools which have been designed to help practitioners to develop the skills required to locate and make sense of research evidence, which in turn is designed to help to transfer research knowledge into practice. For further information on approaches to critical appraisal, *see* for example, Booth (2006) and Pearson *et al.* (2007).

In some practice settings, journal clubs and multidisciplinary critical appraisal programmes have been established, with varying degrees of success; these adopt similar strategies to those outlined above and are dependent in part on skilled facilitation if the exercise is to bring about effective learning (Mayor *et al.* 2004; Carroll-Johnson 2005). There is accumulating evidence that these approaches to working with research in practice are viewed positively by practitioners, result in increased understanding of the evidence base for practice and can bring about improvements in service provision (McQueen *et al.* 2006; Milne *et al.* 2007). The now extensive body of research which has examined barriers to research utilisation within nursing has identified a variety of reasons why nurses and other healthcare professionals do not find it easy to read and understand research papers (Funk *et al.* 1991; Closs *et al.* 2000; Freeman and Sweeney 2001; Bryar *et al.* 2003). These include the way in which the research is reported, practitioners' confidence in understanding and interpreting statistical data and the culture of the workplace and support of managers for research- and evidence-based practice. Structured research educational programmes and practice-based journal clubs provide opportunities to address and overcome some of these barriers (Milne *et al.* 2007).

CONSOLIDATED EVIDENCE SOURCES: LITERATURE REVIEWS, SYSTEMATIC REVIEWS AND META-ANALYSIS

As has been indicated earlier, it is very difficult for the average health professional to keep up to date with all of the research evidence in their field; this is as true for researchers as it is for practitioners. This problem has been recognised for some time and there are now a number of consolidated sources of reviewed research evidence which health professionals can draw upon. The majority of these resources can be accessed via the information gateway provided by the NHS Evidence.

First, a word about literature reviews. A key element of most research reports is the literature review. It is essential that researchers demonstrate that they have critically examined the available literature relating to their proposed research question. The justification for the proposed research is normally based on identification of gaps or areas of continuing uncertainty in our existing knowledge base (Hart 1998). Traditional literature reviews summarise the available literature and should evaluate the methodological quality of existing research. These reviews can contribute to our understanding of a particular topic area, but they can also be highly selective in terms of the evidence reviewed and there is no agreed standard for the scope and rigour of literature reviews (Dickson 2005; Beecroft *et al.* 2006). As a result, published literature reviews may or may not provide a comprehensive examination of the quality of the available research in a given area. Because the purpose of a literature review may be to justify a new study, then clear summaries of the effectiveness of a particular practice or intervention may not be included.

In contrast to the sometimes selective and narrow focus of the traditional literature review, systematic reviews represent a rigorous and structured process designed to locate and then review all of the available evidence relating to the effectiveness of a particular intervention or treatment. The Centre for Reviews and Dissemination (2009: v) stated that systematic reviews are required to:

'Identify, evaluate and summarise the findings of all relevant individual studies, thereby making the available evidence more accessible to decision makers.'

Single research studies often provide a partial or limited picture of a particular issue. Systematic reviews attempt to bring together all of the available research evidence, published and unpublished, and so represent valuable consolidated reviews of available research which can help healthcare professionals, service managers and patients to determine objectively what treatments are effective. Systematic reviews of multiple randomised controlled trials are now considered as the 'gold' standard for assessment of effectiveness of treatments or interventions (Muir-Gray 2001; Khan *et al.* 2004). These reviews are important to the decisions made by the National Institute for Health and Clinical Excellence (NICE) in the development of clinical guidelines and approval of interventions for use in the National Health Service in the UK. The notion of a 'gold' standard in terms of research is related to the hierarchies of evidence which have been developed and which are used in various forms in National Service Frameworks and clinical guideline documents to indicate the strength of research evidence which underpins a specific standard. Table 10.3 provides an example of such a hierarchy of evidence; it should be noted, however, that these hierarchies can differ in the emphasis placed on particular forms of evidence.

TABLE 10.3 The strength of different types of evidence

I	Strong evidence from at least one systematic review of a multiple well-designed randomised controlled trial (RCT)
II	Strong evidence from at least one properly designed RCT of appropriate size
III	Evidence from well-designed trials without randomisation, single group pre/post, cohort, time series or matched case control studies
IV	Evidence from well-designed non-experimental studies from more than one centre or research group
V	Opinions of respected authorities, based on clinical evidence, descriptive studies or reports of expert committees

Source: Muir-Gray 2001.

The two main sources of access to systematic reviews in the UK are the Cochrane Library and the Centre for Reviews and Dissemination at York University (CRD). A similar resource is available in Australia at the Joanna Briggs Institute (Pearson *et al.* 2007). The conduct of systematic reviews is very similar to the process of undertaking any research study. However, relatively few health professionals will conduct systematic reviews of the kind published by the Cochrane Library and the CRD. A detailed account of the processes involved in the design and conduct of a systematic review has been reported by Khan *et al.* (2004); detailed guidance is also provided by the CRD and the Cochrane Library. It is important to recognise that the focus of systematic reviews has mainly been on effectiveness and thus existing reviews have been almost exclusively based on reviewing multiple randomised controlled trials (RCTs). More recently there has been increasing recognition of the necessity for systematic review of non-experimental and qualitative research and the inclusion of qualitative research in traditional systematic reviews (Flemming and Briggs 2006; Flemming 2007).

Briefly examining existing systematic reviews relating to breast cancer included in the Cochrane Reviews Library will help to illustrate the kind of evidence currently available and some of the decisions made by reviewers based on this evidence.

Over thirty Cochrane reviews can be found relating to breast cancer, four will be briefly highlighted here to illustrate differences in the evidence reviewed and conclusions drawn. Gibson *et al.* (2007) compared aromatase inhibitors to other endocrine therapy for the treatment of advanced breast cancer. These authors identified 30 RCTs which met their inclusion criteria, they were able to include 25 in their review and, following pooled analysis of the data from these studies, concluded that aromatase inhibitors showed a survival benefit for women with advanced breast cancer when compared with other endocrine therapy. Pavlakis *et al.* (2002) conducted a similar review of multiple RCTs, in this case in relation to the effectiveness of biphosphonates in treating symptoms associated with bone metastases. These are examples of 'gold' standard evidence in this area. In another review to determine whether prophylactic mastectomy reduced death (from any cause) in women who had never had breast cancer and in women with a history of breast cancer in one breast, Lostumbo *et al.* (2004) could not find any RCTs addressing this issue and therefore included only observational studies (cohort, case control and case series), 23 such studies in all. In their conclusions, Lostumbo *et al.* (2004) noted that while the studies reviewed demonstrated that bilateral prophylactic mastectomy was effective in reducing incidence of and death from breast cancer, more rigorous prospective studies (ideally RCTs) were needed. This represents level 3 evidence in the Muir-Gray (2001) hierarchy and is clearly less robust evidence of effectiveness; nevertheless it represents the current best evidence for clinical practice in this field.

However, some important practice questions remain for which systematic review evidence is not currently available. Lockhart *et al.* (2007) intended to assess the effectiveness of different methods used to communicate the primary diagnosis of breast cancer. These authors sought to review RCTs examining these issues but were unable to locate any such studies. In contrast to Lostumbo *et al.* (2004), these authors in accordance with their stated selection criteria, chose not to review non-experimental studies and concluded that it was not possible to answer the review question at this time. These examples illustrate the valuable contribution which systematic reviews can make to health professional practice, but hopefully they also illustrate the current limitations of the available evidence and the choices which researchers have to make when conducting such reviews. Dickson (2005) reminds us that the findings of systematic reviews, in common with any other research study, should not be accepted without critical appraisal of the review (*see* the CASP framework for appraisal tools for systematic reviews, PHRU 2006).

Meta-analysis is sometimes confused with systematic review, but while a meta-analysis may be included in a systematic review, this does not mean that a meta-analysis is the same thing as a systematic review (Dickson 2005). The National Library for Medicine (2007) defined meta-analysis as:

> '*Systematic methods that use statistical techniques for combining results from different studies to obtain a quantitative estimate of the overall effect of a particular intervention*

or variable on a defined outcome. This combination may produce a stronger conclusion than can be provided by any individual study.'

Cornish *et al.* (2007) provide a good example of the use of meta-analysis in a study which is not a systematic review. The authors combined the results for 1443 patients from eleven studies to compare patients' quality of life following abdominoperineal excison of rectum (APER) with that after anterior resection (Cornish *et al.* 2007: 2056). Contrary to existing beliefs about the perceived beneficial effect of avoiding a permanent stoma on quality of life following rectal cancer, Cornish *et al.* (2007) were not able to identify from the pooled data analysis any difference in quality of life post procedures.

This section has reviewed the nature of these consolidated sources of evidence in order to highlight their importance in terms of developing information literacy. These sources are examples of *synthesis* of evidence which can *create* new knowledge or new understanding of existing evidence (SCONUL 1999). These represent a key form of evidence which health professionals must be aware of and use to underpin their clinical practice with research evidence. However, as Sackett *et al.* (1996) and others have pointed out, even the best evidence available must be used alongside clinical judgement and expertise and should, as far as possible, take account of patient preferences and the resources available.

DEVELOPING THE SKILLS TO CONDUCT RESEARCH

This chapter has attempted to demonstrate that developing research knowledge and skills is a progressive and not a once-and-for-all activity. Developing information literacy represents an important process in achieving competence in locating, appraising and disseminating research evidence. These skills are a fundamental requirement for the development of the more advanced skills required to participate in research on a sustained basis or to progress to a career in research. Table 10.1 outlined, in the final column, the skills and knowledge required to undertake research independently, or as is now increasingly common, as part of a multidisciplinary group. The earlier stages of learning about and using research will have examined the ways in which researchers have displayed and documented their use of these skills, and therefore the strategies outlined in Table 10.1 contribute directly to the development of advanced research knowledge and skills. Recent debates surrounding the need to build research capacity in nursing and other health professions suggests that these advanced skills will mainly be developed as part of specific post-qualifying training in research or in combination with postgraduate research training programmes (DoH 2006; UKCRC 2008). Table 10.4 provides an example of how research skills can be developed in a targeted way across academic levels or, in short, focuses on time-limited programmes. It is clear that, while there is a need to develop research career opportunities and to fast track clinical research training, not all health professionals will wish to pursue research careers. However, it is also clear that now more than ever before, health professionals must become information and research literate.

TABLE 10.4 Research teaching and learning: progression across academic levels or within time-limited programmes

Foundation skills and knowledge	Intermediate skills	Application and utilisation	Advanced skills	
	Level 1	Level 2	Level 3	Masters	Doctoral
Progression can be based on academic level – each level requires some degree of revision or prior knowledge and skills	Level 1	Level 2	Level 3	Masters	Doctoral

Progression from basic to advanced competence in information retrieval, critical appraisal and research skills

OR

Within time-limited programmes of study, the majority of the elements are likely to require focused revision and application based on the nature of the programme and students' individual needs. For example:

	Foundation knowledge and skills	Intermediate knowledge and skills	Application and utilisation	Advanced knowledge and skills
Postgraduate Certificate	Individual appraisal and revisit if necessary	Development	Focus	
Postgraduate Diploma		Development	Focus	
Masters Degree		Further development	Focus	Target development
Professional Doctorate		Revisit and further develop	Development	Target competence
PhD		Revisit and further develop	Development	Target competence

KEY POINTS

■ Research generates the evidence used to ensure that clinical practice is effective; therefore understanding research is central to providing appropriate services in cancer and palliative care.

■ Information literacy and skills are now part of the competencies required by all healthcare professions; these skills are transferable and form a key part of professional lifelong learning.

■ Despite a significant increase in the availability and quality of research evidence, practitioners must develop skills in critical appraisal if they are to use evidence judiciously and for the benefit of individual patients.

■ Developing skills in information and research literacy should be a collaborative and work-based activity supported by clinicians and educators.

CONCLUSION

This chapter has explored a range of factors influencing teaching and learning about research and concluded that the concern to base clinical practice on sound evidence of its effectiveness has encouraged more and more healthcare professionals to see the necessity of understanding and using research evidence in their practice. This appreciation of the importance of research has led to increased interest in finding effective ways to learn about and teach about research. This chapter has outlined some key elements in progressing from basic to advanced competence in information literacy, including establishing the importance of critical appraisal and consolidated evidence sources. Developing skills in research represents a continuum which encompasses core skills required of all practitioners in cancer and palliative care and also the more advanced skills required to design and conduct research which will be required of a much smaller number of health professionals. Research need no longer be perceived as a specialised activity conducted and reviewed by a select few; it should be understood as an integral part of modern healthcare provision.

IMPLICATIONS FOR THE READER'S OWN PRACTICE

The issues raised in this chapter should have made readers ask the following questions:

1 Do I and my colleagues at work understand the nature of the information provided for us by the NHS Evidence and INTUTE?

2 Can we change NHS Evidence and INTUTE from icons on the computer screen to resources that we routinely use?

3 Should we work with clinical educators to determine the current level of information literacy skills in our workplace?

4 In conjunction with local higher education providers, can we design participatory and work-based learning activities which will engage staff in examining and understanding key research evidence underpinning current practice?

REFERENCES

Association of College and Research Libraries (1998) *A Progress Report on Information Literacy: an update on the American Library Association Presidential Committee on Information Literacy: Final Report*. Chicago: Association of College and Research Libraries. Available at: www.ala.org/ala/ProductsandPublications/Products_and_Publications.htm

Beecroft A, Rees A, Booth A (2006) Finding the evidence. In: Gerrish K, Lacey A, editors. *The Research Process in Nursing*. 5th ed. Oxford: Blackwell Science.

Black J (1995) On medical research. *Daily Telegraph*. 11 December.

Booth A (2006) Critical appraisal of the evidence. In: Gerrish K, Lacey A, editors. *The Research Process in Nursing*. 5th ed. Oxford: Blackwell Science.

Bowling A (2002) *Research Methods in Health: investigating health and health services*. 2nd ed. Buckingham: Open University Press.

Bowling A, Ebrahim S, editors (2005) *Handbook of Health Research Methods: investigation, measurement and analysis*. Maidenhead: Open University Press.

Bryar R et al. (2003) The Yorkshire BARRIERS project: diagnostic analysis of barriers to research utilisation. *Int J Nurs Stud*. **40** (1): 73–84.

Bundy A, editor (2004) *Australian and New Zealand Information Literacy Framework: principles standards and practice*. 2nd ed. Adelaide: Australian and New Zealand Institute for Information Literacy.

Burns N, Grove SK (2005) *The Practice of Nursing Research: conduct, critique, and utilisation*. 5th ed. St Louis, MO: Saunders.

Carroll-Johnson RM (2005) Reading on the job. *Oncol Nurs Forum*. **32** (2): 221.

Castells M (1996) *The Rise of the Network Society*. Oxford: Blackwell.

[NHS] Centre for Reviews and Dissemination (2009) *Systematic Reviews: CRD's Guidance for undertaking reviews in health care*. 3rd ed. York: Centre for Reviews and Dissemination, University of York. Available at: www.york.ac.uk/inst/crd/

Cheater FM, Closs SJ (1988) The relationship between clinical audit and research. In: Roe B, Webb C, editors. *Research and Development in Clinical Nursing Practice*. London: Whurr.

Closs SJ et al. (2000) Barriers to research implementation in two Yorkshire hospitals. *Clin Effect Nurs*. **4** (1): 3–10.

Committee on Nursing (1972) *Report of the Committee on Nursing*. London: HMSO.

Corner J, Bailey C, editors (2001) *Cancer Nursing: care in context*. London: Blackwell.

Cornish JA et al. (2007) A meta-analysis of quality of life for abdominoperitoneal excision of rectum versus anterior resection for rectal cancer. *Ann Surg Oncol*. **14** (7): 2056–68.

Council on Undergraduate Research (2007) *Learning through Research*. Available at: www.cur.org/index.html (accessed 20 October 2007).

Cullum N, DiCenso A, Ciliska D (1998) Evidence-based nursing: an introduction. *Evid Base Med*. **3** (2): 37–8.

Davidoff F, Haynes B, Sackett D, Smith R (1995) Evidenced-based medicine: new journal to help doctors identify the information they need. *BMJ*. **310**: 185–6.

Department of Health (1993) *Research for Health: a research and development strategy for the NHS*. London: DoH.

Department of Health (1995) *A Policy Framework for Commissioning Cancer Services: a report by the expert advisory group on cancer to the Chief Medical Officers of England and Wales*. London: DoH and the Welsh Office.

Department of Health (1996) *Promoting Clinical Effectiveness: a framework for action in and through the NHS*. London: DoH.

Department of Health (1999a) *A First Class Service: quality in the new NHS*. London: DoH.

Department of Health (1999b) *Guidance for General Practitioners and Primary Care Teams: improving outcomes in gynaecological cancers*. London: DoH.

Department of Health (2000a) *The NHS Plan: a plan for investment, a plan for reform*. London: DoH.

Department of Health (2000b) *The NHS Cancer Plan: a plan for investment, a plan for reform*. London: DoH.

Department of Health (2000c) *National Service Framework for Coronary Heart Disease*. London: DoH.

Department of Health (2001a) *National Service Framework for Older People*. London: DoH.

Department of Health (2001b) *Manual of Cancer Services Standards*. London: DoH.

Department of Health (2004) *Building on the Best: end of life care initiative*. London: DoH.

Department of Health (2006) *Best Research for Best Health: introducing a new national health research strategy*. London: DoH.

Department of Health (2007) *Getting it Right for People with Cancer: clinical case for change*. London: DoH.

Department of Health (2008) *High Quality Care for All: NHS next stage review final report*. London: DoH.

Dickson R (2005) Systematic reviews. In: Hamer S, Collinson G, editors. *Achieving Evidence Based Practice: a handbook for practitioners*. 2nd ed. Edinburgh: Ballière Tindall.

Doll R, Peto R (1981) The causes of cancer: quantitative estimates of avoidable risks of cancer in the United States today. *J Natl Canc Inst.* **66** (6): 1191–308.

Fallowfield LJ, Jenkins VA, Beveridge HA (2002) Truth may hurt but deceit hurts more: communication in palliative care. *Palliat Med.* **16** (4): 297–303.

Flemming K, Briggs M (2006) Electronic searching to locate qualitative research: evaluation of three strategies. *J Adv Nurs.* **57** (1): 95–100.

Flemming K (2007) Research methodologies: synthesis of qualitative research and evidence-based nursing. *Br J Nurs.* **16** (10): 616–20.

Freeman AC, Sweeney K (2001) Why general practitioners do not implement evidence: a qualitative study. *BMJ.* **323**: 1100.

Funk SG, Champagne MT, Wiese RA, Tornquist EM (1991) Barriers: the barriers to researcher utilisation scale. *Appl Nurs Res.* **4** (1): 39–45.

Garland GA (2005) Audit. In: Hamer S, Collinson G, editors. *Achieving Evidence Based Practice: a handbook for practitioners*. 2nd ed. Edinburgh: Ballière Tindall.

Gerrish K, Lacey A, editors (2006) *The Research Process in Nursing*. 5th ed. Oxford: Blackwell.

Gibson LJ, Dawson CL, Lawrence DJ, Bliss JM (2007) Aromatase inhibitors for treatment of advanced breast cancer in postmenopausal women. *Cochrane Database Syst Rev.* **1**: CD003370. DOI: 10.1002/14651858.CD003370.pub2

Hamer S, Collinson G, editors (2005) *Achieving Evidence Based Practice: a handbook for practitioners*. 2nd ed. Edinburgh: Ballière Tindall.

Hart C (1998) *Doing a Literature Review: releasing the social science imagination*. London: Sage.

Healthcare Commission (2007) *The Annual Health Check 2006/2007: a national overview of the performance of NHS trusts in England*. London: Healthcare Commission.

Holloway I, Wheeler S (2002) *Qualitative Research for Nurses*. 2nd ed. Oxford: Blackwell Science.

Hopkinson JB, Wright DNM, Corner JL (2005) Seeking new methodology for palliative care research: challenging assumptions about studying people who are approaching the end of life. *Palliat Med.* **19** (7): 532–7.

Huggins R, Jenkins A, Scurry D (2007) *Developing Undergraduate Research at Oxford Brookes*

University: recommendations and models for future development. Discussion Paper from Oxford Brookes University/ University of Warwick Centre for Excellence in Teaching and Learning and the Reinvention Centre for Undergraduate Research. Available at: www2. warwick.ac.uk/fac/soc/sociology/research/cetl/ugresearch/

Jenkins A, Healy M (2007) *UK Based Undergraduate Research Programmes.* Discussion Paper from the University of Warwick Centre for Excellence in Teaching and Learning and the Reinvention Centre for Undergraduate Research. Available at: www2.warwick.ac.uk/fac/soc/ sociology/research/cetl/ugresearch/

Johnson M (2006) *Building and Sustaining Research Capacity in Community Practice, Midwifery and Nursing: report of an expert colloquium.* Convened by the Research Collaborative of the Community Practitioners and Health Visitors Association. The Royal College of Midwives, the Royal College of Nursing. London: RCN.

Khan K, Kunz R, Kleijnen J, Antes G (2004) *Systematic Reviews to Support Evidence Based Medicine.* London: Royal Society of Medicine.

Lockhart K, Dosser I, Cruickshank S, Kennedy C (2007) Methods of communicating a primary diagnosis of breast cancer to patients. *Cochrane Database Syst Rev.* **3**: CD006011. DOI: 10.1002/14651858.CD006011.pub2

Long AF, Godfrey M (2004) An evaluation tool to assess the quality of qualitative research studies. *Int J Soc Res Meth.* **7** (2): 181–96.

Lostumbo L, Carbine N, Wallace J, Ezzo J (2004) Prophylactic mastectomy for the prevention of breast cancer. *Cochrane Database Syst Rev.* **4**: CD002748. DOI: 10.1002/14651858.CD002748. pub2.

Malone DE (2007) Evidence based practice in radiology: an introduction to the series. *Radiology.* **242**: 12–14.

Mayor P, Boyle P, Price L (2004) How a research network developed a multidisciplinary journal club. *Prof Nurse.* **19** (6): 308–9.

McQueen J, Miller C, Nivison C, Husband V (2006) An investigation into the use of a journal club for evidence based practice. *Int J Ther Rehabil.* **13** (7): 311–17.

Milne DJ, Krisknasamy M, Johnston L, Arande S (2007) Promoting evidence based care through a clinical research fellowship programme. *J Clin Nurs.* **16** (9): 1629–39.

Muir-Gray JA (2001) *Evidence Based Healthcare.* 2nd ed. Edinburgh: Churchill Livingstone.

Nail-Chiwetalu BJ, Ratner NB (2006) Information literacy for speech-language pathologists: a key to evidence based practice. *LSHSS.* **37**: 157–67.

National Library for Medicine (2007) *HTA 101: III. Primary data and integrative methods: meta-analysis.* Available at: www.nlm.nih.gov/nichsr/hta101/ta10105.html

Pavlakis N, Schmidt RL, Stockler M (2002) Bisphosphonates for breast cancer. *Cochrane Database Syst Rev.* **1**: CD003474. DOI: 10.1002/14651858.CD003474.pub2

Pearson A, Field J, Jordan Z (2007) *Evidenced Based Clinical Practice in Nursing and Healthcare: assimilating research, experience and expertise.* Oxford: Blackwell.

Pilgrim Projects (2007) *Patient Voices: getting the balance right.* Available at: www.pilgrim.myzen. co.uk/patientvoices/hip.htm

Polit DF, Beck CT (2006) *Essentials of Nursing Research: methods, appraisal, and utilisation.* 6th ed. Philadelphia, PA: Lippincott Williams and Wilkins.

Public Health Resource Unit (2006) *Critical Appraisal Skills Programme* (CASP). Available at: www.phru.nhs.uk/pages/phd/resources.htm

Ratner NB (2006) Evidence based practice: an examination of its ramifications for the practice of speech-language pathology. *LSHSS.* **37**: 257–67.

Romer PM (1990) Endogenous technological change. The problem of development: a conference of the Institute for the Study of Free Enterprise Systems. *J Polit Economy.* **98** (5): 2. S71–S102.

Sackett D *et al.* (1996) Evidence based medicine: what it is and what it isn't. *BMJ.* **312**: 71–2.

Shilling V, Jenkins V, Fallowfield L (2003) Factors affecting patient and clinician satisfaction with the clinical consultation: can communication skills training for clinicians improve satisfaction? *Psychooncology.* **12** (6): 599–611.

Society of College, National and University Libraries (1999) *SCONUL Seven Pillars Model for Information Literacy.* London: SCONUL.

Trinder L, Reynolds S, editors (2000) *Evidence Based Practice: a critical appraisal.* Oxford: Blackwell Science. *See* Chapter 1 in particular.

United Kingdom Central Council (1986) *Project 2000: a new preparation to practice.* London: UKCC.

United Kingdom Clinical Research Collaboration (2006) *Developing the best research professionals. Qualified graduate nurses: recommendations for preparing and supporting clinical academic nurses of the future.* London: UKCRC.

United Kingdom Clinical Research Collaboration (2008) *Clinical Academic Careers for Nurses, Midwives and Allied Health Professionals.* Available at: www.ukcrc.org/workforcetraining/nursesmidwivesahp.aspx (accessed 2 February 2009).

USEFUL WEBSITES

The Cochrane Collaboration: www.cochrane.org

The Critical Appraisal Skills Programme (CASP) tools: www.phru.nhs.uk/pages/phd/resources.htm

The Information Gateway, INTUTE: http://intute.ac.uk/

The Joanna Briggs Institute of Evidence Based Nursing in Australia: www.joannabriggs.edu.au

The NHS Centre for Reviews and Dissemination at the University of York: www.york.ac.uk/inst/crd/

NHS Evidence: www.evidence.nhs.uk/

The National Institute for Health and Clinical Excellence: www.nice.org.uk/

National Institutes for Health Research – Research Capacity Development Programme – Clinical Academic Training Pathway for Nurses, Midwives and Allied Health Professions: www.nccrcd.nhs.uk/nursesmidwivesandahp

The National Library of Medicine (USA): www.nlm.nih.gov/

Patient Voices: www.pilgrim.myzen.co.uk/patientvoices/hip.htm

The Public Health Electronic Library: www.phel.gov.uk/

The Reinvention Centre for Undergraduate Research, Centre for Excellence in Teaching and Learning, Warwick University: www2.warwick.ac.uk/fac/soc/sociology/research/cetl/

RDInfo (part of the National Institute for Health Research; contains a wide variety of useful research-related resources and information): www.rdinfo.co.uk/

The Scottish Intercollegiate Guidelines Network (SIGN): www.sign.ac.uk

Social Care on Line (similar to NLH): www.scie-socialcareonline.org.uk/

The UK Clinical Research Collaboration: www.ukcrc.org

11

Memoirs from a parallel universe: Dr Who and the cybernurse – compassion or competence?

Lorna Foyle

'Each of us in our own way can try to spread compassion into people's hearts. Western civilizations these days place great importance on filling the human "brain" with knowledge, but no one seems to care about filling the human "heart" with compassion.'

Dalai Lama (1989)

AIM

The aim of this chapter is to look at the reflections of a mature nurse educator and discuss what relevance this may have on the education of future healthcare professionals.

LEARNING OUTCOMES

By the end of this chapter, the reader should be able to:

- explore the impact of historical influences on present day and past learning
- debate the importance of compassion and competence in the delivery of high-quality cancer and palliative care
- explore ways that the teacher might promote discussion about compassion and competence
- share some personal experiences in the specialities of cancer and palliative care, clinically and educationally
- stimulate readers to chronicle some of their experiences in order to expand professional horizons and continue the process of lifelong learning.

INTRODUCTION

The title of this chapter sounds intriguing if some what puzzling. It originated when I was invited to talk at a national conference to celebrate the opening of a brand new oncology building in Hull in 2008. I was asked for the title well in advance in order to assist the conference planning group in their organisation of the conference. Well, for some time I have had an interest in the changing face of healthcare delivery and the way different healthcare professionals' roles have changed to accommodate the constant change imposed by a multitude of policy initiatives.

At that time I was becoming aware that these changes and new responsibilities were impacting on different healthcare inter-professional relationships and multi-disciplinary team workings. I gave the conference planning team the basic title 'Dr Who and the cybernurse' (indulging my own passion for science fiction); a few months later, I added the question: compassion or competence? If I was delivering this session again, I suspect that this title would metamorphose once more. For the purpose of this chapter, I have added the memoirs from a parallel universe element as some of the material originates from my own personal experiences and, with retirement rapidly approaching, this provides an opportunity to reflect on issues that have been and remain important to me and may be of interest to you as readers.

BACKGROUND

Unfortunately, for those of you who are Dr Who fans, and are anticipating exploration of his many adventures in this chapter, you will be disappointed. However, many of the challenges that face him seem to parallel the issues we are facing in modern oncology and palliative care delivery The title 'Dr Who and the cybernurse' was intended to draw an analogy about changes to the traditional roles of doctors and nurses in the acute healthcare setting alongside the changing roles of a Time Lord and his trusty and courageous assistants.

The reduction of doctors' hours has meant that many aspects of their work have been adopted by other healthcare professionals. Nurses have by default been the ones to adopt the additional responsibilities and duties relinquished by doctors. By accepting these responsibilities, nurses are in danger of losing their professional identity at the very least, and more importantly of devaluing caring which is considered the very essence of nursing. Caring and compassion are the very qualities that drew them into the profession originally. This aspect of advanced nursing practice is eloquently discussed in Chapter 8.

This thought prompted me to pose the question: compassion or competence? So, reader, which of these qualities should dominate our clinical practice in our healthcare professional roles? More importantly which of these qualities should be the driving force in our delivery of healthcare and palliative care, and which should be nurtured in the education of the healthcare workforce?

When we think of Dr Who, we recall the faces of the many actors who have portrayed him. Which one springs to your mind? What is it about this doctor that appeals to you? Those of you who are of a certain age, like me, will remember them all and may find that each has his own unique appeal. The face of the doctor may have changed over time, but surely he is the same Time Lord with the same value systems that have propelled him on his various journeys and sustained him in times of peril? Being true to one's beliefs and self has always been important, but is as relevant today as it has been in the past. Does this equate to the evolution of doctors of medicine who have adhered to their Hippocratic oath and developed their own values system? It is important to note that while the Dr Who television series has a male doctor in the leading role, we will be aware that many women doctors and male nurses are part of modern healthcare delivery. The analogy was created merely to assist in visualising the concepts of change in these professions.

The cybermen in the Dr Who series are regular adversaries of the doctor. The purpose of their existence is to rule the world and they will sacrifice anyone (doctor or human) who stands in their way. In order to prevent this, the doctor will often appeal to them at a deeply emotional level, delivering a profound and measured oration. This discourse is usually in vain as they are robots and are depicted as being devoid of any feeling. They go for what they want in a totally robotic manner, entirely disregarding human appeals. They remove all obstacles before them to achieve their universal goal of world domination. It is not intended to compare current nursing motivation to that of the cybermen. However, it has struck me that there are some similarities. In the milieu of advancing medical technology, nurses have been forced to embrace many of these technologies while advancing their practice. In this process, has nursing sacrificed some of the more humanistic aspects and qualities of its caring role? Furthermore, are we becoming cybernurses?

If nurses focus on achieving competence in the technological aspects of nursing, will they lose the ability to connect with patients, carers and other healthcare colleagues?

Although these aspects of nursing may be disappearing, it is often not by design but in response to increasing demands from policymakers and mandatory professional regulation. Paradoxically, caring may be relegated by healthcare professionals to meet patients' expectations and government targets. Sometimes these changes in roles have been subtle but they have had an immense impact on patients and professional relationships. Take for example the recent development of nurse prescribing in the specialities of oncology and palliative care. Many patients are confused about who the doctor is and who the nurse is; they cannot distinguish between the disciplines. Patients expect doctors to prescribe and nurses to administer the medication. This expectation emanates from societal stereotyping and is further promulgated by media coverage of modern healthcare delivery.

Which of these professionals should they trust and believe? The answer will of course be 'all healthcare professionals', but who is pivotal in the professional–patient relationship? This is a thorny problem for patients when they are at a most vulnerable time in their illness experience. There are no doubt many advantages to the supplementary prescribing role but nurses may be losing a golden opportunity to interact with junior medical colleagues and contribute to their expanding knowledge and continuing professional development.

In busy oncology and palliative care units, this expansion of their role can cause an intrinsic conflict for nurses as they try to balance both technical and human aspects of caring. Prioritising interventions becomes harder as nurses juggle between supporting patients and carers through critical points in their pathway, while meeting the demands of policymakers and organisations to achieve statutory requirements and targets. Similarly, while inter-professional working has become the norm in oncology and palliative care, the change in relationship and workload responsibilities between professions is rarely recognised. The need for focused team-building activities becomes imperative. This is discussed in Chapter 19.

This has led to the dispersion of some areas of conflict between professions while several unanticipated tensions may emerge. Inevitably as changes are implemented, some questions are answered while more evolve.

The change in medical and nursing relationships may have repercussions on the patient–professional relationship. Just how has the relationship changed over time?

Has our ability to be compassionate increased or decreased as a response to integrating modern technology into care delivery? Has striving to achieve clinical competence impacted on our interpersonal relationships with patients, carers and colleagues?

Figure 11.1 represents a discussion between a doctor and nurse about which quality, compassion or competence, is the most important in caring for the patients in the specialities of cancer and palliative care. Two cartoons were commissioned by me for the conference which were produced by a friend's talented daughter, Suzanne Trickett.

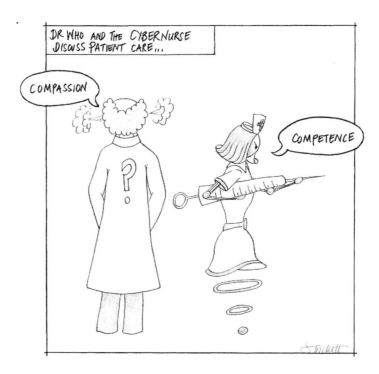

FIGURE 11.1 Which quality is the most important: compassion or competence?

In fact, which of the qualities of compassion or competence do healthcare profession-als value the most? More significantly, which of these abilities do patients and carers prefer? Is it compassion or is it competence? The literature describes competency and compassion in equal measure, although few authors have debated the merits of each quality in the same context.

Before continuing this debate, it is useful to look at definitions of competence and compassion.

COMPETENCE DEFINITIONS

The *Oxford Dictionary of English* defines competence as 'the *ability* to do something successfully'. Boyatzis (1982), who linked competency to effective performance and the achievement of results, provided the following definition:

> '*Competence should be viewed as a person's ability to perform, and their competency as their total capability, that is, what they can do, not necessarily what they do.*'

This definition of competence can differentiate superior performance from average or poor performance by focusing on the person who does the job well and the charac teristics and qualities that enable a person to do a superior job – rather than matching competence to the job itself. Is this how healthcare educators interpret competence or is an average standard of competence assumed? Building on the above definitions, Epstein *et al.* (2002) suggest that professional competence is:

> '*the habitual and judicious use of communication, knowledge and technical skills, clin-ical reasoning, emotions, values, and reflection in daily practice for the benefit of the individual and community being served.*'

Competence can often depend on individual attitudes which should include a willing-ness to cognitively self-explore. This requires clinicians to be attentive and cautiously curious, and to demonstrate presence in unfolding clinical activities. By its very nature clinical competence will always be developmental, transient and context dependent. As one level of competence is achieved, the practitioner will be expected to move to the next level by working through a hierarchy of competencies developed by each profes-sion and medical speciality. Comparing the performance of experts and novices as they achieve competence provides a method of understanding how expertise develops (Benner 1984). It is therefore important to help novice nurses to work through this hierarchy of competencies to attain expertise in the clinical setting without causing distress to themselves and their patients during the learning process (Taylor 2002).

The UK National Vocational Qualification (NVQ) perspective stresses the job, not the person, and focuses on minimum standards rather than superior performance. In addition, its focus is more on skills and performance in the workplace rather than knowledge, which some would say is an essential of competence. Competence is argued to be something that a person working within an occupational area should be able to do (Mansfield and Mitchell 1996). It is associated with certification and licensing and protecting public safety. Frameworks can provide an educational tool to mark the progress of a learner as they progress through a range of occupational standards and criteria. Performance criteria within frameworks can provide an assessor with statements by which judgements about an individual's ability to perform a specified activity to an acceptable level can be made. This can be viewed as a subjective activity. Conversely, performance criteria within frameworks can provide clinicians with the opportunity to demonstrate that they have the knowledge, judgement, skills, energy, experience and motivation required to respond adequately to the demands of their professional responsibilities (Roach 1992: 61). Most professions have developed a range of competencies that their students must achieve before they qualify. Rarely do students get the opportunity to discuss competence. Here is an exercise that has proved both to stimulate discussion and deepen students' understanding.

Exercise 11.1

Give the students a few academic definitions of competence.
● How would the students define competence and how is this similar or different to the definitions provided?

Put the students' responses on a flip chart. You can discuss these immediately or later in the session.
    Tell the students a case study that has a successful outcome because of a clinician's competence. Then ask them to reflect on how they felt about this successful outcome.
● Can they think of scenarios when a clinician's competence has achieved a positive outcome?

Next, tell them a case study that has a negative outcome because of a clinician's incompetence. Ask them to contrast this with the positive scenario and to identify contributing factors that make clinicians incompetent.
    This can lead to some lively discussions which can in turn lead to a further exercise if the teacher asks:
● What prevents us from achieving competence in everyday practice?

Bob Becker (2007), in the second book of this series, writes extensively about competency and its application to palliative care. It is recommended that readers consult his work as part of your further reading around this topic area.

COMPASSION DEFINITIONS

Having looked at competence definitions in the context of this chapter, our attention should turn to our definitions of compassion in relation to the provision of cancer and palliative care. Compassion is defined comprehensively in the *Oxford Dictionary of English* (1989): the word owes its derivation to Latin *com* (together with) and *pati* (to suffer). Further definitions are laid out as follows:

1   Suffering together with another, participation in suffering; fellow-feeling, empathy. A feeling of deep sympathy and sorrow for another who is stricken by misfortune, accompanied by a strong desire to alleviate the suffering.
2   The feeling of emotion, when a person is moved by the suffering or distress of another, and by the desire to relieve it; pity that inclines one to spare or to succour.
3   Sorrowful emotion, sorrow, grief.

Synonyms for compassion are listed as: commiseration, mercy, tenderness, heart and clemency. For those of you that teach about compassion in the future, as I hope you will, there follows a very simple exercise to elicit definitions and feelings that surround compassion. Used in conjunction with telling a story (*see* Chapter 3), this exercise can have a very powerful and profound effect on students' attitudes.

Exercise 11.2

Give the students a few academic definitions of compassion. Then ask the students:
● What other words stimulate you to think of compassion and how are they similar or different to the definitions?

Put these on a flip chart. You can discuss these immediately or later in the session.
    Tell the students a story that they can connect with and ask them what feelings the story evoked and which of the words on the flip chart best describes how they are feeling.

Then get the students to reflect on when they last had similar feelings in the clinical area and discuss what stops these emotions from emerging on a regular basis.
    This can lead to some lively discussions, which in turn can lead to a further exercise if the teacher asks:
● What inhibits us from displaying compassion in everyday practice?

Compassion is often understood as an emotion. In understanding compassion as an emotion, Oakley (1992) refers to it as the emotional component that provokes feelings from our inherent spirituality. It can be understood in terms of an emotional presence that affects us and characteristically permeates our perceptions, our humanity and our subsequent actions in ways which rest in the depths of our subconscious mind (Sabo 2006) and are not always visible. This emotional presence suggests that compassion affects our lives over extended periods of time, not just in the moment, and can exist in the conscious mind and be described as an absence of feeling. For example, *'the clinician who exhibits compassion will therefore not simply respond with feelings at the time of the patient's suffering, but will care for the patient in an ongoing way that might not always be expressed in terms of feeling'* (Pask 2003).
    Empathy is a synonym often most closely associated with compassion and in the literature is interchangeable. Definitions of empathy include:

> *'Accurate empathy involves more than just the ability of the therapist to sense the client's 'private world' as if it were his own. It also involves more than just the ability of the therapist to know what the client means. Accurate empathy involves the sensitivity to current feelings and the verbal facility to communicate this understanding in a language attuned to the client's feelings.'* (Truax 1961).

Empathy requires that the individual perceive the world as the other, be non-judgmental, understand the other's feelings and communicate this understanding (Wiseman 1996). Sometimes the sheer effort of providing empathy and demonstrating compassion to our patients, carers and colleagues places an incalculable cost on self. This to the point where it is more comfortable for many of us to focus on being a competent practitioner than on exposing ourselves to the pain of connecting with and caring for our client group, resulting in preferring detachment over attachment and loss.

To ensure the effectiveness of caring, practitioners should have the ability to empathise, understand and help the client. In this scenario, empathy becomes a double-edged sword for the clinician. On the one side, empathy promotes caring work and emotional labour; on the other side, the act of caring leaves the clinician vulnerable to its very act:

> *'We all feel or have felt the distress and the isolation. Ultimately, I believe, there is no solution to the problem. All of us who attempt to heal the wounds of others will ourselves be wounded; it is, after all, inherent in the relationship.'* (Hilfiker 1985: 93)

Lastly, what distinguishes compassion from empathy is its intrinsic, emotion-packed effect. That is to say, compassion compels and empowers people to not only acknowledge, but also to act towards alleviating or removing another's suffering or pain. In the early 1980s, McNeill *et al.* (1982: 4) were already discussing what compassion entails:

> *'Compassion asks us to go where it hurts, to enter into places of pain, to share in brokenness, fear, confusion, and anguish. Compassion challenges us to cry out with those in misery, to mourn with those who are lonely, to weep with those in pain. Compassion means full immersion into the condition of being human.'*

Along with acknowledging our fellows' suffering comes the urge to intervene and abate it. To exercise compassion, however, is no small undertaking. As Dietze and Orb (2000: 169) comment, *'at its heart compassion requires us to transcend traditional boundaries and distinctions . . . compassion suggests that any sense of differentiation between people is removed'*.

They also distinguish compassion from pity, observing that compassion *'does not define one person as being weak, inferior or lesser in any way against another'* whereas *'pity is a feeling which conveys condescension and dissociation'* (ibid.).

It would appear that compassion is incited by the recognition of suffering. That is to say, for compassion to occur, suffering must be identified and acknowledged.

In the clinical setting, at best, is it sympathy rather than compassion that is evoked?

And how has compassion and competence affected healthcare provision over time? Have these qualities remained constant or have they really changed? If compassion and competence have changed, how have they changed? As this chapter sits in the middle of this book, I can travel forwards and backwards, just like a Time Lord. Similarly I can explore history to reveal the relationship between compassion and competence in caring for the sick.

THIRTEENTH-CENTURY HEALTHCARE

To start this historical review let us turn the clock back to medieval times and go to the city of Norwich in England. Was compassion and competence prevalent when looking after the sick in the thirteenth century? One of the first recorded hospitals in England, which has been caring for sick people for over 700 years, is the Great Hospital, or St Giles as it was then known, in Norwich. It was founded by Bishop Walter de Suffield in 1249. The bishop was moved to establish it as he witnessed the pain and suffering of the poor menfolk on the streets of Norwich. Surely, this is the act of a compassionate man? St Giles' was established and enjoyed the relative comfort of 30 beds with 'mattresses and sheets and coverlets for the use of the infirm poor' (www.greathospital. org.uk/history.shtml).

There were quite a few rules and regulations, but most of the sick were dealt with by the master, the religious brethren and sisters. Four of these rules are relevant to our discussion. They are:

> there are to be at least three or four women, aged over fifty, who are to change the sheets and take care of the sick
> everyone has to get up at dawn to say prayers
> the sisters were to sleep in a separate dormitory
> no women were allowed to stay in hospitals as patients.

For more information on the rules and regulations, a visit to the listed website is well worthwhile.

As was the custom of the time, the resources were shared. The hospital gardens produced vegetables and herbs that were frequently used in the kitchens. Flowers and herbs were also grown for the production of scented candles; and, during the fourteenth century, surplus apples, pears, leeks, garlic, onions and honey were sold on the open market for a modest profit.

Unlike today, patients in a medieval English hospital generally had to rely on herbal preparations rather than expensive drugs, and there were no surgeons to operate on patients. In fact, the latest academic research has found that most medieval hospitals were religious institutions where spiritual health was given precedence over bodily health. Of course, this made perfect sense in a world where sin and disease went hand in hand. If you treated the soul, then you treated the body. Indeed, spiritual medicine was thought to be very effective, and it did not require any professional doctors.

Religious sisters and lay nurses played a vital role in providing patients with a package of holistic care, even if their contribution has not always been fully appreciated by historians.

For a start, nurses not only made the beds but laundered the bedding and also:

'[took] good charge and care of all the infirm and other sick lying there. They shall change the sheets and other bed clothes as often as necessary, and serve them humbly in necessary things as far as they are able.' (www.greathospital.org.uk/history.shtml)

It can be seen that the care of the sick in those days was dependant on many factors, including the compassion and piety of the fathers of the church and the competence of the nursing sisters. Crude as this care was, it was innovative and life-changing for the select few. Compassion drove the church leaders to give care to the sick of Norwich and the nursing sisters delivered care in a competent fashion, particularly in those chaotic times.

If you are ever in Norwich, the Great Hospital is well worth visiting and additionally the memorial to Edith Cavell is situated in the grounds of its magnificent cathedral.

EIGHTEENTH-CENTURY HEALTHCARE

Let us travel forward a few centuries in time to the eighteenth century and see how the face of medicine has changed. Poor health was no longer treated with herbal preparations alone. People were also treated using surgical procedures, such as bleeding and the removal of limbs. Cancer had been identified and was treated mainly with herbal remedies.

The famous Scottish surgeon, John Hunter (1728–93), was the first surgeon in the UK to suggest that some cancers might be cured by surgery. If the tumour had not invaded nearby tissue and was 'moveable', he said, 'then there is no impropriety in removing it' (www.rcseng.ac.uk/museums/history).

Hunter had many qualities, including humility that remained even when he acquired prosperity, as well as the strength to endure adversity when he was poor, in his early years of medicine. He had a rough exterior but was considered very kindly. The poor could call upon his services more successfully than could the rich; it is said that he would rather treat a diligent labourer than look after a member of the aristocracy. He clearly had a number of motivations, and financial reward was not always the dominant one among them. Was the type of treatment he delivered driven then by a deep sense of compassion? Unfortunately, in that period nurses were sullied with an unsavoury reputation and were labelled as drunks and as soldiers' whores. Surgeons particularly consigned them to undertake menial work, such as cooking and cleaning for the patients. The nurses were not encouraged to interact with patients.

NINETEENTH-CENTURY HEALTHCARE

Having stopped very briefly in the eighteenth century, I shall move forward to the nineteenth century and examine nursing again. In those days, nursing was a career with a poor reputation, filled mostly by poorer women, 'hangers-on' who followed the armies. In fact, nurses were equally likely to function as cooks.

However, one woman was to change the face of nursing: Florence Nightingale. She single-handedly raised the public opinion of nursing from that of sordid and squalid to respectable.

She gained her reputation for success by changing the care procedures for the wounded in the Crimean War. Driven by compassion for the brave British soldiers who were suffering intolerable losses, she travelled to Inkerman and instituted a strict regime of cleanliness and care. She ensured that nursing care was delivered to a high standard, thereby reducing mortality on the battlefront by 50% (www.florence-nightingale.co.uk). Her exploits were reported widely in the press and public affection for her grew. She returned to England and public opinion was reflected in the donations that poured into the Nightingale Fund.

In 1860, using the public subscriptions to the Nightingale Fund, she established the Nightingale Training School for nurses at St Thomas' Hospital. Probationer nurses received one year's training, which was mainly practical ward work interspersed with occasional lectures. On completion of their training, Florence Nightingale rewarded her trainees by giving them books and inviting them to tea. Trained nurses were then sent to hospitals at home and abroad to establish similar nurse training schools. In 1860 her best known work, *Notes on Nursing*, was published. Florence Nightingale could be described as the personification of the compassionate and competent health professional. Yet despite the elevation of nursing which she had effected in the eyes of the public, the relationship between nursing and medicine continued to be quite tense. Surgeons and physicians were still remembering the tawdry past of nursing and some were unwilling to change this perception to match the changing reality. In order to progress this debate, let us move forward to the twentieth century.

THE SWINGING SIXTIES

In particular, let us explore healthcare delivery in the 1960s. An eighteen-year-old starts her nursing career in a hospital in Birmingham.

> 'Nurse Fuller was placed on the toughest female surgical ward in the hospital after her preliminary training school (PTS). Student nurses were consigned to the sluice when consultants did their ward rounds. They were told that they should definitely be seen and not heard. Unfortunately she was heard more often than she should have been, as she developed a severe bout of "clumsitis" every time a consultant or the ward sister came into sight. It was an era of crisp white beds often remade on sister's orders, screens on wheels and sterilisation of equipment on the ward. Patients with cancer had a fifty-fifty chance of recovering. Radical mastectomy was the order of the day for patients with breast cancer and the patients were regularly instructed to used rolled-up bandages to pad out their bras to form crude temporary prostheses, which more often than not became a permanent arrangement.
>
> The consultant and sister parried regularly to attempt to get the best deal for the patients. Sister ran a tight ship and she was one of the most competent ward sisters that Nurse Fuller ever worked with. In the 1960s, the dying cancer patient's pain management was a hit or miss affair and the medication of choice was the ubiquitous Brompton's cocktail.

The first dying patient encountered by Nurse Fuller was a 28-year-old married woman with metastatic breast cancer. She was the mother of two young children and, as she drifted in and out of consciousness, she let out high-pitched, almost ethereal screams induced either by pain or the medication. Nurse Fuller became uneasy when dispatched to undertake nursing care for this dying lady. She became scared and frightened; the clumsy syndrome seemed to take on a life of its own when she was expected to care for this particular patient. But sister rarely left first "warders" alone for too long with this young woman and her family. The formidable ward sister became the most sensitive of carers, ensuring that no effort was spared in the provision of care given to the patient and her family. The vision of her placing a supportive arm around the husband and children when the patient finally died is ingrained in Nurse Fuller's memory. After the bereaved family had left, the sister went around all her ward staff to ensure that team members were coping, even the lowly first warders. It had been a particularly harrowing death to witness. I know because I was that first "warder". It was an era when we were discouraged from showing feelings and actively encouraged to be emotionally detached.' (Menzies-Lyth 1988)

I was struck then and still am by the image of this indomitable ward sister wiping away a gentle tear of compassion when she thought no one was watching her. She was a perfect role model in the blending of compassion and competence.

THE LATE TWENTIETH CENTURY

Moving forward to the 1990s but across the Atlantic, I want to draw your attention to a moving account of oncology nursing that journalist Suzanne Gordon poignantly wrote to explore what nurses do in the delivery of modern healthcare. She embodies this in a description that she entitles 'the tapestry of care'. The way she describes Nancy Rumplik's role in the care of oncology patients does ring true for those of us who are still involved in the provision of that care and the education of clinicians who deliver such care. The extract below from Gordon's book, *Life Support*, has been adapted slightly to maintain the cancer and palliative care focus of this chapter.

'It is four o'clock on a Friday afternoon. The Haematology/ Oncology Clinic at Boston's Beth Israel Hospital is quiet, almost becalmed. Nancy Rumplik is starting to administer chemotherapy to a man in his mid-fifties who has colon cancer.

Nancy is forty-two and has been a nurse on the unit for the past seven years. Her brown, straight hair is cut in a short bob. Her eyes are a pale, almost indistinguishable hazel, the bridge of her nose a wide track that crooks slightly to the left at its tip. Her soft voice is muted by the weariness of a long day.

She stands next to the wan-looking man and begins to hang the intravenous chemotherapy that will treat his cancer. Dressed in black jeans and a T-shirt that accentuates his pallor, he seems apprehensive about the treatment but does not verbalise his concerns. Nancy, who wears a white lab coat with a stethoscope dangling around her neck, reminds him of the purpose of every drug that is going into his system. As the solution drips through the tubing and into his vein, she sits by his side, watching to make sure that he has no adverse reaction.

Even though she concentrates on her own patient, Nancy's eyes constantly sweep the room to check on the remaining patients. She focuses for a moment on a heavy-set African American woman who is sitting in the opposite corner. The woman, in her mid-forties, is dressed in navy trousers and a brightly coloured shirt. Her sister, who is notably younger and heavier, is by her side. The patient seems fine, so Nancy returns her attention to the man next to her. Several minutes later, she looks up again, checks the woman, and stiffens. There is a look of anxiety on the woman's face she did not see before. Leaning forward in her chair, she stares at the woman.

"What's she getting?" she mouths to another nurse.

Looking at the patient's chart, the other nurse names a drug that causes a number of severe allergic reactions. In just that brief moment, as the two nurses confer, the woman suddenly clasps her chest and her look of anxiety returns to terror. Her mouth opens and shuts in silent panic. Nancy leaps up from her chair, as do other nurses, and sprints across the room.

"I can't breathe", the woman splutters when Nancy is at her side. Her eyes bulge and she grabs Nancy's hand; she tightens her grip and her eyes roll back as her head slips to the side. Realising that the patient is having an anaphylactic reaction – her airway swelling and closing shut – Nancy immediately turns a small spigot on the IV tubing to shut off the drip. At the same instant, a nurse calls a physician and the team responsible for responding to medical emergencies in the hospital. By this time, the woman is struggling for breath.

An oxygen mask is slipped over the woman's head and a blood pressure cuff placed around her arm. A nurse administers an antihistamine and cortisone to stop the allergic reaction and to decrease the inflammation blocking her airway. An oncology physician arrives within minutes. He assesses the situation and then notices the woman's sister standing, paralysed, watching the scene. "Get out of here!" he furiously commands.

The woman moves away as if she has been slapped. Then, with practiced synchronicity, no one leading or following, Nancy continues to work with the nurses and physician to stop the reaction and stabilise the patient.

Just as the emergency team arrives, the woman's breathing returns to normal and the look of abject terror fades from her face. Grasping Nancy's hand, she looks up and repeats, "I couldn't breathe. I just couldn't breathe." Nancy gently explains that she has had an allergic reaction to a drug and reassures her that it has stopped.

After a few minutes, when he knows the patient is stable, the physician and an emergency team walk out of the treatment area, but the nurses continue to comfort the terrified woman. Nancy then crosses the room to talk with her male patient who is ashen-faced at this reminder of the potentially lethal effects of the medication he and others are receiving. Responding to his unspoken fears, Nancy says quietly, "It's frightening to see something like that. But it's under control."

He nods silently, closes his eyes, and leans his head back against the chair. Nancy goes over to the desk. One of the nurses comments about the physician's treatment of the patient's sister. She goes into the waiting room, where the woman is sitting in a corner, looking bereft and frightened. Nancy sits down next to her. She explains what happened and suggests that the patient could probably benefit from some overnight company. Then she adds, "I'm sorry the doctor talked to you like that. You know, it's a very anxious time for all of us."

At this gesture of respect and recognition, the woman smiles solemnly. "I understand. Thank you." Nancy Rumplik returns to her patient.

Nurses like Nancy Rumplik are constantly engaged in what appear to be simple interactions – administering a medication, giving a bath, emptying a bedpan, checking a patient's medication box, making sure his home refrigerator is well stocked. But there is nothing simple about these exchanges. They are some of the threads with which their tapestry of care is woven and are critical to nurses' knowledge of and relationships with patients. These encounters allow nurses to develop a sense of patients that they refer to as the patient's "baseline". This permits them to know, often at a glance, when an important change in the patient's condition has occurred even before that change is registered in a falling blood pressure, rising temperature or laboured breathing.

In a cancer ward, nurses catch a serious reaction to medication almost before it happens. In an operating room, nurses make sure the right patient is being operated on, or that the right procedure is being performed on the right limb or organ. On an ICU [intensive care unit] or in a home care, nurses question why a patient is getting another painful diagnostic test that may reveal little useful information; why adequate pain medication is not given following surgery; why a patient is being discharged too quickly; whether someone is available to take care of the patient in the home; and at the end of life, why expensive, heroic treatment that will only prolong death is presented as the only option.

In the self-enclosed world of the high-tech hospital, where ordinary men, women and children are confronted with people who wear alien costumes, adhere to peculiar customs, and even speak their own language, nurses help patients deal with their fears and anxiety – not only of their diseases but of the people who are supposed to cure them. Watch Nancy, and you see how important this is to frightened patients and family members. In our high-tech medical system, nurses are the ones who care for the body and the soul. No matter how sensitive, caring, and attentive physicians are, in both the hospital and home nurses are often closer to patients' needs and wishes than physicians. That's not because nurses are inherently more caring than doctors, but because they spend far more time with patients and know them better. This investment of time and knowledge allows nurses to save lives. But nurses also help people adjust to the lives they must live after they have been saved. And when death can no longer be delayed, nurses help patients confront their own mortality with at least some measure of grace and dignity.

But what nurses do for those individuals will rarely be mentioned. It was a nurse who bathed a cardiac patient and comforted this grown man while he struggled with the terror of not knowing if he would live or die. It was a nurse who held the plastic dish under the cancer patient's lips as she was wracked with nausea and who wiped a bottom raw from diarrhoea.

Because we would prefer to forget the realities of illness, we grasp the fantasy that medicine can triumph over the human condition. In defining health care as medical care, we've come to think of illness as an event. You get sick. You go to a doctor. He or she gives you a diagnosis and treatment plan. You follow it and hopefully you are cured.

But illness is a process, not an event – one that requires care both before, during, and after medical encounters that punctuate it. Rather than forcing nursing into the biomedical model of diagnosis, treatment, and cure, think of nursing as a tapestry of care woven from countless threads into an intricate whole.

The fact that nurses' work is interspersed with many so-called menial tasks that don't demand total attention is not a reason to demean their work or, as is happening today, to replace nurses with less skilled workers. It's this hands-on care that allows nurses to explore patients' physical condition and register their anxiety and fear. It's this that allows them to save lives and to ascertain when it is appropriate to help patients die. And it is only in watching them weave the tapestry of care that we grasp its integrity and intent.' (Gordon 1997: 3–7, 19–20)

I feel that Suzanne Gordon has truly captured the essence of modern cancer nursing and for those of you who may have connected to this passage as I did, may I recommend that you read this book. It looks at other nurses' caring work and issues that are equally as poignant and evocative. In fact, as educationalists you can recommend your students to read it and discuss how relevant the stories and vignettes are to modern nursing, and to cancer and palliative care specialities. This book can, most certainly, be used in a teaching session focusing on the 'compassion or competence' debate. This book is so rich in teaching materials. Nurse Rumplik demonstrated that competence and compassion, when integrated with high-tech care, can provide outstanding,

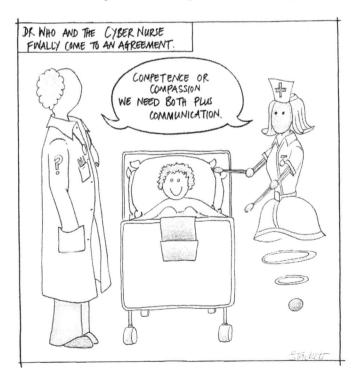

FIGURE 11.2 Dr Who and the cybernurse achieve an understanding

high-quality care. Figure 11.2, which was also created by my friend's daughter, depicts the contemporary relationship between doctor and nurse working in harmony with compassion and competence to ensure the highest standard of care for the cancer and palliative care patient. It would appear that balancing and sustaining caring and compassion are essential qualities, required by all healthcare professionals in twenty-first-century healthcare.

KEY POINTS

- Compassion and competence have many definitions and there are many interpretations of those definitions.
- History lessons can be useful in teaching healthcare students about competence and compassion.
- The nurse–doctor relationship is constantly changing.
- Nursing and medicine should work harmoniously for the best possible patient outcomes.
- Patients need clinicians who have been educated to achieve competency and demonstrate compassion, particularly in oncology and palliative care.
- Education is pivotal to all aspects of healthcare provision.

CONCLUSION

> 'By 2011, computers will learn and reason better than humans. By 2012, they'll memorize, recognize, and learn in a human fashion. By 2013, health care professionals will view them as colleagues rather than tools. Health care will finally grasp the gold ring of precision as computers eliminate the guesswork, eradicate the deadly errors, and usher in the age of accuracy.' (Simpson 2001)

The future is a challenge as technology and science advance. The above quote about healthcare in the next decade alarmed me. I do want competent care delivered with compassion. I became a patient shortly after delivering this session. I was unexpectedly taken seriously ill. I was cared for by doctors and nurses who embodied compassion and competence. As I was hooked up to several machines, it was the turning of my pillows and the quiet reassuring messages from my carers that sustained me during this period. The thought of communicating with machines, as the above quote suggests, is daunting. What will they be programmed to say? They may become competent but will they ever be able to show compassion when patients are terrified and facing their darkest moments. The greatest challenge for all healthcare professionals as they move towards the future is to maintain that finely poised balance between compassion and competence. It is not a case of either compassion or competence. We need both qualities combined with the art of reliable and sensitive communication to deliver high-class care. It is not the responsibility of any one discipline because, in contemporary oncology and palliative care, it is essential that all healthcare professionals deliver competent care intermingled with compassion.

IMPLICATIONS FOR THE READER'S OWN PRACTICE

1 How do you know when you have been compassionate and competent?
2 How did you feel when you read the extract from life support?
3 What creative teaching methods could you use to teach your students about com-passion and competence?
4 In what ways will the history of nursing and medicine help you to become a better teacher in the future?
5 How will you learn more about this in the future?

REFERENCES

Becker R (2007) The use of competencies in cancer and palliative education. In: Foyle L, Hostad J, editors. *Innovations in Cancer and Palliative Care Education*. Oxford: Radcliffe Publishing.

Benner P (1984) *From Novice to Expert*. London: Addison-Wesley.

Boyatzis RE (1982) *The Competent Manager: a model for effective performance*. New York: Wiley.

Dietze EV, Orb A (2000) Compassionate care: a moral dimension of nursing. *Nurs Inq*. **7**: 166–74.

Elliott J (1991) Competency-based training and the education of the professions: is a happy mar-riage possible? In: Elliott J, editor. *Action Research for Educational Change*. Milton Keynes: Open University Press: 118–34.

Epstein RM, Edwards M, Hundert MD (2002) Defining and assessing professional competence. *JAMA*. **287**: 226–35.

Gordon S (1997) *Life Support*. Boston, MA: Little, Brown and Company.

Hilfiker D (1985) *Healing the Wounds: a physician looks at his work*. New York: Pantheon Books.

Mansfield B, Mitchell L (1996) *Towards a Competent Workforce*. Aldershot: Gower.

McNeill DP, Nouwen HJM, Morrison DA (1982) *Compassion: A reflection on Christian life*. New York: Doubleday Books.

McClelland D (1973) Testing for competence rather than intelligence. *American Psychologist*. **28**: 1–14.

Menzies-Lyth I (1988) A case study in the functioning of social systems as a defence against anxiety. In: Menzies-Lyth I. *Containing Anxiety in Institutions: selected essays*. London: Free Association Books.

Oakley J (1992) *Morality and Emotions*. London: Routledge.

Pask EJ (2003) Moral agency in nursing: seeing value in the work and believing that I make a difference. *Nurs Ethics*. **10**: 165–74.

Roach S (1992) *The Human Act of Caring: a blueprint for the health professions*. Rev. ed. Ottawa, ON: Canadian Hospital Association Press.

Sabo BM (2006) Compassion fatigue and nursing work: can we accurately capture the conse-quences of caring work? *Int J Nurs Pract*. **12**: 136–42.

Simpson RC (2001) Compassion meets the computer age. *Nurs Manag*. **32** (1): 13–14.

Skelton G (1989) Assessment and profiling of clinical performance. In: Bradshaw P, editor. *Teaching and Assessing in Clinical Nursing Practice*. London: Prentice Hall.

Soanes C, Stevenson A, editors (2005) *The Oxford Dictionary of English*. Rev. ed. Oxford: Oxford University Press.

Taylor C (2002) Assessing patients' needs: does the same information guide expert and novice nurses? *Int Nurs Rev.* **49** (1): 11–19.

Truax C (1961) *A Scale for the Measurement of Accurate Empathy* [discussion paper]. Madison, WI: University of Wisconsin Press.

Wiseman T (1996) A concept analysis of empathy. *J Adv Nurs.* **23**: 1162–7.

USEFUL WEB ADDRESSES

www.greathospital.org.uk/history.shtml
www.rcseng.ac.uk/museums/history
www.florence-nightingale.co.uk

12

The teaching of hope and suffering in palliative care education

Robert Becker

Hope is the thing with feathers
That perches in the soul,
And sings the tune – without the words,
And never stops at all,

And sweetest in the gale is heard;
And sore must be the storm
That could abash the little bird
That kept so many warm.

I've heard it in the chillest land,
And on the strangest sea;
Yet, never, in extremity,
It asked a crumb of me.

Emily Dickinson

AIM

The aim of this chapter is to examine teaching approaches to hope and suffering as a key component of cancer and palliative care education.

LEARNING OUTCOMES

By the end of this chapter, the reader should be able to:
- understand the concepts of hope and suffering as a lived experience for the dying and their families
- offer opportunities to challenge learners' attitudes and skills by

---

> utilising a range of creative approaches in the classroom to enhance learning about hope and suffering
> • to view hope and suffering as core underpinning concepts in the teaching of cancer and palliative care.

INTRODUCTION

The opening poem by Emily Dickinson (Franklin 2005) is an apt reminder of the nature of hope and suffering to humanity and its context within palliative care. She uses the metaphor of a bird to define hope and then uses the storm to represent suffering, while acknowledging that hope is ever present and can help in even the most extreme of situations.

There are very few subjects which are taboo within good palliative care education. Experienced educators in the field are used to tackling sensitive topics like sexuality, and spiritual care, and do so with enthusiasm, creativity and vigour, yet despite this it is rare to find the topics of hope and suffering given explicit curriculum time. The assumption is often made that these areas are so integral to an understanding of the nature of palliative care and crop up in discussion in so many taught subject areas that they are implicit and contiguous in the teaching, therefore there is no real need for them to be explicit. This chapter will challenge this precept and argue that a clear conceptual grasp of the fundamentals of the complex nature of hope and its close bedfellow, suffering, is a core foundation to successful palliative care education. Practitioners of every healthcare profession deal with life in crisis as a basic tenet of their job, therefore all have encountered both physical and psychological suffering and the need to promote hope as part of the healing process as an integral component of professional practice.

THE CONCEPTS OF HOPE AND SUFFERING

Hope is an elusive quality that, like faith and courage, is acknowledged as an important facet of our humanity, but remains difficult to explain in terms of the life of an individual. When Dante (1265–1321) used those immortal words 'abandon hope all who enter here' to describe the entrance to hell, he was attempting to say that everything that is of importance to life itself is left behind at this point (*Encyclopaedia of Philosophy* 1967). In terms of health, hope has been intrinsically linked with caring and the professional roles of caregivers (Cutcliffe and Herth 2002).

Suffering is perhaps not so tangible and has been examined from both the first and third person perspective, as a philosophical concept and as a paradox of medicine, which defies scientific enquiry by virtue of its very subjectivity (Nyatanga and Astley-Pepper 2005).

Attempted definitions: hope

Much of the generic literature available which studies hope has definitions that are similar in nature and content – for example, 'A desire accompanied by expectation' (Frank and Fromm 1968), 'A confident leap into the future' (Alfaro 1970) and 'A conviction that a good future is possible' (Smith 1983). Implicit within most of these definitions are several common denominators:

> the expectation of a better future
> the strong affective component
> the desire for something which is good and positive
> life experience and relationships with others.

Hope therefore would seem to be neither desire, nor optimism, expectation, nor even wishful thinking, although most of these notions do play their part. Hope can be seen as an active, not passive characteristic, which is expressed in emotional terms through a process of both conscious and unconscious reasoning. From a developmental perspective, hope has been identified as an essential part of early human development (McGee 1984; Erikson *et al.* 1975).

Within the realms of healthcare, there have been a number of attempts to arrive at a meaningful definition. Of these, Menninger (1959) would appear to have been one of the first to address this issue in any depth, when he identified hope's relevance to the treatment of patients with psychiatric disorders. Beck and Weissman (1974) likewise associated hope with the effectiveness of psychiatric intervention, and more recent work by Cutcliffe (1998) and Moore (2005) confirm its continuing relevance in a mental health context. Hope has been studied as a variable in the occurrence of, and recovery from, cancer (Hickey 1986; Hinds and Martin 1988; Herth 2000) and also in relation to adaptation to chronic illness (O'Malley and Menke 1988). More recently it has been studied in relation to the elderly (Duggleby and Wright 2005), family members of the terminally ill (Benzein 2005) and informal caregivers (Holtslander *et al.* 2005).

Frankl (1963) wrote about hope and suffering from a very spiritual perspective, relating his experiences within the Nazi concentration camps, and talked at length about people finding a sense of meaning as a survival tactic when faced with and surrounded by death. He found that fellow captives who had a reason or purpose to live often appeared to fare better than those who found the dreadful suffering overwhelming. Menninger (1959) also details similar experiences of doctor/prisoners in Buchenwald concentration camp. To ascribe a meaning to something therefore demands an affective and cognitive process, which is dependent on values, culture, beliefs and previous experience. Hope is seen today as a multidimensional concept, encompassing not only earthly goals, actions and relationships, but also eternal spiritual goals, actions and relationships with a divine being, neither of which are mutually exclusive.

Many of these definitions represent confident yet empirical attempts at conceptualising hope. Those authors who have researched hope tend to confine their work to certain age groups, or to life-threatening pathological conditions, and usually the latter. Work in this area from well populations is rare and represents a major gap in the existing literature. An exception is Turner (2005), who looked at hope from the perspective of well young Australians and found that relationships, choices, motivation and belonging were the key dimensions to their lives. Insights such as this can give us a normality baseline on which to make judgements of hope and suffering alongside more illness-focused research.

If hope in the context of palliative care is to be more clearly understood, then any definition should encompass a broad holistic perspective which endeavours to involve not just the individual but also their loved ones. As well, it should be rigorous enough to address both the normalistic and pathological ideologies of palliative care.

Attempted definitions: suffering

There is a commonality of meaning evident within the few definitions of suffering that have been offered by authors, which is helpful to our understanding, but all agree that the personal, subjective experience of suffering will always defy full analysis (Frankl 1963; Cassell 1992; Rodgers and Cowles 1997; Van Hooft 1998). These authors describe suffering as essentially a negative experience involving distress, discomfort and endurance. Perhaps of most relevance is Nyatanga's (Nyatanga and Astley-Pepper 2005) observation that the healthcare professions involved in palliative care argue that the relief of suffering is part of their job and it is clearly spelt out in the internationally accepted WHO definition of palliative care (2002), yet currently there is no clear view of what suffering is, how to assess it and what will alleviate it.

DEVELOPMENTAL TOOLS AND INVENTORIES

Empirical and anecdotal evidence tells us much about hope and suffering, but the development of testable and reliable tools, which can be used in a palliative care setting to both assess these concepts and contribute towards actively inspiring hope, so as to reduce perceived suffering, are now coming to the fore.

Erikson (1975), Hinds (1984), Nowotny (1989) and Miller (1988) have all developed scales to measure hope and hopefulness. Perhaps the best current example is Herth's Hope Index (1992). It conforms to the idea that hope is a multidimensional phenomenon and the design reflects this. Herth's Hope Index is in Likert format (1–4 scale) and is based on three factors:

> an inner sense of temporality and the future, i.e. having goals or fearing for the future

> an inner positive readiness and expectancy, i.e. believing that life has value and worth

> an interconnectedness with self and others, i.e. feeling all alone or having a faith that comforts.

The 12-item index has consistent reliability and is seen as a practical and effective tool to screen adults for different levels of hope (Herth 1992, 1993, 2000). There are a number of elements in Herth's work which are not evident in earlier scales, such as the more global, non-time-oriented approach, an emphasis on relationships rather than self and the continued presence of hope despite difficult or absent interpersonal relationships. Its primary advantage would seem to be that it is concise, clear and, in use, does not seem to induce fatigue in the patient, which can distort the assessment.

TEACHING APPROACHES

There are some subjects that can cause an audience to mentally switch off in seconds if not approached in the correct manner, and the teaching of hope and suffering can potentially be one such topic. The inherent abstraction and subjectivity of the subject matter may do little to raise curiosity and facilitate motivation. It is incumbent on the teacher therefore to introduce a variety of approaches which will challenge the audience to think, reflect and at times analyse hope and suffering in the context of, first, their own lives and, by extension, the lives of their patients. Learning conducted in this way via a mix of both experiential and didactic approaches has the potential to strongly influence attitudes as well as to enhance knowledge and skills (Farley 2005). The safety factors of well-established ground rules, which include confidentiality and support of each other, are essential if this is to succeed. Much relies on the honesty of the participants if they are to maximise the benefit of the exercises used and there is the potential for participants to become emotional at times, as triggers from past events come forward. For this reason, it is important that the teacher should be experienced at handling the sensitive dynamics that may present themselves and a team-teaching approach is advised so that a colleague can be there for such eventualities.

It is suggested that a mix of self-study, group work and case study work can work well. Clearly the make-up of the audience and the numbers being taught will influence the choice of teaching technique. If faced with a room full of 150 junior students, the more didactic approach takes precedent. A carefully crafted PowerPoint presentation with selected bullet points and some interesting graphics to demonstrate both hope and suffering will always have good impact.

QUESTIONS FOR DISCUSSION

There are a number of paradoxes and contradictions that exist when examining such difficult concepts as hope and suffering and which merit exploration. A clear examination of these can form the basis of useful discussion and debate, either in the classroom, or within a seminar context, or even as possible assignment topics.

➤ How can an essentially forward-looking concept such as hope ever be realistically reconciled with the process of a life reaching its conclusion?

➤ If palliative care is a representation of enhancing a normal life process, as put forward by several definitions (NCHSPCS 2001; WHO 2002; EAPC 1989; NICE 2004), then the behaviours and emotions exhibited in this time of crisis which are described as hope and suffering could be seen as a telescoping of normal life, sandwiched into an undetermined but short time span. Is it realistic or even desirable, therefore, to view these concepts as a pathology examined within a predominantly medical model?

➤ We have little valid research into how well populations view hope and suffering in the context of their lives, therefore where is the normality baseline from which to make judgements on levels of hope and suffering?

➤ If suffering is a subjective first person-defined experience which varies between individuals and their given circumstances, then by definition it is not amenable to rigorous scientific enquiry. How then can the palliative purport to understand and alleviate it?

CLASSROOM EXERCISES
The short story

Vignettes are a powerful strategy which enhances learning and can have a high impact as a reflective learning tool for the author, listener or reader. Their use in the context of palliative care is well established. Tapping into the rich vein of clinical experiences that are part of the daily life of the palliative care professional can have profound results. Stories enable us to visualise a captured moment of real significance, image by image and word by word. They help us to use our imagination to safely project our thoughts and emotions into an alternate snapshot of life (Becker 2005).

The emotive language used in such stories can be seductive, therefore in order to achieve a more academic stance participants can be asked to consider the professional and ethical dilemmas posed by the scenarios. Use can be made of codes of professional conduct and ethical frameworks combined with rigorously researched hope-fostering strategies, such as those put forward by Herth (1990), in order to assess, plan, implement and evaluate care. The vignettes suggested below are aligned to fit in with Herth's strategies and can be used to stimulate discussion in groups, or indeed the audience can create their own with suitable guidance.

Interpersonal connectedness

> There she was hidden nearly by the crisp white sheet pulled up to her nose. Two withered hands gripped tightly to the edge of the sheet. Two soft bright eyes appeared from the abyss looking at me. 'Got a minute, nurse? Hold my hand, please?' she said. I asked her, 'Are you frightened?' 'No', she replied, then silence. After about a minute she looked at me and said, 'I had forgotten what life felt like.'

Lightheartdness

> Alex was a young man who was dying and he knew the score. His family was with him. I went in to see if anyone wanted a drink. Alex came out with the usual corny joke and some cheeky comment. I answered back, 'Any more of that, mate, and you're dead meat.' I just wanted the ground to open up and swallow me, but Alex laughed like a drain.

Personal attributes: courage and serenity

> Jenny is strong, focused and in control of her life and illness. She began to talk about her family, especially her husband who had not come to terms with things. Jenny felt she should be strong for him and not let him see her cry. I paused and said, 'It's okay to cry, you know.' She went silent and the tears began to flow.

Attainable aims

I have a tumour in my spine. Haven't been out of bed for four weeks and the nurses insist on using a hoist. Why, for God's sake? I can use my legs now. Explanations echo in my ears. I am desperate to get home and my wife will never manage a hoist. Then this nurse with a sliding board and a determined smile arrives and takes over. The others don't like it, but three attempts and 40 minutes later I'm sat in a chair. No contraptions, just a shiny board. Now I can go home. I could have hugged and kissed her.

Spiritual base

Dawn is breaking. My guardian angels will soon arrive with my tablets, washed down with God's wine. Same vibes, different voices, another day. 'So this is why the cream curdles and the flowers never smell sweet in this room.' I sleep, then wake up and the pain is there again. Head, heart, stomach, everywhere. My family look on, bemused, worried and unsure what to do. More tablets and God's wine. A kiss, a prayer – maybe tonight?

Affirmation of worth

John had a degenerate illness and still had all his mental faculties, though he could not communicate well. His love of music shone through this and he loved to play his 1970s and 1980s music, much to the frustration of his family. He knew this, but he said to me one day, 'This is my way of saying I am still here, reach out and touch me, hug me, and kiss me if you dare. I'm still here.'

The case study

The longer case study can be used with a range of questions, both to consolidate learning and to encourage analysis and synthesis of ideas. Ian's story has many identifiable strands that link closely with current literature.

Ian is 48. Nine months ago he had an epileptic fit. Extensive investigations revealed a brain tumour. After surgery, Ian, his wife and family were told that the surgery could only be palliative. When asked, 'How long have I got?' his doctor indicated that it was unlikely that Ian would live for more than six months. Before Ian became ill, he was the manager of a car salesroom with a turnover in excess of £5 million per year. Ian loved his work, describing it as his second passion next to his wife Jenny and his two boys, aged 25 and 23. He enjoyed the friendship he shared with his colleagues and prided himself on his relationship with his customers, many of whom came back time and time again.

Ian's third passion was running. In hospital, part of his morning ritual was to put on his London Marathon Medal. He loved to tell the staff about the many fun runs he had entered and how he had willingly raised money for various cancer charities. 'I never thought that I would ever get any of it back', he would often say. The laughter hid his pain. His family loved to celebrate his running achievements by showing off his medals and photographs. Ian asked one of the nurses to 'hide the bloody things before anyone else sees what I was and what they want back'. Ian believed in facing facts and making the best of things. This was his way of coping, or as he said 'hoping that it was all a bad dream'. In his more intimate moments with the staff, he would 'indulge in a few tears', as he put it, but never when Jenny or the boys were about. He said, 'They have so much to go through and after all, my pain will soon be over. Crying in front of them would be self-indulgent.' When asked what his hopes were, he said, 'I know that I won't know anything about it, but I just want to be remembered as a good husband, a good father and a good mate. Nothing else really matters to me.'

➤ What coping strategies did Ian employ to maintain his hope in the face of such difficulty?
➤ Beneath the public face was a man who was suffering deeply – what hope-fostering strategies can we use as health professionals with people like Ian and his family?

Self-reflection exercises

These are immensely powerful and need to be used with caution. The experience of placing oneself in a fictional scenario and responding to this can potentially be cathartic for some members of an audience. The bonus is that, if done well, the learning achieved can be profound. As mentioned before, the use of supportive ground rules, team-teaching and skilled facilitation is central to success with this approach. The scene presented below focuses on hope and personal mortality.

The fictional scenario

Imagine yourself to be the person in this mini case study. Consider the questions asked carefully and be as honest as you can in your responses.

> You have just returned from an outpatient appointment at your local hospital where the consultant you saw told you that the tests confirm that you have an advanced cancer that has spread to different sites in your body. He confirms that your likely life expectancy is only about four weeks at best. Amid the feelings of shock and fear that race through your mind will be thoughts about the future life you had planned that will no longer happen.

➤ What hopes have been taken away from you by this devastating news?

Feedback
➤ How did it feel knowing that you may have only a few weeks to live?
➤ Did any themes emerge in your answers?

Follow-up question
➤ What will your hopes be for the short time you have left?

Feedback
Option 1: Discuss these hopes with the person next to you and look for any common denominators that crop up.

Option 2: This exercise can be conducted using small groups who feed back to the class via flip chart. Done this way, it is less threatening for individuals and can be a more successful strategy with less experienced staff.

Follow-up question
➤ Now look back over the list you have just made and prioritise two hopes that you could realistically achieve over the next month.

It is hoped that a range of helping strategies will come forward from the use of these teaching exercises. Some of the more relevant, evidence-based ones are given below.
➤ Develop an empathetic understanding of patients' and families' worries, fears and doubts and a willingness to try to alleviate these feelings where possible and to help families build upon their strengths (Egan 2004). The emotions expressed may well be both positive and negative and fluctuate across a whole spectrum of behaviours.
➤ The need to look towards realistic, attainable goals is important to our patients and is closely linked to their emotional state. Poncar (1994) believed that hope of attaining an important goal influences the affective state, i.e. the greater the goal, the greater the positive feelings experienced.
➤ Laughter is an emotion which is a fundamental part of care within a palliative setting, yet it rarely seems to be acknowledged for its relevance in terms of hope maintenance. It is also a very healthy emotion and, when culturally and contextually acceptable, helps to foster positive attitudes, comforts relatives and more significantly is very normality based (Becker 2003). Herth (1990) alludes to this when she talks of 'playfulness'.
➤ The key element of relationships underpins the very essence of good palliative care. By working directly with families, a close therapeutic rapport can be developed with the patient (Smith 2004). This participation implies that goals are worth striving for and can be achieved with co-operation. It also helps to dispel the sense of helplessness and guilt, which is often there.
➤ Allowing opportunities for families to be alone is crucial, so that they are not overshadowed by the system (Herth 1993).
➤ It would seem to be the willingness of others to share part of themselves through their affirmation, reassuring presence, encouragement, willingness to listen attentively, to touch and to share hopes and feelings that makes all the difference (Le May 2004.) Work by Benner and Wrubel (1989) has shown clearly that the ability to use human presence in a way that acknowledges our shared humanity may in some way directly or indirectly restore the person-

centred dignity and affirmation of being that is necessary for the emergence of hope.

➤ The relevance and importance of maximising life's aesthetic experiences as a strategy is mentioned by Miller (1985), Herth (1990) and Poncar (1994). The range of these is infinite and highly personal in context and can include such simple things as observing a sunrise or sunset, taking a walk at some favoured beauty spot, enjoying a taste of wine, coffee, or a special food, listening to inspiring music or poetry, viewing art, reading a book, receiving a visit from a much-loved pet, or having a new hairstyle (Becker and Gamlin 2004).

➤ Other strategies can include distraction activities, confronting the problem, redefining the problem, reminiscence work and helping the person to renew his or her spiritual beliefs.

KEY POINTS

■ Hope and suffering are rarely taught as explicit topics in palliative care courses.

■ Both the concept of hope and that of suffering are now seen as multidimensional, dynamic and embodying goals, actions, relationships and meaning with a strong spiritual component.

■ While there is an increasing body of literature that attempts to define and refine hope into a range of conceptual models and assessment tools, it is unlikely that such tools will become commonplace in everyday practice.

■ There is a dearth of literature available which looks at hope from the perspective of the well person.

■ Inspiring hope in the dying is both complex and challenging and demands self-insight, confidence and maturity if it is to be done well.

■ The teaching of hope within the classroom needs to be done by using a variety of approaches which demand of the audience a reflective and analytical stance.

CONCLUSION

Our understanding of the concept of hope has moved a long way in the last 30 years, while suffering has received little academic attention. Hope is now almost universally seen as a multidimensional concept, with common elements related to a person's meaning, anticipation of events, thoughts, feelings, behaviours and relationships, coupled with a positive future orientation, grounded in the present, but linked to the past (Stephenson 1991). This may sound like a comprehensive definition, but the very breadth of it creates problems when attempting to individualise it in clinical practice.

It is contended that most of the hope-inspiring strategies detailed are implicit in everyday practice and are being done under the auspices of 'good' palliative care, founded in the commonly accepted philosophical beliefs and definitions which already exist (WHO 2002; NICE 2004; NCHSPCS 2001). It is simply that it is not thought of in the context of hope. Controversy will always surround our attempts to pin down to absolutes such complex human dimensions as hope and suffering. Rigorous research of a qualitative nature has shed some light onto our understanding, but equally it has raised as many perplexing questions as it has attempted to answer.

Hope and suffering, it can be argued, are fundamental to life and humanity and should not be pigeonholed into academic, clinical or theological corners. When we attempt to inspire hope and reduce suffering, this begins as soon as the patient and family become active participants in care. Considerable responsibility lies therefore on all care professionals to shape this by their strategies and interventions.

Qualitative dimensions of care, such as the hope and suffering, despite their subjectivity have the potential to become subject to standard-setting and audit if the use of assessment tools becomes commonplace. The dying can't come back to tell us how effective our care was, but what better judgement of the true value and efficacy of palliative care to present to commissioners and purchasers of services than accurately collated, reliable evidence of hope maintenance and alleviation of suffering throughout the dying process? The evidence-based healthcare culture so prevalent in Western society is increasingly demanding such evidence to justify its continued funding and existence. Palliative care practitioners need to ask themselves whether the development of such tools is wise or not.

The converse argument is perhaps more realistic. The practical reality is that such detailed evidence is unlikely to be forthcoming outside of a small number of specialist palliative care facilities where staffing ratios and operational philosophy make it a feasible option. Most people do not die in such facilities (ONS 2003) and assessment tools that challenge the status quo away from the predominant medical model of care towards a more eclectic behavioural, cognitive, existential and psychosocial model are unlikely to become widespread in mainstream healthcare.

In the UK, the End of Life project (EOL 2006) initiated by the government in 2003 has seen the introduction of integrated care pathways for the dying in acute environments which are multi-professional in orientation and purport to provide an evidence-based, client-centred framework for the last few days of life (Ellershaw and Wilkinson 2003). Sitting alongside this in the primary care sector is the Gold Standards Framework (Thomas 2003), which provides a similar structure for community-based staff to help them plan care for the dying in their own home. Both these initiatives include elements of psychological care, spiritual care and family support within them, but make no clear reference to the maintenance of hope and alleviation of suffering as perceived by the patient. The integration of a few simple questions oriented this way would be eminently feasible and could potentially yield a rich vein of information to inform more patient-centred care.

Hope and suffering are powerful concepts and, as such, will remain challenging subjects to teach to any audience. They are at the heart of our very existence and in times of crisis help to define our well-being. It is not unreasonable therefore to suggest that we should emphasise them more in undergraduate and postgraduate curricula. All healthcare practitioners need to ask themselves whether they subscribe to a belief that inspiring hope and mitigating suffering is important to them and how they can use their skills, knowledge and compassion to convey the positive messages contained therein. The role modelling of such skills in practice is perhaps the most powerful mode of learning there is and can help to shape the attitudes and behaviours of future professionals in ways that are impossible in the classroom. We would do well to examine our policies and directions in palliative care education so that such opportunities are captured and utilised to maximum advantage.

IMPLICATIONS FOR THE READER'S OWN PRACTICE

1 How often do you teach hope as an explicit topic in palliative care?
2 How can you ensure that the multidimensional concepts of hope and suffering are embedded in the educational and clinical setting?
3 Can any of the models or assessment tools be adapted as an exercise in teaching hope and suffering?
4 In what ways will you know you have achieved the confidence and maturity to teach about hope and the dying?

REFERENCES

Alfaro J (1970) Christian hope and the hopes of mankind. In: Duquac C, editor. *Dimensions of Spirituality*. New York: Herder & Herder: 59–69.

Beck AT, Weissman A (1974) The measurement of pessimism: the hopelessness scale. *J Consult Clin Psychol.* **42** (6): 336–40.

Becker R (2003) Have you heard the one about . . . [editorial]. *Int J Palliat Nurs.* **9** (9): 372–3.

Becker R (2005) Short stories [editorial]. *Int J Palliat Nurs.* **11** (2): 52.

Becker R, Gamlin R (2004) Spiritual care. [Chapter 10.] In: *Fundamental Aspects of Palliative Care Nursing*. Salisbury: Quay Books.

Benner P, Wrubel J (1989) *The Primacy of Care*. London: Addison Wesley.

Benzein E (2005) The level of and relation between hope, hopelessness and fatigue in patients and family members in palliative care. *Palliat Med.* **19**: 234–40.

Cassell EJ (1992) The nature of suffering: physical, psychological, social and spiritual aspects. In: Starck P, McGovern J, editors. *The Hidden Dimensions of Illness: human suffering*. New York: National League for Nursing Press.

Cutcliffe JR (1998) Hope, counselling and complicated bereavement reactions. *J Adv Nurs.* **28** (4): 754–61.

Cutcliffe JR, Herth K (2002) The concept of hope in nursing 1: its origins, background and nature. *Br J Nurs.* **11** (12): 832–40.

Dufault K, Martocchio B (1985) Hope: its spheres and dimensions. *Nurs Clin North Am.* **20** (2): 379–91.

Duggleby W, Wright K (2005) Transforming hope: how elderly palliative patients live with hope. *Can J Nurs Res.* **37** (2): 71–84.

Egan G (2004) *The Skilled Helper: a problem management and opportunity development approach to helping*. Florence, KY: Wadsworth.

Ellershaw JE, Wilkinson S (2003) *Care of the Dying: a pathway to excellence*. Oxford: Oxford University Press.

Encyclopaedia of Philosophy (1967) Dante Alizheri 1265-132. Basingstoke: MacMillan Publishing Company: 291–3.

End of Life Care Programme. Available at: http://eolc.cbcl.co.uk/eolc (accessed 2 October 2006).

Erikson R, Post R, Paige A (1975) Hope as a psychiatric variable. *J Clin Psychol.* **31** (2): 324–30.

European Association of Palliative Care (1989) *European Association of Palliative Care By-laws.* Milan: EAPC National Cancer Institute.

Farley G (2005) Death anxiety and death education: a brief analysis of the key issues. [Chapter 6.] In: Foyle L, Hostad J, editors. *Delivering Cancer and Palliative Care Education.* Oxford: Radcliffe Publishing.

Frank J, Fromm E (1968) *The Revolution of Hope.* New York: Harper & Row.

Franklin RW (2005) *The Poems of Emily Dickinson.* Cambridge, MA: Belknap Press.

Frankl VE (1963) *Man's Search for Meaning.* Boston, MA: Beacon Press.

Herth K (1990) Fostering hope in terminally ill people. *J Adv Nurs.* **15**: 1250–9.

Herth K (1993) Abbreviated instrument to measure hope: development and psychometric evaluation. *J Adv Nurs.* **17** (10): 1251–9.

Herth K (1993) Hope in the family caregiver of terminally ill people. *J Adv Nurs.* **18**: 538–48.

Herth K (2000) Enhancing hope in people with a first recurrence of cancer. *J Adv Nurs.* **32** (6): 1431–41.

Hickey S (1986) Enabling hope. *Cancer Nurs.* **9** (3): 133–7.

Hinds P (1984) Introducing a definition of hope through grounded theory methodology. *J Adv Nurs.* **9** (4): 357–62.

Hinds P, Martin J (1988) Hopefulness and the self sustaining process in adolescents with cancer. *Nurs Res.* **37** (6): 336–40.

Holtslander L, Duggleby W, Williams A, Wright K (2005) The experience of hope for informal caregivers of palliative patients. *J Palliat Care.* **21** (4): 285–91.

Le May A (2004) Building rapport through non verbal communication. *Nurs Resid Care.* **6** (10): 488–91.

McGee RF (1984) Hope: a factor influencing crisis resolution. *Adv Nurs Sci.* **6**: 34–44.

Menninger K (1959) Hope. *Am J Psychiatry.* **116**: 481–91.

Miller JF (1985) Inspiring hope. *Am J Nurs.* **85**: 23–5.

Miller JF (1988) Development of an instrument to measure hope. *Nurs Res.* **37** (1): 6–10.

Moore SI. (2005) Hope makes a difference. *J Psychiatr Ment Health.* **12**: 100–5.

National Institute for Clinical Excellence (2004) *Improving Supportive and Palliative Care for People with Cancer.* [*See* Chapter 5.] London: NICE.

National Council for Hospice and Specialist Palliative Care Services (2001) *What Do We Mean by Palliative Care?* [discussion paper] Briefing No. 9. London: NCHSPCS.

Nowotny M (1989) Assessment of hope in patients with cancer: development of an instrument. *Oncol Nurs Forum.* **16** (1): 57–61.

Nyatanga B (2005) The concept of suffering: a hidden phenomenon. (Chapter 5.) In: Nyatanga B, Astley-Pepper M. *Hidden Aspects of Palliative Care.* Salisbury: Quay Books.

Office of National Statistics (2003) *Mortality Statistics: review of Registrar General on deaths in England and Wales 2003.* Series DH1 36. London: ONS.

O'Malley PA, Menke E (1988) Relationship of hope and stress after myocardial infarction. *Heart Lung.* **17** (2): 184–90.

Poncar PJ (1994) Inspiring hope in the oncology patient. *J Psychosoc Nurs.* **32** (1): 33–8.

Rodgers BL, Cowles KV (1997) A conceptual foundation for human suffering in nursing and research. *J Adv Nurs.* **25**: 1048–53.

Smith MB (1983) Hope and despair: keys to the socio-psychodynamics of youth. *Am J Orthopsychiatry.* **53** (3): 388–99.

Smith P (2004) Working with family care givers in a palliative care setting. In: Payne S, Seymour J, Ingleton C, editors. *Palliative Care Nursing: principles and evidence for practice.* [Chapter 15.] Maidenhead: Open University Press.

Stephenson C (1991) The concept of hope: revisited for nursing. *J Adv Nurs.* **16**: 1456–61.

Thomas K (2003) *Caring for the Dying at Home: companions on the journey.* Oxford: Radcliffe Publishing.

Turner dS (2005) Hope as seen through the eyes of 10 Australian young people. *J Adv Nurs.* **52** (5): 508–17.

Van Hooft S (1998) Suffering and the goals of medicine. *Med Health Philos.* **1**: 125–31.

World Health Organization (2002) *WHO definition of palliative care.* www.who.int/cancer/ palliative/definition

13

The challenges and importance of teaching law relating to the end of life

Anne Leach

'Whatever the human law may be, neither an individual nor nation can commit
the least act of injustice against the obscurest individual without having to pay
the penalty for it.'

Henry David Thoreau

AIM

To explore the implications of UK law in end-of-life care and the challenges
for teaching and incorporating aspects of law into cancer and palliative care
educational programmes.

LEARNING OUTCOMES

By the end of this chapter, the reader should be able to:
- have an awareness of the legal framework for practice for all
  professionals
- describe some of the legal processes involved in UK law
- examine aspects of law as they relate to the healthcare of patients
- identify specific topics which need to be covered currently, in cancer
  and palliative care studies
- explore a variety of innovative teaching and facilitative methods to
  enhance students' knowledge and skills about the legalities in cancer
  and palliative practices.

INTRODUCTION

Decision-making in end-of-life care for those with advancing disease, those who may
have a life-limiting condition, or those in the terminal phase of their illness, has both

an ethical and legal dimension in its processes. The law as with many other aspects of medical care has great influence in the care and treatment of those patients who are terminally ill. Dimensions of prima facie medical ethics, beneficence justice, respect for persons and autonomy suggest a framework for moral dilemmas. These are generally understood and utilised in multiprofessional cancer and palliative practices. Moral justification often underpins decisions around continuing, withdrawing or cost of treatment, patient and family choices, disclosure of information, consent, confidentiality and quality-of-life issues. There are those in society who challenge these decisions within legal circles, with an aim to protect public interest from a wider perspective. In other words, the laws governing society often decide the moral conduct, freedom and choices that are acceptable and those that are not, setting standards for regulation of this conduct which aim to reflect a general public consensus (Kennedy 1984). Within cancer and palliative care, there are also *moral* rules governing practice, which are based on a single or multiple principles. Not surprisingly, these are bound up within the patient–practitioner relationship.

As in all professional practice, *duty, obligation, truth-telling, privacy, rights* and *protection from harm* are core values, even when there is a conflict of interests. Traditionally the law has respected the relationships of the medical profession and their treatment decisions. As a consequence, the law has not always posed the question 'Do doctors always act in the best interests of their patients?'

Moral direction for health professionals emanates from public policy which incorporates regulations and guidelines. These guidelines are promulgated by government agencies and accepted by public bodies in society. Some guidelines are legally enforceable within law, and other policies which protect the public do so in a more conventional sense. This interface between law, ethics and policy is crucial for decision-making in clinical and judiciary (courts) settings.

Many difficult and controversial medical situations are now being referred to the courts, as clinical decision-making with patients, families and carers becomes more transparent and challenging, i.e. when there is a conflict of interests by those involved. Some of those issues are increasingly about judgements around rights to treatment, to consent/refusal of treatment, to killing and letting patients die. The courts not only look at the legal picture but also at the clinical scene as it is presented. In society, every individual has the right to choose and voice their wishes by law but those deemed unable to do so, for whatever reason, are seen by the court as vulnerable members of society. The law is specific on who can give a valid consent and considers children under the age of 14 years (minors) and those with temporary or permanent mental incapacity as being unable to fully consent in law. These individuals must be protected against the decisions of others. Although medical cases are few in comparison to other types of court cases, they do highlight a very difficult task for the judiciary when courts are seen as courts of law and not, as some suggest, courts of medicine. Judges do, however, try to sensitively deal with issues around life and death, upholding the law while striving to maintain some impartiality for the human distress which is often presented.

There appears to be a more of a *culture* of litigation generally in society as the public seek answers, retribution and recompense for what befalls them at the hands of another. This can be seen, for example, from the many medical negligence cases which are increasing, from the lack of appropriate information and from the refusal of Trusts to pay for expensive medical drugs. Doctors as well as patients are generally much more aware of patients' rights and are now working more closely within the boundaries of their professional practice.

PALLIATIVE PHILOSOPHY

Traditionally the patient with a terminal illness was seen to be the cancer sufferer whose disease was advancing and incurable, therefore care of the dying patient focused on the 'terminally ill cancer patient'. It is important to remember that a cancer diagnosis is not now synonymous with an early demise and people are living longer with their condition or completely recover.

With the developments of the hospice movement and advances in cancer care, palliative care became firmly established as an approach and model, as did the developments of palliative medicine. Taking this philosophy, palliative care principles and practices are now afforded to the care of non-cancer patients where their medical care is non-curative, needing palliation of symptoms. In other areas of medicine, doctors treat patients who may have short-term or long-term critical need, cases where the life of one or more is threatened (childbirth or miscarriage), the mentally ill and those with profound physical and mental difficulties. Palliative care principles and philosophies are very applicable to these care settings, affording much more rigorous decision-making processes.

End-of-life care is becoming increasingly more medicalised as some palliative interventions take a more technical/medical approach while physicians try to maintain 'humaneness' as a basic value. Palliative care educators must strike a balance when teaching the science of symptom management, the art of managing death, dying and bereavement care. While medical care is a core dimension, the management of end-of-life care is predominantly undertaken by nurses working within a multiprofessional team (Ingham and Coyle 1997). All professionals within the team must respect the law in relation to patient and family care and therefore education programmes should incorporate these aspects to a greater or lesser extent, depending on the nature of practice.

The British legal system is very often criticised as being unjust, out-of-date and complex when there appears to have been an unsatisfactory outcome for those concerned. For example, prosecutions for those attacks in the name of protecting one's property may seem unjust, as may the outcome of cases where death lies clearly at the hands of another but the case is dismissed because the correct legal processes have not been followed. Alternatively for those who feel that justice and fairness have prevailed, a satisfactory outcome may make them feel fully supported by the legal system. For example, the life sentence for death by gross medical negligence or murder, or the release with caution of someone who has committed the mercy killing of a spouse with longstanding, intractable pain. Many of these kinds of views and opinions can seem to suggest a challenge to the moral codes of rights, wrongs and feelings of those within our society and challenge personal liberties and freedom of choice. However challenged those in society may feel, UK law aims to protect the very body of that society, particularly vulnerable individuals who may find themselves compromised by the actions of others. In essence, *law* is a form of social control, playing an important part in the maintenance and creation of this social order, offering a formal mechanism to deal with conflict and *dis-order* as it arises. In this chapter, the author seeks to highlight those areas in society and healthcare which have strict rules and regulation in law but have the potential for alternative judgements and outcomes. Health practitioner/students have a responsibility to gain some level of knowledge about the law as they study concepts of health from sociopolitical, cultural and economic perspectives. While many legal aspects may be seen to be managed by lawyers, it is essential that health professionals have some understanding of the legal implications and position on many clinical issues today. Providers of education and continuing professional development have therefore a responsibility to address the needs of students in these areas as they may be faced with moral and legal dilemmas. Although law and ethics are inextricably linked, this chapter is primarily concerned with those legal principles, doctrines and categories of law which constitute the legal framework for the public, health providers and students within British society and its healthcare system.

IMPORTANT AREAS OF LAW IN HEALTHCARE

Medical law is a comparatively new subject. It has emerged in English law over the last two decades as a distinct area both in legal practice and academic circles (Kennedy and Grubb 2001). It is essentially concerned with relationships between patient and practitioner, and although it affects all those delivering healthcare it does focus heavily on the decisions made by doctors. Medical law is made up from other areas of law – for instance, family law; the law of tort, which is common or civil law where any individual can bring a case against another if they feel they have a grievance; and criminal and public law.

Dimond (2008) and other eloquent writers provide us with application of the law to healthcare situations in a number of books and articles, both in legal and healthcare journals, using the various categories of law with an ease of interpretation for the reader. Teachers must remind their students of those particular categories that affect both their personal and professional life. Good practice is to remind students of the sources of UK law, these being:
➤ government (the political party of the time), legislative executive
➤ judicial independence (judge-made law).

The relationship between the above two provides some interesting thinking and debate in legal circles as the government can legislate after due processes, as it chooses. This begs the question of to what extent, if any, the judiciary can legitimately oppose the wishes of the legal supremacy afforded to government, expressed in its legislation, or the extent of interference with the pursuit of those wishes. The judiciary therefore has the role in interpreting government legislation, and making decisions on individual cases and changes seen through case precedent. These powers have been greatly enhanced by the passage of the Human Rights Act 1998, although rights of individuals have always been a fundamental principle in UK law. Since its introduction, the

Human Rights Act 1998 deploys the rights and freedoms of the European Convention of Human Rights, and UK jurisdiction is obliged to uphold any violation of these rights (Makkan 2000). Over the last five years there has been an increase in the number of such cases presented.

In understanding what affects health professional practice, it is important to recognise that when we step outside the boundaries of rules and regulations, we must be aware of the ensuing consequences and take responsibility and account for our actions. Although the areas of law have been stated already, there are two main categories of law predominantly affecting healthcare.

➤ Civil or common law – where one person may take out action against another. Usually judges made decisions in settling such disputes and the judges have discretionary powers to compensate or award damages. These cases may or may not be of a criminal nature; they might, for example, concern complaints involving hospital care, doctors' decisions or information given and when harm was seen to have been done at the hands of another. Many of these cases are resolved without going to court through NHS complaints procedures, but those taken to court are judged on facts, principles of law, fault, causation and the resulting 'harm', e.g. *Wilsher v. Essex Area Health Authority* (1988).

➤ Criminal law – where there has been a breach of the criminal law which can be followed by a prosecution in the criminal courts. For example, in cases of theft of equipment or drugs, inappropriate administration and overdosing of preparations to patients and withdrawing statutory services. Some of these negligent actions can result in death, e.g. *R v. Adomako* (1994).

PRACTITIONER ACCOUNTABILITY

Healthcare professionals must remind themselves of the two broad categories of law in terms of accountability but they also have employer and professional accountability within this legal framework. This therefore entails a duty to protect oneself and those we care for; a duty to our employer to act appropriately and a duty to be guided by our professional bodies for good, safe practice.

So far we have focused on sources and categories of the law which may impact on general healthcare applicable to both cancer and palliative domains. Any legal decisions made can affect the quality of life and the quality of death for both individuals and their families. UK law is also concerned with understanding death, how death is brought about, the nature of causation and how we as a society deal with our dead. Although rites of passage, mourning practices and disposal of the deceased are bound up in religious and cultural beliefs (Walters 2003), laws are there to protect the wider society from those death practices seen to be unacceptable within that society. For example, there is no legal rule on where a burial takes place, but the Health and Safety Act 1974 sets out criteria in order to protect public health. According to these criteria, burials in the UK could not take place in, say, back gardens and neither would it be acceptable to hold the public cremations that are the norm in some other cultures. Death studies aim not only to explore death in society, and its impact on health professionals; teaching death and dying can also serve to develop students' knowledge and skills in critical thinking, creativity and personal growth (Farley 2004) around these areas.

LEGAL TOPICS IN CANCER AND PALLIATIVE CARE EDUCATION

We have acknowledged so far that the law does govern what happens in healthcare and society using sources of law. In relation to cancer and palliative care specifically, the law's application via a number of legal procedures, together with factual information and sources, reminds us about life, quality of life and death.

The patient–practitioner relationship requires both to enter into a 'contract' and as a result a 'duty of care' exists from the practitioner, a legal duty in professional practice. This involves, for example, a duty to provide pain management where statutory laws govern medicines, to obtain the patient's consent to receiving drugs, to offer information about medication and its side-effects, to adhere to standards of prescribed medication and to ensure confidentiality and recording of those drugs (Dimond 2008). The government's drive for supportive care in cancer and palliative care requires a level of knowledge, skills, service development, patient and family information systems in medical treatment and bereavement support during and after death. Patients and their families face a number of distressing events needing accurate, informative and necessary information and support from professionals along the dying trajectory, in death and in what to do after the death. Professionals need to have a range of information to give to patients and relatives but also to respond to those questions which may be asked in privacy. Many issues that are important to patients when they want to 'put their affairs in order', or to let someone know about their wishes, have a legal implication requiring practitioners to have some legal understanding to respond appropriately and may involve the medical team or family.

Patient and family care issues which may have legal implications

➤ making treatment choices, consenting or refusing treatment
➤ withdrawing treatment
➤ requests to end life or advance directions (living wills)
➤ making of a will for property and assets
➤ delegating power of attorney for legal consent by another in cases of incapacity
➤ donation, retrieval and storage of organs or tissues after death
➤ funeral arrangements.

Many of these issues are crucial to quality and dignity at the end of life, as they are very real life issues when patients have little time left and families may need some guidance. The accuracy of information from a practitioner alongside as to who to contact for legal advice – and one who can use common sense to act quickly – is the essence of good supportive care.

Legal requirements after death

There are a number of legal requirements after death which may or may not involve the relatives, and professional awareness is crucial if families and carers are to understand

what may happen next. Those areas usually involving families are:
- registration of the death with the death certificate
- consent to organ donation, retrieval or storage, if the patient has not had the opportunity to make known any wishes they may have
- funeral arrangements.

Those areas of law relating to death where relatives may *not* directly be involved, but where they may need sufficient understanding of some legal processes, should they be requested to do so, are:
- establishment of the exact time of death (in an investigation about the death)
- cause of death (if unknown or suspicious)
- requests for post-mortem
- coroner inquests
- disposal of the deceased
- property rights, which may even include the body
- releasing the body for burial/cremation
- funeral arrangements
- diagnosing death from a legal and clinical perspective, where life is being prolonged by artificial methods
- death occurring outside the UK.

Practitioners in the field of cancer and palliative care, while supporting the patient and family until death, need to appreciate the importance of 'after-death care' and the legal requirements facing carers and families.

Legal requirements during a phase of illness
The law relating to treatment
The law is concerned with the basic premise of:
- what constitutes 'treatment'
- consent by the individual to that treatment.

Medical treatment: Although the law has made no concrete definition of medical treatment and still relies heavily on the discretion of the medical professional to administer what is a right and proper intervention, it does, however, question medical competence to do so. The nearest legal definition of treatment was found in the Medical Treatment (Prevention of Euthanasia) Bill in 1999, although that Bill did not in fact pass the parliamentary hurdle and so has no standing in current UK law. The definition of treatment provided by the failed Bill is nonetheless of some interest:

> 'any medical or surgical treatment, including the administration of drugs or use of any mechanical or other apparatus for the provision or support of ventilation or of any other bodily function.'

Notably, the Bill did not have any regard for treatments – either medical or otherwise – which may be given in the best interests of patients to relieve distress – for example, sedating the seriously ill newborn, or offering nursing care (*R v. Arthur* 1981) which can be seen as supporting quality rather than quantity of life or the last dose of radiotherapy to reduce pain and swelling of an affected limb. Further to this definition and understanding, Beauchamp and Childress (2007) make a more moral distinction between *ordinary* and *extraordinary* treatment, recognised as appropriate in law, as follows:

> 'Ordinary means are all medicines, treatments and operations which offer a reasonable hope of benefit and which can be obtained and used without excessive expense, pain or other inconvenience. Extraordinary means are all medicines, treatments and operations, which cannot be obtained or used without excessive expense, pain or other inconvenience or which if used, would not offer a reasonable hope of benefit.'

The legal position would therefore be that those treatments deemed as ordinary would be a legal requirement, but that the doctor is not bound to prescribe those treatments deemed as extraordinary.

Most cancer and palliative 'treatments' currently rest with weighing up the benefits against the burden; they are heavily influenced in decision-making on the doctrine of 'best interests' and, in most cases, on consent to treatment. 'Best interests' can be an acceptable justification in law if the practitioner is deemed competent and the consent by the patient is questionable. The British Medical Association goes further to suggest that food and water constitute medical treatment (as in the case of Tony Bland) and their understanding of those treatments which provide comfort and the alleviation of pain and other distressing symptoms is wide enough to include palliative care.

Other legal principles and justifications in law around decisions to treat or not to treat are listed in Table 13.3. When courts are required to make decisions around the lawfulness of treatment, they do consider ethical standpoints and the interpretation of these into legal principles when deciding the outcome.

Consent

Any action (treatment or care) to another without consent would be unlawful and would amount to trespass, possibly leading to a criminal charge of assault or battery under the Offences Against Person Act (1861). To complicate issues further, battery can also be dealt with as a civil matter in the law of tort. In making a valid consent in law the person must be deemed competent, be adequately informed and give this consent voluntarily. Consent can be withdrawn legally any time after it has been given. The general consensus is that treatment which the patient is consenting to is 'therapeutic'. The capacity to consent relies on the patient's understanding the 'broad nature' and 'purpose' of the treatment or care and being able to understand the likely or possible effects or consequences. It is not possible to explore capacity in this chapter, but suffice to acknowledge that this is a huge area for the courts in determining a satisfactory outcome. Many practitioners are acutely aware of those factors affecting a patient's capacity – for example, drugs, pain, shock, confusion, mental illness, drowsiness, misconceptions of reality and the impact of loss, all within the clinical situation.

TABLE 13.1 Topics in cancer and palliative care on consent

- refusal of treatment
- withdrawal of treatment
- request for treatment
- request for euthanasia/assisted suicide
- withholding treatments
- research and clinical trials

The law is very clear on these issues by the competent, consenting individual in decision-making and a number of cases have been argued where there has been a conflict of interests. The case of *Re C* (1994), involving capacity to make a valid consenting decision, has become the 'test' now used in law and, in a somewhat modified form, is the basis for assessing incapacity in the Mental Capacity Act 2005. This legislation has also codified the law on advance directives (now known as directions) and the creation of powers of proxy decision-making by persons who may be aware that they will lose capacity (e.g. lasting powers of attorney).

TABLE 13.2 Other topics needing legal consideration

- statutory provision of health and social care
- allocation of resources, including cancer drugs and life-sustaining measures
- complementary therapies, in relation to standards, safety, consent and conflict with doctors
- personal and organisational liability, including health and safety and product liability
- confidentiality
- record-keeping

Implications for cancer and palliative care educators

For any teacher in cancer, palliative and terminal care – the novice and the experienced educator alike – medical law is a huge subject to tackle and yet it is an important area to address. It is not sufficient to teach ethics without some understanding of the law. It does remain difficult to untangle them, as many arguments are based on both moral and legal principles (*see* Table 13.3).

TABLE 13.3 Moral and legal doctrines around decision-making

- sanctity of life
- autonomy/rights
- necessity
- best interests
- duty and obligation
- justice and fairness
- intentions

Teaching aspects of law requires the teacher to have, if not legal training in medical law as taught by a lawyer, then at least knowledge of:
➤ statutory and non-statutory health and social care provision
➤ statutes governing services, treatment, actions and standards of care
➤ the interface between ethics and law in decision-making processes by the courts
➤ the application of certain legal requirements to areas of practice for learners
➤ subject matter to a level of expertise within planned teaching timetables as appropriate
➤ how best to provide the learner with opportunities for debate, discussion and reflection
➤ legal research, sources of information and where to direct the learner
➤ appropriate sources of legal material.

TABLE 13.4 Sources of legal material

• www.dh.gov.uk
• www.homeoffice.gov.uk
• www.tso.co.uk
• www.official-documents.gov.uk
• www.statutelaw.gov.uk

SOURCES AND OPPORTUNITIES TO ADDRESS LEGAL ASPECTS IN CANCER AND PALLIATIVE CARE

It is not always necessary to formalise education opportunities, but many teachers would see a formal presentation as an appropriate method to deliver key aspects of law on a number of topics highlighted so far. This can be very time consuming on an already tight curriculum or education schedule. The following section may highlight for the reader where legal aspects may be incorporated into educational venues, taking opportunities to enhance the needs of learners/practitioners.
➤ *Hospice education:* many hospices have well-established education and training departments. Some of these are linked to national organisations such as the Marie Curie Cancer Care; some have designated education and training personnel; some have their education programmes accredited with local universities; some offer short courses, modules, study days or evenings and are often on a rolling programme basis (Hostad *et al.* 2004). These are ideal for 'in house' continuing professional development and for exploring end-of-life issues with local multiprofessional groups. Palliative care physicians and specialist nurses are in an ideal position to address topics for their immediate colleagues within the hospice. Education and training strategies could identify training and development needs relating to legal aspects of cancer and palliative care along with statutory/mandatory training in moving and handling, fire, health and safety etc.
➤ *University education:* many universities provide formal undergraduate programmes incorporating legal aspects to a larger or lesser degree, depending

on timetables and time available, as well as offering pre-registration, post-registration and postgraduate studies for a variety of professionals in cancer and palliative care. Some of these programmes are linked to local hospices or other palliative care education providers. More in-depth study of the law is often a matter of personal choice, where practitioners and educators continue to develop their expertise. If an in-depth course is required, some universities offer specific courses on the law and healthcare.

➤ *NHS education and training:* many hospitals and primary care Trusts have education and training departments, again providing opportunities on 'in house' topics around 'topical' issues of law relating to aspects of practice. These can be done as full-day or half-day study sessions, workshops or seminars taught by both 'in house' and external speakers, if organised well. Indeed, the larger cancer centres around the UK tend to have integral education facilities or at least an educationalist who might be offering, or who is able to produce, an appropriate course relating to legal aspects, if the demand is there.

➤ *Public and lay carer education:* many health professionals are involved in public education at some level, helping patients and carers to deal with issues of concern, whether implicitly or explicitly (Hostad *et al.* 2004), prior or during treatment or even around after-death care issues. Hostad and colleagues demonstrate that by making information more available and accessible to the public, we can enhance the autonomy, empowerment and coping strategies of individuals for optimum health and well-being in advancing disease and the terminal phase of life. Addressing legal issues with patients and carers can add some quality dimensions to certain difficult dilemmas and choices. These can be incorporated into hospice programmes, lay carer support groups, bereavement groups, and either informal or formal talks on many issues highlighted. Carer groups are ideal in identifying particular topics where essential information may be required. The public domain remains a key area to flag some controversial issues and offers opportunity for the legal position to be explained, particularly via television soaps or documentaries, radio programmes or debates, published writings and video materials.

➤ *Professional networks:* these remain excellent sources via which the legal position of specific clinical situations can be explored. Such exploration can take the form of seminars, conference papers or presentations, master classes or invited speakers to professional group meetings. A common thread in all is that specific topics will be analysed in some depth from both ethical and legal perspectives, for specialist practice.

INTEGRATION AND TEACHING LEGAL ASPECTS OF CANCER AND PALLIATIVE CARE

There is no easy way to teach legalities in palliative and cancer care. However, there are some interesting and creative ways of delivering some aspects of this topic while taking in the range of opportunities already mentioned. In most instances, legal issues appear on courses, modules, curriculae and study days combined with ethics. This reminds students and other professionals that there are limitations in law to the moral maze of decisions made in practice.

The law can be seen as being very complex, and its use of professional terminology and jargon only reinforces this popular perception. Educationalists do have a responsibility to try to 'simplify' the language to help reduce confusion and provide clarity.

Most education and training programmes for health professionals include some aspects of law. Parts of the pre-registration curriculum would be designed to raise awareness among those in the early stages of basic training of how the law aims to protect practitioners throughout their working lives. UK law can therefore provide a protective framework for clinical practice, which can be built upon as healthcare changes and clinical situations become more challenging. Lifelong learning is proposed in a number of government initiatives (DoH 2001) and it is the role of all practitioners to impart and keep up to date with the changing nature of medical law. But the significant question is: where and how do we do this?

FACILITATION OF LEGAL MATTERS IN EDUCATION: WHO SHOULD DO THIS? WHERE IS THE BEST PLACE AND WHEN?

The teaching and learning process requires both teacher and learner to engage in a number of strategies, both cognitive and behavioural, in meeting goals and objectives in the acquisition of knowledge (Curzon 1990).

Most educators address legal aspects while teaching ethics, providing some study direction, or by engaging an external legal person (the lawyer) to facilitate learning and assist students to understand legal positions. There are a number of methods which the educator can use to address legal issues, ranging from the formal lecture to a clinical situation of a patient and family discussion. Often the latter are instigated by the patient or a family member.

There needs to be a combination of personnel involved in teaching, ranging from members of the multiprofessional team to benefits and advice agencies, local authority agencies, solicitors, lawyers and legal teams if necessary. It is important for educators to recognise the wide range of sources available, although clearly there will be cost implications with a number of these options.

Due to the amount of legal material governing cancer and palliative practice, there are limitations to topics which can be studied in any depth. Due to time and programme constraints within formal education, it is often left to the teacher to be selective about which areas will be covered, particularly with specialist palliative and cancer care practitioners. Depending on the competency level required and the length of the course, basic legal principles and the legalities during and after death should be addressed. Other selected aspects of palliative, cancer and end-of-life issues may be integrated into other taught sessions such as: 1) communication and information-giving; 2) breaking bad news and confidentiality; 3) pain management. Students can be given directed or self-directed learning opportunities around further legal topics of clinical importance.

Useful methods and tips in the classroom setting
The formal lecture
As most teachers will recognise, the lecture style usually promotes one-way communi-cation, is structured and requires the teacher to know the audience, plan objectives and consider some audiovisual material. The lecture style is demanding on teacher time but can be a very useful way of delivering large amounts of material around a topic. Rather than students rigorously taking notes, it can be more productive to provide them with a written handout of the lecture; students can then follow the teacher more attentively, making additional notes and comments for personal use. The handout will contain a summary of the legal aspects to be covered in, for example, a one-hour or two-hour sessions. A useful tip for teachers is that, while progressing through the handout, they should stop at critical points, elaborate, give examples and allow the students to ask questions or to ask for clarification of issues explored.

Examples of teaching topics

1   Incapacity and consent: elaborate on the arguments for acting in the best interests of the patient and provide some cases for the students to comment on.
    Useful cases in this context might include *Airedale NHS Trust v. Bland*, and *Re H (Adult Incompetent)* (1990). The latter concerns a brain-damaged individual about whom decisions were made just to provide hydration and nutrition.
2   Consenting competent patients: elaborate on issues around refusing, withdrawal, and requests for treatment.
    Useful cases in this context might include *R v. Cox* (1992), involving mercy killing, and *R v. Pretty* (2001), involving the aiding of death by request. Similarly the controversial Assisted Dying for the Terminally Ill Bill 2004 could be discussed.
3   Legal requirements after death: succinct information can be provided on post-mortems, registration of death when a patient dies in hospital, at home or in a hospice, Coroners' Courts and the disposal of bodies.

Time may be tight in these lectures but the sessions will cover important areas and raise debate and thinking for students around the principles of law in the cases signalled and on why the courts rule on and in a certain way.

The seminar
The nature of the seminar differs greatly from the above lecture style. Seminars require considerable skill of the teacher to prepare, control and understand group dynamics (Curzon 1990). Teachers using this strategy almost need to 'mediate' the interactions of the group as they explore a topic, endeavour to understand it, learn from each others' ideas and arguments and speak freely, listen and observe. Whether discussion is teacher led or student led, there must be clear objectives and, if possible, some pre-requisite knowledge by the group in preparation for the seminar. This can be done by giving the students some factual information – for example, a specific piece of legisla-tion or a case study on which the seminar will be based and which may provide some basic understanding of the topic.

The seminar can be presented by the teacher, providing a balance of views and opinions and posing a number of questions and challenges for the group. This requires the teacher to be in control, aware of individual and group emotions, and to bring discussions back on track if they stray. The teacher also needs to be aware of not playing devil's advocate too obviously as this will make the group feel manipulated and convey the impression that the 'teacher conclusion' is the right one. Silences can be a challenge for teachers, but good preparation will ensure that you have alternative questions and approaches. To get group discussion underway, breaking into smaller groups may help, then reconvene or have a natural tea break. Silences can be a thinking time but, if responses are slow, asking the group about a clinical/practical issue will usually get a response.

Examples of topics for seminars

1   The Mental Capacity Act (2005) could offer teacher-led material around the attempts made by the Act to provide a statutory framework to empower and protect vulnerable people. Consent by another can be explored here, and what 'capacity' means – including that unwise decisions do not provide evidence of lack of capacity – as well as the requirement that decisions under the Act must be made in the best interests of the individual. The Act offers a good opportunity to explore lasting power of attorney and to ask students their views on advanced directions and on the restraining of people under the legislation. Sections of the Act which relate these aspects need to be pointed out during the seminar.

2   Seminar materials can include video excerpts on topical issues such as physician-assisted suicide and euthanasia. This allows students to engage in debate after the presentation of ideas by the teacher and can help to inform and crystallise their personal and professional standpoints while ensuring that the patients' wishes and choices are respected.

    Television documentary recordings are valuable visually to complement the spoken-word focus of the seminar. Asking the students to write their thoughts and opinions while watching any teaching video work is essential, as it will prompt them in subsequent debate. A topic for such debate might be: Can there be any justification for assisted suicide?

    The Voluntary Euthanasia Society (VES) Dignity in Dying programme has large amounts of material for students to access.

Group debates and discussion

These strategies for teaching legal topics differ again from the seminar approaches in that group work is structured into the lesson. Group work has advantages of social interaction and facilitation, and it can be more accurate in clarifying judgments than those resulting from an individual examination of an issue. Group work/discussion often benefits those students whose views may need clarifying; it also has the advantage of developing lively debate involving a clinical perspective.

Group work can take the following forms:
➤ Case studies for students to discuss and analyse. These could be from a critical incident, a real patient scenario, a major current issue or they could take a role-play format.

Examples of case studies

David has had motor neurone disease for two years. He has had numerous hospital and hospice admissions and is now on a ventilator in hospital. His condition is deteriorating and he has asked the physician to let him die. The doctor has a dilemma, as he is required to respect the patient's wishes and yet he cannot act unlawfully to do this. David has applied through his lawyer for an injunction against the hospital so that he can lawfully be removed from the ventilator, even though the certain result would be death.

The group discussion would have to highlight issues around consent and capacity, acts and omissions of the doctor, the right to switch off and all this in relation to the competent and incompetent patient.

John was admitted to hospital with abdominal pain. He had been suffering from indigestion for some months and thought he had an ulcer. Further investigations diagnosed an inoperable stomach malignancy and the surgeon felt that an open approach to telling John was his only option. This was in conflict with John's wife's and daughter's wishes and they pleaded with the nursing staff not to let the doctor tell John. Support for the family is a crucial and moral imperative for staff. So what were they to do?

• How do the legal and ethical standpoints emerge in these two cases? What are the issues around patient's rights?

➤ Other types of group activity work well with some topics and can be structured in the form of a debate where 'for' and 'against' arguments are presented by two people and the remainder of the group discusses their interaction. Teachers must be mindful of who is doing all the work and modify this approach by making the arguments a collective consensus. There need to be well-prepared materials, so students need one or two weeks to research, get together and prepare material for class.

Examples of legal issues which would make suitable topics for debate

• hydration and nutrition
• passive euthanasia
• legal definitions of death
• the right to treatment or not
• current issues where the law has changed recently or where it has a direct impact on patient choices and decisions, e.g. rationing treatments, using patient scenarios
• the principle of double effect in pain management in palliative care
• quality of life v. quality of death – the legal choices people and families can make

Tutorials

Tutorial work usually convenes within a formal course programme and can be done on a one-to-one basis or in groups, but it does require the size of the group to be small, i.e. 14 students. Tutorials can be useful for skills teaching, remedial work, post-lecture or in preparation for a lecture, and to supervise course work. Tutorials are usually student led or group led.

Examples of legal issues suitable for tutorial work

- a critical incident from a practice situation, shared with the group
- a piece of reflective practice, again shared and discussed in the group
- a piece of legislation and its application to clinical practice
- dealing with patient and family requests which may need legal consideration, including exploration of appropriate communication skills for achieving this

---

Web-based learning

This is an ideal medium for students to work through directed pathways, case studies, legal/factual material or just to browse legal sources for personal interest. Such learning does, however, require the educator to create a whole new dimension for web-based materials and it also relies on the students' computing and IT skills.

Useful methods and tips in the clinical setting

Not all education takes place within a formal setting and clinical environments often have experienced academic clinical educators who provide a wealth of expertise and education to clinical staff. These roles do, however, vary greatly depending on the organisation and education responsibilities. Education can be a combination of:

➤ study day programmes on specific, chosen legal topics
➤ lunchtime seminars at which a relevant invited professional – e.g. a local solicitor, Coroner's officer, funeral director – gives a half-hour or one-hour talk
➤ focus group activity with staff, depending on time and personnel available. These groups focus on one aspect of an issue or explore one topic specific to a particular setting or currently relevant, highlighting a piece of legislation affecting palliative care that might provide a valuable basis for staff discussion.

Example of a topic for focus group activity

Using as a point of departure the Assisted Dying for the Terminally Ill Bill 2004 or requests from families of dying patients to continue or to stop the patient's treatment, the group might explore the broader issues.

Mention would be made of the concept of dying with dignity, with reference to the Voluntary Euthanasia Society. Exploration would cover the ground that if any form of euthanasia is unlawful, then issues of 'ending' and 'not continuing' may look much the same. Debate could take place on acts and omissions of either killing or letting die for those who have unbearable suffering and little quality of life, and on the implications of what would happen if these people were able to choose when death comes, how and by whom.

➤ These small groups can provide value time for all healthcare staff involved in patient care to come together, led by a senior member of staff. These sessions can work very well when health assistants who have little formal education are encouraged to share views and opinions and to learn about the law affecting their practice. Much multiprofessional learning can be achieved by small group discussion in practice.
➤ Teaching at the beside can be challenging. Cancer and palliative care healthcare advocates open, transparent communication between the patient, the family and the multiprofessional team. All the same, some issues may be appropriate for discussion at the beside while others may need to be dealt with elsewhere – at team meetings or clinical handovers – and then discussed with the patient. Staff can be encouraged by senior members and clinical educators to reflect, de-brief and share their learning.

Many of these methods, either formal or less formal, can and do challenge the very core of personal and professional attitudes and philosophies of individuals as well as offering a challenge for educators themselves.

Other sources to investigate and acquire legal information

➤ Local libraries often have a legal section where the public can find cases and legislation.
➤ Obtaining 'reading rights' to a local university library as a clinical educator is worth investigating. There may be a charge for this but it would be a most useful resource to be able to explore the vast amount of legal material available in such an institution.
➤ Internet sources can pose a challenge in terms of finding what educators and students need, but again they can provide very useful sources, particularly for Department of Health material on the NHS and healthcare provision.

KEY POINTS

■ The law provides us with a legal framework for professional practice and seeks to protect society, particularly those vulnerable members of that society.
■ Legal practice is based on intellectual, academic, factual and evidence bases in its application to cases presented.
■ The interface between the law, morals and medical care results in cases being judged on their own merits and applying principle, doctrines and justifications within the categories of law. The courts do not seek to give permission but to propose what is lawful and what is not.

- Palliative care educators have a responsibility to integrate legal issues into education and training programmes in nurturing and developing personal and professional attitudes to many challenging clinical situations.
- There are some interesting and challenging ways to deliver legal topics in cancer and palliative care when limited time and resources are often issues in themselves.
- Education in cancer and palliative care requires practitioners to grasp, analyse, conceptualise and synthesise many challenging and emotive issues and the law is there to guide and protect both practitioners and patients.

CONCLUSION

The English legal system aims to protect the living person but also has rules to protect the dead. The law and morality are inextricably linked, however reluctant the courts are to decide over life and death. While cancer and palliative care practice and education acknowledges the concepts of autonomy, consent and the right to self-determination, the law still imposes limitation to treatment and how an individual dies. Decisions are routinely made by the multiprofessional team, monitoring medical and nursing care, with educators reinforcing and teaching this approach within a legal framework. The media have highlighted a number of situations which have reflected the importance of education in cancer and palliative care. These situations include the Shipman case; use of the breast cancer drug Herceptin; the reading again in the House of Lords of the Assisted Dying Bill; and the cases of those who 'mercifully' end the life of loved ones. Practitioners are faced from time to time with moral dilemmas which have legal and binding protocols, and all are responsible in some way for teaching others within the scope of their practice. For many healthcare professionals, the law may seem less than engaging, but it is crucial in today's modern healthcare environment – with its attendant culture of litigation and with due regard for the rights and choices of patients and families – that they do indeed engage with the legal aspects of healthcare practice. While lawmakers continue to strive for meaningful articulation of the fundamental aims of the legal system, and to consider reforms and the new challenges for the courts, healthcare practitioners continue to protect and enhance the quality of life and death for cancer patients and those with a non-cancer diagnosis who also have palliative care needs.

'The law is reason, free from passion.'

Aristotle.

IMPLICATIONS FOR THE READER'S OWN PRACTICE

1 What legal topics have you explored from a personal and professional perspective?
2 What opportunities are available to you for acquiring legal material and how would you organise this?

3   What innovative ways could you use to build upon the range of teaching methods
    explored in this chapter?
4   In what way can you support students and clinical staff who may have challenging
    and conflicting opinions around care and treatment of patients and quality of life
    and death?
5   How could you ensure that teaching materials are up to date for classroom and
    clinical teaching?

CASES

Airedale NHS Trust v. Anthony Bland [1993] 1 All ER 821
Bolam v. Friern Hospital Management Committee [1957] 2 All ER 118
R v. Adams [1957] CLR 365
R v. Adomako (1994) HL
R v. Arthur (1981)
R v. Cox (1992) 12 BMLR 38
Re C (Adult: Refusal of Medical Treatment) [1994] 1 WLR 290
The Harold Shipman Inquiry – report
The Case of Annie Lindsell – unreported
Wilsher v. Essex Area Health Authority [1988] 1 All ER 87

REFERENCES

Beauchamp T, Childress J (2007) *Principles of Biomedical Ethics*. 5th ed. Oxford: Oxford
    University Press.
Curzon LB (1990) *Teaching in Further Education: an outline of principles and practices*. 4th ed.
    London: Cassell.
Department of Health (2001) *Working Together, Learning Together: a framework for lifelong
    learning in the NHS*. London: DoH.
Dimond B (2002) *Legal Aspects of Pain Management*. London: Mark Allen Publishing.
Dimond B (2008) *Legal Aspects of Nursing*. 5th ed. London: Pearson Education.
Farley G (2004) Death anxiety and death education: a brief analysis. In: Foyle L, Hostad J, editors.
    Delivering Cancer and Palliative Care Education. Oxford: Radcliffe Publishing.
Hockton A (2001) *The Law of Consent to Medical Treatment*. London: Sweet & Maxwell.
Hostad J, McManus N, Foyle L (2004) Public information and education in palliative care. In:
    Foyle L, Hostad J, editors. *Delivering Cancer and Palliative Care Education*. Oxford: Radcliffe
    Publishing.
Ingham J, Coyle N (1997) New themes in palliative care. In: Clark D, Hockley J, Ahmedzai S,
    editors. *New Themes in Palliative Care*. Buckingham: Open Press University.
Kennedy I (1984) The law relating to the treatment of the terminally ill. In: Saunders C, editor.
    The Management of Terminal and Malignant Disease. Oxford: Hodder Arnold.
Kennedy I, Grubb A (2000) *Medical Law*. London: Butterworths.
Makkan S (2000) *The Human Rights Act 1998: the essentials*. London: Callow.
Mason JK, Laurie GT (2007) *Law and Medical Ethics*. 7th ed. Oxford: Oxford University Press.
The Medical Treatment (Prevention of Euthanasia) Bill (1999).
The Mental Capacity Act (2005).

National Institute for Clinical Excellence (2004) *Improving Supportive and Palliative Care for Adults with Cancer*. London: DoH.

The Offences Against Persons Act (1861).

Walters T (2003) Historical and cultural variants on the good death. *BMJ.* **327**: 218–20.

Wicks E (2001) The right to refuse medical treatment under the Convention on Human Rights. *Med Law Rev.* **9**: 17–40.

Williams G (2001) The principles of double effect and terminal sedation. *Med Law Rev.* **9**: 41–53.

USEFUL WEBSITES

Department of Health: www.doh.gov.uk

British Medical Journal: www.bmj.com

NHS Evidence: www.library.nhs.uk

Voluntary Euthanasia Society: www.ves.org.uk

14

Diet and nutrition in cancer and palliative care education

Shupikai Rinomhota

'If we could give every individual the right amount of nourishment and exercise, not too little and not too much, we would have found the safest way to health.'

Hippocrates, 460–377 BC

AIM

This chapter focuses on the relationship between the individual suffering from cancer or any other life-threatening illness and the contribution of diet and nutrition to the general well-being of that individual. In this era of new technological developments in treatment and innovative drug discoveries, the issue of nutrition in care and education for all practitioners is often regarded as secondary, even an afterthought. Educators have an important role to play in helping practitioners to refocus on the central importance of nutrition in cancer and palliative care by emphasising how this aspect of care is enabling to both the patient and the practitioner.

LEARNING OUTCOMES

By the end of this chapter, the reader should be able to:
- discuss the role of diet and nutrition in cancer and palliative care
- reinforce the relationship between nutrition and dimensions of cancer or other life-threatening illness in practitioner education
- highlight the central role that practitioners and educationalists can play in ensuring the best nutritional care of the patient
- challenge misconceptions in relation to nutrition and cancer and palliative care
- understand the importance of ensuring this topic is addressed in the field of cancer and palliative care education.

INTRODUCTION

The last ten years have enriched both my experience and my reflection on the teaching of nutrition in cancer and palliative care due to my increased interaction with many practitioners from a variety of settings involved in cancer and palliative care, both within hospitals and in the community. The experience of seeing my own father dying from prostate cancer, after a significant period of living far away from him, was very humbling to me and gave me pause for reflection. Up to this day I have a vivid memory of a once very fit and robust man who had become emaciated and gaunt but remained emotionally competent and spiritually content. This chapter is born from my experience of seeing and working with cancer sufferers as a nurse, from the time-limited experience of seeing my father die from the disease, my knowledge and understanding of human nutrition and many fruitful classroom/seminar discussions with various experienced practitioners in cancer and palliative care that include nurses and dieticians.

FROM DOUBLE-EDGED SWORD TO COMFORTER AND THERAPY

The interaction of diet and nutrition with cancer could be considered to be like a double-edged sword. This is because in the early stages of the continuum of life, a few food components, although not many, could be considered to be harmful and to possibly lead to the development of cancer. These substances include aflatoxins from poorly stored food substances that may lead to the development of liver cancer and some food additives that are added by manufacturers in processed foods to increase their shelf life. In addition, many people are questioning the use of fungicides and pesticides in vegetables and other food crops and hence the increase in the organic market, certainly within the UK. Epidemiological evidence supports the increased occurrence of certain cancers among some immigrant communities settled in new home countries, due to changed lifestyle and in particular dietary changes. For example, Yu et al. (1991) reported increased cancer rates of the colon, rectum, prostate and breast in Chinese Americans when compared to those Chinese in Shanghai, while Ghadirian et al. (2003) reported lower incidence of gastric cancers but higher incidence of cancer of the breast, colon, pancreas and prostate among Japanese Americans in California and Hawaii when compared with Japanese still residing in Japan. However, the overall benefits of a good diet and healthy nutrition to life and healthy living as well as during ill-health are immense. A summary report by the World Cancer Research Fund (WCRF) and the American Institute for Cancer Research (AICR) (Potter et al. 1997) concluded that while the global incidence of cancer was 10.3 million cases in 1996, this was projected to rise to 14.7 million in 2020, an increase of 42.7%. Such statistics are frightening but one hopes that something can be done to alter the course of events. The authors of the WCRF and the AICR argue that, while the chief causes of cancer are the use of tobacco and inappropriate diets, between 30% and 40% of all cancers can be prevented by appropriately changing one's diet, through physical activity and by maintaining appropriate body weight.

But of course those colleagues who have worked and are working in cancer and palliative care are all familiar with the challenge of trying to coax cancer sufferers to eat adequately, or to eat at all, due to changes in taste of food (dysgeusia) as well as in smell. From an education perspective, ensuring that students and practitioners understand the dimensions of cancer and palliative care as well as how diet and nutrition relate to these dimensions is paramount. These dimensions include the physical, the psychological, the spiritual, the disease process and the treatment process. A few misconceptions are held especially by sufferers of cancer, but also by other members of the general public and a few practitioners, about diets and foods that work in cancer. It becomes even more important to ensure that these misconceptions are discussed in the classroom in seminars with students and practitioners, so that the correct information is disseminated. It is the role of educators to ensure that the role played by diet and nutrition in cancer is not simplistically a case of asking such questions as: Does taking a certain food cause cancer? Does taking certain vitamins prevent or reduce cancer? Indeed while these questions are useful and important to ask, practitioners need to understand aspects of the process of carcinogenesis, the antagonistic, synergistic and additive effects of diet with other lifestyle factors such as smoking and excess alcohol consumption.

Prasad *et al.* (1998) reviewed the relationship of diet with other factors and highlighted the reasons why such a question as the important role of diet in cancer cannot be answered simplistically. They hypothesised that, for example, when considering the issue of human carcinogenesis alone, a four-stage model of mutations that encompasses many facets could be given. They proposed that the first stage in carcinogenesis is a random mutation of the normal cell which may be due to increased exposure to mutagens, deficiency in natural repair mechanisms and/or deficiency protective substances. All of these causative factors could be a result of poor dietary intake, an important facet that educators need to emphasise. The second mutation proposed by Prasad *et al.* (1998) is in the differentiation gene, which results in the continued proliferation of the cell without differentiation and subsequent apoptosis. Apoptosis is programmed cell death that is lacking in cancer cells, which become immortal. These same authors proposed that the third mutation is that of random accumulation of additional genetic mutations in the hyperplastic cells coupled by activation of certain oncogenes, while the fourth mutation involves continual random mutation of cancer cells resulting in the aggressive cellular behaviour that is seen with some of the cancers that have metastases.

However, in terms of cancer risk reduction, Prasad *et al.* (1998: 197) suggest that an important question for researchers to ask and for good protocol design may be: 'Does supplementation with multiple vitamins, together with diet and lifestyle modification, reduce the risk of cancer?' Designing a protocol for humans solid enough to answer this question is not easy. However, there is enough evidence to support the view that high amounts of vitamins in the body may cause tumour cell death, may reduce the expression of certain oncogenes and reduce other growth factors that are believed to stimulate some cancers.

PRACTICAL APPLICATIONS OF NUTRITION TO CANCER AND PALLIATIVE CARE EDUCATION

In order to make the teaching of nutrition in cancer and palliative care relevant, educators need to ensure that the dimensions described earlier in this chapter are fully explored. Since many practitioners have limited nutrition knowledge, due to the fact that nutrition education is not routinely taught to all healthcare professionals, especially nurses and doctors, this means that many practitioners, apart from dieticians and nutritionists, are not confident in discussing diet and nutrition issues with clients. Therefore it becomes the educators' role to clarify this important relationship between diet and nutrition with the dimensions of cancer and palliative care, thus fostering a knowledge base that enables practitioners to feel confident enough to explore nutritional issues with patients and clients, to assess their nutritional status, to recognise the causes of malnutrition within the illness context much earlier than is often the case, and to adopt nutritional supportive measures that encompass all the dimensions of cancer. In all this the sufferer must be actively participating in his or her care. The practical applications of all this emphasise the need for understanding what each dimension brings to the care of the patient. Depending on where the cancer is, the physical dimension manifests itself with dysphagia (difficulty in swallowing), dysgeusia (loss of taste), nausea, vomiting, unusual smells, anorexia, lethargy and exhaustion, to mention but a few. In addition, there are changes in protein and fat metabolism as well as in energy expenditure due to pathophysiological changes as a result of the carcinogenesis and inflammatory process (Deans *et al.* 2009). Indeed a recent review and study by these same authors (Deans *et al.* 2009) supports the view that not only does the production of pro-inflammatory cytokines such as interleukin 1, interleukin 6 and tumour necrosis factor lead to altered metabolism but also that serum acute phase protein concentrations are correlated with both total weight loss and rate of weight loss. Therefore, there is a need to understand how these factors lead to malnutrition and cachexia, and how the effects of dietary and nutritional support affect patient outcomes. Cancer cachexia is a multimodal problem (Fearon 2008) and is very challenging to practitioners and patients alike.

The multimodal approach of cancer management involving polychemotherapy, radiotherapy and surgery (Allum *et al.* 2002; Enzinger and Mayer 2003; Odelli *et al.* 2005) usually leads to poor nutritional status that requires nutritional support (Mekhail *et al.* 2001; Bidoli *et al.* 2002). In the last century, Dewys *et al.* (1980) noticed that the length of hospital stay was increased, and response to therapy and indeed survival rates of cancer patients were affected by malnutrition, while in the same period Burt and colleagues (1984) confirmed the latter two findings. During the same decade Robinson *et al.* (1987) and in subsequent years Ottery (1995) demonstrated the association of increased length of hospital stay in cancer patients with increased complications, reduced healing rate, higher healthcare costs and higher rates of mortality. Amazingly all these issues are still observable today, thus suggesting that the important issues relating diet and nutrition with cancer care have not yet been internalised by healthcare professionals to a level that, as yet, makes a significant difference. The use of gastrostomy feeding tubes such as percutaneous endoscopic gastrostomy (PEG) tubes to support patients in head and neck cancers has been discussed by several workers

(Tyldesley *et al.* 1996; Lee *et al.* 1998; Scolapio *et al.* 2001; Piquet *et al.* 2002; Lin *et al.* 2005). Generally these studies support the view that aggressive nutritional intervention has been found to be helpful in reducing weight loss and dehydration during chemoirradation and in improving the quality of life. It is important to consider other metabolic changes that occur due to nephrotoxicity resulting from a combination of therapies. For example, in the study by Lin *et al.* (2005) it was observed that during induction chemotherapy, there were no statistically significant changes in the weight, blood urea nitrogen (BUN) and creatinine. However, during chemoirradiation statistically significant, higher levels of BUN and creatinine as well as loss in weight were found when compared to pre-chemoirradiation levels. In addition, albumin, magnesium, potassium and sodium were decreased. These metabolic changes are important, as potassium and magnesium are intracellular ions while sodium and calcium are extracellular ions. Albumin is the most important colloid in influencing the osmotic pressure of body fluids.

One very important aspect that educationists need to consider in their discussion with practitioners is the issue of cancer-related fatigue, a recent review of which has been completed (Prue *et al.* 2006). In their review, different factors have been associated with cancer-related fatigue. From a nutritional perspective, it is not surprising that an association was found between fatigue and loss of appetite (Ahlberg *et al.* 2005); between fatigue and nausea and vomiting (Stone *et al.* 2000; Stone *et al.* 2001; Holzner *et al.* 2002); and between fatigue and diarrhoea (Stone *et al.* 2001; Holzner *et al.* 2002; Ahlberg *et al.* 2005). Loss of appetite, nausea, vomiting and diarrhoea all result in decreased food intake and reduced energy levels. But this is not the whole story. Malnutrition will result in inadequate minerals and vitamins, both of which are needed for various anabolic (synthetic) and catabolic (breakdown) pathways involved in protein and energy metabolism. An adequate intake of iron, for example, leads to low haemoglobin levels which has been associated with fatigue by several authors (Kallich *et al.* 2002; Hwang *et al.* 2003; Respini *et al.* 2003; Tchen *et al.* 2003; Jacobsen *et al.* 2004; Wratten *et al.* 2005). Prue *et al.* (2006) cite as many as 14 studies that found an association between anxiety and/or depression with fatigue. This is not surprising either, as both anxiety and depression, in relation to the disease process if not the prognosis, would lead to decreased food intake and reduced energy levels. Indeed although it is generally accepted that some people eat for comfort during depressed episodes, it is unrealistic to expect that this would occur in cancer patients.

MULTIPROFESSIONAL IMPLICATIONS

The scale of the challenge in communicating the issues that relate food, nutrition and cancer is such that it is unreasonable to expect individuals trained in a single discipline to teach the issues adequately. This suggests the need for a multiprofessional approach to teaching all the relevant aspects of cancer and palliative care in an integrative way within cancer care modules and programmes. This does not imply having all the multiprofessional team members in one room at the same time but that the approach taken needs to allow the practitioner to see how and where all the relevant information fits into his or her practice in terms of cancer care and to be able to relate it to practice. The active involvement of nutritionists and dieticians in communicating the issues of diet and cancer to practitioners is such an example. In this way, instead of treating many issues as peripheral or Cinderella topics, better integration of information could take place. So how should multiprofessional team members communicate this information? It is the author's view that when teaching about food and nutrition in cancer care, focus should not just be on current issues of how to manage diet and nutrition in cancer sufferers but also on ensuring that practitioners are fully aware of the causes of cancer and how to prevent or reduce risk. This is the whole notion of the double-edged sword. For example, it is important to communicate that it is not just the total fat and the saturated animal fat that is implicated in the causation of cancers of the breast, colon, endometrium, lung and prostate, but that methods of cooking such as grilling and barbecuing should be reconsidered as well.

Indeed the most pressing issue for most practitioners will be the need to know how to deal with the here and now in order to improve or maintain the quality of life. This brings us to the nature of food and diet that is consumed and is required to improve the current status.

NUTRITIONAL THERAPIES AND DIETARY MANAGEMENT

There are many unproven theories and misconceptions about which diets work in cancer although, indeed, some investigations on alternative diets have been done. Therefore, it is paramount for educationists to discuss dietary plans and ensure that accurate information is communicated to cancer sufferers by practitioners. Furthermore it is important to reinforce the fact that the choice to follow any dietary plan by patients is empowering and needs to be accepted.

The Bristol diet

The Bristol diet (Forbes 1984) recommends that fresh fruit, fresh fruit juices, fresh vegetables or fresh vegetable juices should be consumed for a limited period of time, with the rationale being to allow a period of detoxification that will facilitate physical, spiritual and general welfare improvement. The diet recommends avoiding caffeine, dairy products including milk and milk products such as cheese and yoghurt, sugar, salt and red meat. In addition, it recommends the consumption of produce that is organically grown and other whole foods such as organic fish, poultry and eggs. The Bristol diet was developed at the Cancer Help Centre in Bristol.

The Bristol diet has been criticised by practitioners for its emphasis on omitting foods that are considered important in diet and nutrition, such as dairy products and red meat; for removing components that add zest and taste to foods, such as salt and sugar; and for promoting organic produce that adds additional cost to the family budget. Ironically, although the diet was proposed over two decades ago, the important role of organic produce and whole grains in diet and nutrition is ever becoming more recognised by nutritionists and medical scientists. Whatever the shortfalls of the diet, its proponents recommend that the diet can be made to suit each individual and that adjustments need to made slowly – something one would feel is sensible advice.

The Gerson diet

The Gerson diet or therapy was developed by Max Gerson in the 1940s, initially to treat tuberculosis and later to manage cancer and degenerative diseases. The theoretical perspective and rationale was to focus on those factors that would facilitate the restoration of health and well-being, such as the role of enzymes, hormones, minerals and other dietary components. A review of the Gerson diet (McCarthy 1981) suggests that, in spite of methodological criticism of no proper trials and a lack of controls, testimonies from other medical practitioners before the Senate Select Subcommittee hearing in 1945 on cancer research support the view that the Gerson diet produced positive results of tumour regression, with one medical practitioner acknowledging his observation of severe pain relief in approximately 90% of cases. The Gerson diet places its emphasis on the consumption of raw fruit and raw vegetables together with their juices and recommends avoiding all processed foods, canned foods, dairy products, fats and spices. It also recommends consumption of a diet high in potassium and low in sodium. Thus, there is a high potassium-to-sodium ratio in the Gerson diet. Gerson increased the potassium content of his diet by potassium supplementation. One suggestion was that this diet might stimulate the production of aldosterone, a mineral-corticoid hormone produced by the adrenal cortex. A diet low in sodium triggers the release of aldosterone, which facilitates sodium reabsorption within the distal convoluted tubules and collecting ducts of the nephron and excretion of potassium. McCarthy (1981) hypothesises that aldosterone release may have immunostimulant or palliative properties that enhance host resistance to tumour growth. In Addison's disease, aldosterone is known to prevent vascular collapse by sensitising vascular muscle

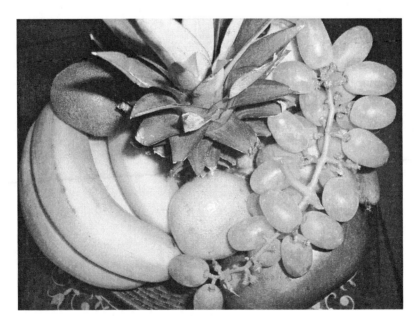

FIGURE 14.1 Several diets strongly promote the consumption of fresh fruit and fresh fruit juices for the health benefits these provide

to the catecholamines adrenaline (epinephrine) and noradrenaline (norepinephrine). In their studies with rats, Woodbury and Kock (1957) suggested that aldosterone increased intracellar potassium while lowering intracellular sodium in some tissues (brain and muscle), and (Hegyvary 1977) argues that aldosterone may regulate serum electrolytes. McCarthy (1981) argues that this decrease in intracellular water may be associated with the relief in pain reported by some patients taking the Gerson diet.

The consumption of a diet high in fresh fruit and vegetables (Figure 14.1 and Figure 14.2) means that the Gerson diet is high in both beta carotene and vitamin C as well as many other protective nutrients such as phenolic compounds that include flavenoids and eicosanoids. Certainly the eicosanoids, which are synthesised from omega-3 fatty acids, have lesser potent inflammatory and immunological effects on tissues, with the result that the immunological, inflammatory and oxidative stressors are reduced (Wahle *et al.* 2003). From a preventative perspective, the epidemiological evidence to support the view that high intakes of fruit and vegetables are associated with a reduction in various cancers of the gastrointestinal tract (oesophagus, gastric and colorectal) and of other organs (prostate, cervical, pancreatic and bladder) has been found to be consistent (Margetts and Buttriss 2003).

In addition, this diet possesses fewer toxins, free radicals or reactive oxygen species due to the absence of additives. One would have to accept that cancer cells generate many free radicals and endotoxins that require the combined effort of antioxidants to mop them up, admittedly with great difficulty since malignant cancers are vicious diseases.

The Macrobiotic diet

The Macrobiotic diet has been well described by Kushi *et al.* (2001) and Maritess *et al.* (2005). Developed in the 1960s by George Ohsawa, a Japanese philosopher, the diet is a lifestyle philosophical approach to healthy living incorporating not only healthy eating but also exercise, meditation, reduction of stress and minimising exposure to pesticides.

TABLE 14.1 Macrobiotic diet recommendations

Encouraged foods	Discouraged or eliminated foods
Complex carbohydrates – organically produced	High-protein foods
Cereal grains (40–60%)	Meat
Brown rice, barley, millet, oats, buckwheat	Poultry
Vegetables – organically produced (20–30%)	Animal fat
Beans (5–10%)	Dairy products
Chickpeas, lentils, tofu	Eggs
White meat, fish	Refined sugars
Fruit, seeds and nuts	Processed foods
	Pesticide-sprayed vegetables

Source: based on Maritess *et al.* 2005.

One misconception is that a macrobiotic diet is used to treat cancer. A macrobiotic diet is high in complex carbohydrates but low in animal protein and in fat. It recommends organically grown foods as well as a minimum of processed foods.

Kushi *et al.* (2001: 3058S) gave macrobiotic dietary guidelines that refer to the 'Great life pyramid' in which they highlight the foods that need to be consumed regularly (daily), occasionally (weekly) and optionally or infrequently or transitionally (monthly), to use their own terminology, while Maritess *et al.* (2005) have suggested components for an eating plan that may contain 40–60% cereal grains, 20–30% vegetables and 5–10% beans (Table 14.1). Thus, in addition to other treatment modalities, dietary changes could be used to prevent further development of the cancer (Pierce 2007).

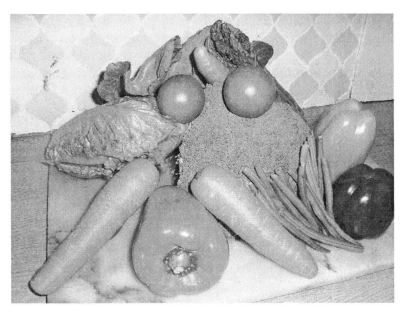

FIGURE 14.2 Several diets strongly promote the consumption of organically grown fresh vegetables for the health benefits these provide

Other characteristics that include age, gender, activity level, cultural food patterns, environmental food availability and traditional diet are all taken into account when formulating a diet or eating plan. It must be remembered that there are problems when formulating such a diet plan due to the additional expense of organic foods and the extra preparation time that is needed. Another challenge for many people is adhering to the diet plan. There is also the issue that some important nutrients such as calcium, protein, vitamin B12 and possibly energy may be deficient where both food planning and preparation may not be intensive enough. Furthermore in adolescents reduced bone mass (Parsons *et al.* 1997) and cobalamin (vitamin B12) deficiency (van Dusseldorp *et al.* 1999) have been highlighted. Thus, adopting these diets can be ill-informed where a limited nutrition knowledge base and inadequate dietary preparation are the order of the day.

The Gonzalez therapy

The Gonzalez therapy has its basis in offering an aggressive nutritional programme to individuals suffering from advanced cancer as well as other debilitating conditions such as chronic fatigue syndrome and multiple sclerosis (Gonzalez and Isaacs 2007). The therapy has its main basis in the use of pancreatic enzymes (amylase, trypsin and lipase) from a pig source that are taken orally by the cancer sufferer together with a dietary regime whose three main facets encompass individualised diets on a continuum ranging from raw vegetarian food to red meat-based diets; individualised supplement protocols that include micro elements, macro elements as well as vitamins; and intensive detoxification including the use of coffee enemas (Gonzalez and Isaacs 2007). These same two authors describe a rich history relating to the use of enzyme treatment in cancer going back over 100 years, which was first proposed in 1902 by Professor Beard at Edinburgh when he suggested trypsin as a powerful cancer inhibitor. Trypsin digests proteins in the duodenum but it is secreted in an inactive form as chymotrypsin by exocrine cells of the pancreas and activated by hydrochloric acid from the stomach, while amylase digests carbohydrates and lipase digests fats or lipids in the form of triglycerides. Gonzalez and Isaacs (2007) describe, very clearly, that their therapy is a progression of that used by Kelly in the 1960s in the USA. As is always the case with new therapies that do not fit the norm, Kelly was ostracised for his innovative approaches by his colleagues due to a lack of understanding of how the therapies work. Needless to say, many patients fail to improve and die while taking conventional drugs in mainstream hospitals. It would have been interesting to have discussed diet and nutritional issues relating to end-of-life and to patient and carer psychological well-being. Due to space constraints, this cannot be pursued here.

Future developments

The important role of antioxidants and the consumption of fresh foods and vegetables in the diet in whatever acceptable form to the individual will continue to be debated. However, more recently the debate on the role of functional foods (Webb 2006) and whole grains (Marquart *et al.* 2007) has commenced and there is prolific activity by scientists and nutritionists trying to clarify how these food substances are beneficial in both health and illness. Functional food or medicinal food is any fresh or processed *food* claimed to have a health-promoting or disease-preventing property beyond the basic function of supplying *nutrients*. The general category of functional foods includes *processed food* or foods fortified with health-promoting additives such as nutritional food supplements given to cancer patients. Both functional foods and whole grains are likely to have a more active role in prevention, including cancer prevention among other disease processes, by inhibiting detrimental pathophysiological pathways and mopping up free radicals that are damaging to cells.

HOW TO TEACH THE NUTRITION–CANCER RELATIONSHIP

Practitioners who wish to teach the relationship between nutrition and cancer need to consider the following approaches:

➤ seminar discussions that foster an understanding of the role of diet and nutrients

➤ use of case-based scenarios
➤ reflective practice on efficacy of conventional versus alternative (nutritional) therapy
➤ reflection in patient choices
➤ discussion on treatment/therapy options
➤ e-learning – encouraging students and fellow practitioners to access relevant web pages.

KEY POINTS

■ Cancer is a multidimensional problem that requires a multimodal management approach.
■ There is a nutritional basis for cancer prevention, cancer causation and cancer management.
■ Recognition of the interaction between cancer disease processes and nutrition is paramount in the management of cancer.
■ The important role of natural produce that includes fresh fruit, fresh vegetables and whole grains is underestimated.
■ Relevant education on the role of diet and nutrition is an imperative in cancer care and management.

CONCLUSION

Both educationists and practitioners alike must reflect on the observation that the increase in the incidence of certain cancers is consistent with a decrease in the consumption of fresh produce and an increased consumption of processed and refined foods. The complexity of cancers suggests that it is unlikely that nutrition and diet alone will be adequate to cure cancers. However, it is logical to argue that a diet high in natural fresh produce and with no additives must be of therapeutic value to the individual suffering from cancer and must have beneficial protective effects to the healthy individual. Just as Hippocratic medicine showed humility and passivity by believing in nature's healing powers, it is very relevant today, two and a half thousand years after Hippocrates, for educators, practitioners and patients to take stock and reflect on the important role of diet and nutrition both in health and in cancer. The sceptics need to accept that it is neither practical nor realistic to run large-scale dietary randomised control trials on individuals with terminal illness without withholding other treatment modalities.

IMPLICATIONS FOR THE READER'S OWN PRACTICE

It is important that the reader asks the following questions and attempts to answer them as honestly as possible for herself or himself.
1 What is your understanding of the role of diet and nutrients in health and disease?
2 How will you teach diet and nutrition differently as a result of reading this chapter?

3   How important is nutrition as a therapy option in your own practice area?
4   How might you actively involve the patient/client to increase dietary intake?
5   What plans do you have for incorporating these topics into your educational activities/portfolio in the future?

REFERENCES

Ahlberg K, Ekman T, Gaston-Johansson F (2005) The experience of fatigue, other symptoms and global quality of life during radiotherapy for uterine cancer. *Int J Nurs Stud.* **42**: 377–86.

Ames BN (1983) Dietary carcinogens and anti-carcinogens. *Science.* **221**: 1256.

Allum WH, Griffin SM, Watson A, Collin Jones D (2002) Guidelines for the management of oesophageal and gastric cancer. *Gut.* **50** (Suppl V): 1–23.

Bidoli P *et al.* (2002) Ten-year survival with chemotherapy and radiotherapy in patients with squamous cell carcinoma of the oesophagus. *Cancer.* **94**: 352–61.

Burt ME, Brennan MF (1984) Nutritional support of the patient with oesophageal cancer. *Semin Oncol.* **11**: 49–51.

Deans DAC *et al.* (2009) The influence of systemic inflammation, dietary intake and stage of disease on rate of weight loss in patients with gastro-oesophageal cancer. *Br J Cancer.* **100**: 63–9.

Dewys WD *et al.* (1980) Prognostic effect of weight loss prior to chemotherapy in cancer patients. *Am J Med.* **69**: 491–6.

Enzinger PC, Mayer RJ (1984) Oesophageal cancer. *New Engl J Med.* **349**: 2241–52.

Fearon KC (2008) Cancer cachexia: developing multimodal therapy for a multidimensional problem. *Eur J Cancer.* **44** (8): 1124–33.

Forbes A (1984) *Bristol Diet.* London: Ebury Press.

Ghadirian P, Lynch HT, Krewski D (2003) Epidemiology of pancreatic cancer: an overview. *Canc Detect Prev.* **27**: 87–93.

Gonzalez NS, Isaacs LL (2007) The Gonzalez therapy and cancer. A collection of case reports. *Alt Therapies.* **13**: 1–3.

Hegyvary C (1977) Effects of aldosterone and methylpredinisone on cardiac- (sodium-potassium ion) dependent ATPase. *Cell Mol Life Sci.* **33**: 1280–1.

Holzner B *et al.* (2002) The impact of haemoglobin levels on fatigue and quality of life in cancer patients. *Ann Oncol.* **13**: 965–73.

Hwang SS *et al.* (2003) Multidimensional independent predictors of cancer-related fatigue. *J Pain Symptom Manag.* **26**: 604–14.

Jacobsen PB *et al.* (2004) Relationship of haemoglobin levels to fatigue and cognitive functioning among cancer patients receiving chemotherapy. *J Pain Symptom Manag.* **28**: 7–18.

Kallich JD *et al.* (2002) Psychological outcomes associated with anaemia-related fatigue in cancer patients. *Oncology.* **16**: 117–24.

Kushi LH *et al.* (2001) The macrobiotic diet in cancer. *J Nutr.* **131**: 3056S–64S.

Lee JH *et al.* (1998) Prophylactic gastrostomy tubes in patients undergoing intensive irradiation for cancer of the head and neck. *Arch Otolaryng–Head Neck Surg.* **124**: 871–5.

Lin A *et al.* (2005) Metabolic abnormalities associated with weight loss during chemoirradiation of head-and-neck cancer. *Int J Rad Oncol Bio Phys.* **63** (5): 1413–18.

Margetts B, Buttriss J (2003) Epidemiology linking consumption of plant foods and their constituents with health. (Chapter 3.) In: Goldberg G, editor. *Plants: Diet and Health.* Oxford: British Nutrition Foundation and Blackwell Science: 49–64.

Maritess C, Small S, Waltz-Hill M (2005) Alternative nutrition therapies in cancer patients, seminars I. *Oncol Nurs.* **21** (3): 173–6.

Marquart L *et al.* (2007) *Whole Grains and Health.* Oxford: Blackwell Publishing.

McCarthy MF (1981) Aldosterone and the Gerson diet: a speculation. *Med Hypotheses.* **7**: 591–7.

Mekhail T *et al.* (2001) Enteral nutrition during the treatment of head and neck carcinoma. *Cancer.* **91**: 1785–90.

Odelli C *et al.* (2005) Nutrition support improves patient outcomes, treatment tolerance and admission characteristics in oesophageal cancer. *Clin Oncol.* **17**: 639–45.

Ottery FD (1995) Supportive nutrition to prevent cachexia and improve quality of life. *Seminars in Oncol.* **22**: 98–111.

Parsons TJ *et al.* (1997) Reduced bone mass in Dutch adolescents fed a macrobiotic diet in early life. *J Bone Miner Res.* **12** (9): 1486–94.

Pierce JP *et al.* (2007) Influence of a diet very high in vegetables, fruit and fibre and low in fat on prognosis following treatment for breast cancer: the women's healthy eating and living (WHELI) randomised trial. *JAMA.* **298**: 289–98.

Piquet M *et al.* (2002) Early nutritional intervention in oropharyngeal cancer patients undergoing radiotherapy. *Supp Care Cancer.* **10**: 502–4.

Potter JD [Chair] (1997) *Food, Nutrition and the Prevention of Cancer: a global perspective.* Washington, DC: World Cancer Research Fund/American Institute for Cancer Research: 1–16.

Prasad KN, Cole W, Hovland P (1998) Cancer prevention studies: past, present and future directions. *Nutrition.* **14** (2): 197–210.

Prue G *et al.* (2006) Cancer related fatigue: a critical appraisal. *Eur J Cancer.* **42**: 846–63.

Respini D *et al.* (2003) The prevalence and correlates of fatigue in older cancer patients. *Crit Rev Oncol Haematol.* **47**: 273–9.

Robinson G, Goldstein M, Levine G (1987) Impact of nutritional status on DRG length of stay. *J Parenter Enteral Nutr.* **11**: 98–111.

Scolapio JS *et al.* (2001) Prophylactic placement of gastrostomy feeding tubes before radiotherapy in patients with head and neck cancer: Is it worthwhile? *J Clin Gastroent.* **33**: 215–17.

Stone P *et al.* (2000) Cancer-related fatigue: inevitable, unimportant and untreatable? Results of a multi-centre patient survey. Cancer Fatigue Forum. *Ann Oncol.* **11** (8): 971–5.

Stone P *et al.* (2001) Fatigue in patients with cancers of the breast or prostate undergoing radical radiotherapy. *J Pain Symp Man.* **22**: 1007–17.

Tchen N *et al.* (2003) Cognitive function, fatigue, and menopausal symptoms in women receiving adjuvant chemotherapy for breast cancer. *J Clin Oncol.* **22**: 4175–83.

Tyldesley S *et al.* (1996) The use of radiological gastrostomy tube placement in head and neck cancer patients. *Int J Rad Oncol Bio Phys.* **22**: 98–111.

Van Dusseldorp M *et al.* (1999) Risk of persistent cobalamin deficiency in adolescents fed a macrobiotic diet in early life. *Am J Clin Nutr.* **69**: 664–71.

Wahle K, Lindsay D, Bourne L (2003) Plant and plant-derived lipids. (Chapter 10.) In: Goldberg G, editor. *Plants: Diet and Health.* Oxford: British Nutrition Foundation and Blackwell Science: 183–208.

Webb GP (2006) *Dietary Supplements and Functional Foods.* Oxford: Blackwell Publishing.

Woodbury DM, Koch A (1957) Effects of aldosterone and desoxycorticosterone on tissue electrolytes. *Proc Soc Exp Biol Med.* **94** (4): 720–3.

Wratten C *et al.* (2004) Fatigue during breast radiotherapy and its relationship to biological factors. *Int J Rad Oncol Biol Phys.* **59** (1): 160–7.

Yu H *et al.* (1991) Comparative epidemiology of cancers of colon, rectum, prostate and breast in Shanghai, China versus the United States. *Int J Epidem.* **20** (1): 76–81.

USEFUL WEBSITES

www.aicr.org/
www.bapen.org.uk/
www.cancer.gov/
www.wcrf-uk.org/
www.food.gov.uk/
www.health.gov/dietaryguidelines/
www.nice.org.uk/
www.nih.gov
www.nutritionsociety.org
www.quotationsbook.com

15

User involvement in palliative care education: beyond rhetoric and tokenism

Anne Bury

'In the medical community it is a time of extraordinary change of attitudes. The concept of "expert patient" is sweeping through the NHS and is fast replacing the concept of "patient as victim".'

Wardle (2002)

'As soon as you're diagnosed, the medical profession sees you as being the illness with a person attached. Actually you an ordinary person with something dreadful that has happened to you, absolutely dreadful. That doesn't mean that all the rest of your life isn't carrying on. Maybe you're going to have to withdraw from some of it because of the physical limits, but things like relationships are still there. So this picture is about how you are viewed: as the illness, a cancer patient in that bed, somebody who's had a colostomy. I don't blame anybody; I'm just saying how it feels.'

Tracy's story (Petrone 1999: 33)

AIM

This chapter will explore the current involvement of users in palliative care education and identify future opportunities to their input into cancer and palliative education.

LEARNING OUTCOMES

By the end of this chapter, the reader should be able to:

- understand the recent history of user involvement in healthcare
- demonstrate a critical understanding of user involvement in healthcare education
- consider the value and importance of involving a user perspective in healthcare and palliative care education
- explore some of the barriers to fully involving users within the educational process, particularly in the field of end-of-life care
- produce a framework for good practice for user involvement in palliative care education.

INTRODUCTION

User and carer involvement in healthcare and healthcare education is not a new concept. The World Health Organization (WHO) identified the importance of patients' involvement in their healthcare over 20 years ago (Flanagan 1999). Users, albeit as passive objects of paternalistic scrutiny and as a medium through which the student learnt, have always been involved in educating student health professionals (Hak and Champion 1999; Stacey and Spencer 1999).

However, the recent drive towards user involvement in healthcare and health education has been driven by a wish for the user to be an active rather than a passive participant.

This chapter will critically examine user involvement in education and suggest that to really involve users in an active way and avoid tokenism, we need to consider and understand the philosophies and rationale underpinning the new push for user involvement and examine the meaning of this for palliative care education. It will then provide an overview of user involvement in education, explore some barriers to effective participation and follow this with discussion of the value, importance and feasibility of involving users in educating professionals in end-of-life care. To conclude, a framework for good practice will be developed.

Reflecting upon and remembering our own experiences as users is encouraged, as those with a foot in both camps might be able to make 'a special contribution' (Wardle 2002).

I invite you to leave your comfort zone and be critical and questioning of palliative care and education, to be reflective about your own practice and experience. User involvement may assist us in own educational practice as we strive to encourage students to develop critical questioning, creative thinking, and self-awareness through reflective practice. It may also assist us to explore the value of the therapeutic relationship and self-care, and to facilitate interprofessional learning and team working.

USER INVOLVEMENT: WHO ARE USERS?

The term 'user involvement' is used as an umbrella term to describe a range of users and different degrees of involvement, which is often confusing for both service users and professionals. Taylor *et al.* identified five categories of service user, ranging across direct users, indirect users such as carers, potential users, excluded users, and proxy users such as persons or organisations advocating on behalf of users (Taylor *et al.* 1992). It is important to consider all of these in palliative care and also to include our own experience.

THE POLICY AGENDA: HEALTHCARE AND USER INVOLVEMENT IN EDUCATION

The late 1990s saw a number of policy initiatives recommending the involvement of users in the planning, development and evaluation of health and social care services at local, regional and national levels (DoH 1997, 1998, 1999a). Within these there was an explicit expectation that there should be increased patient and carer involvement in education programmes at all stages of the process from curriculum design to delivery and through to assessment (DoH 1999, 1999c; UKCC 1999; ENB 1996). Although recent policy documents recommend user and carer involvement in nurse education programmes, there has been little guidance as to how this could be achieved (Masters *et al.* 2002).

Since then there has been a plethora of further legislation, resulting in the development of the Patient Advice and Liaison Services (PALS) and Patient and Public Involvement Forums (PPI Forums) to identify views of local people about local health issues. A recent White Paper, *Our Health, Our Care, Our Say* (DoH 2006), actively consulted with users to establish what developments they would like to see and these are reflected in the future plans for primary care provision.

User involvement has been integral within recent policy initiatives for cancer and palliative care: *Calman Hine Report* (DoH 1995); *NHS Cancer Plan* (DoH 2000) and *Guidance on Cancer Services* (NICE 2004). In 2001 the Cancer Partnership Project was set up to implement and support the development of patient involvement in NHS Cancer Services.

The early hospice movement originally sought to involve users as partners in planning and delivery of services (Small and Rhodes 2000) and this continues to be a key recommendation in recent guidance from the National Council for Hospice and Palliative Care (2008).

Despite the apparent success of some initiatives and a recognition of the need for a cultural and organisational shift within the healthcare system, the user agenda is at present more 'rhetoric' than 'reality'.

Education of health professionals as well as users is seen as a key mechanism for success (Tritter *et al.* 2003). It is argued that all staff need training about what a user is and what user involvement is, and about the range of ways that might be deployed to involve users and the process by which it might be achieved (Tritter *et al.* 2003). Beresford argues that it is only through training that professionals will learn the skills required to work with users and develop user-centred practice (Beresford 1994).

USER INVOLVEMENT IN EDUCATION: A CRITIQUE

In April 2006 I attended a study day at St Christopher's Hospice, which included a debate on user involvement in palliative care. The motion was:

> 'It is a myth that user involvement in palliative care improves services or patients lives. It is instigated by governments intent on pushing a dubious public and patient involvement agenda in health care.'

Interestingly the majority present took the side opposing the motion. This provided me with a stark reminder of the need for critical questioning in palliative care. The motion was not against user involvement but questioned the value base and motivation behind it, thus helping us to understand the lack of success so far.

There are two distinct camps pushing the user agenda forward, and they hold conflicting philosophies, value bases and agendas (Croft and Beresford 1990).

One is the government-led agenda which purports that users as consumers should be at the centre of healthcare, with documents outlining a user-led agenda promoting a system shaped around the needs of the user rather than the other way around (Small 2003). It can be argued, however, that the focus of recent policy is primarily on the regulation of health professionals and soaring NHS costs, and on the need to create efficiency through the ever-increasing march of bureaucracy, financial constraints, devolved management and technological advances (Small and Rhodes 2000). In this context, it is argued, user involvement is 'consumerist rhetoric' which diverts attention away from the policy push and the reduction of patient–health professional therapeutic encounters in everyday practice. Furthermore, it masks structural inequalities and hierarchical institutional and professional practices (Small 2000). The introduction of consumerism, participation and empowerment is being used to justify contradictory ideological standpoints and realities (Ramon and Sayce 1993). Users are not being given real power to change the system but only to tweak elements about which they have been given a say (Small 2003).

The other driver of the user agenda is underpinned by the politics of empowerment, a collective and proactive approach in which power relations are reversed and whereby users are given control of their care and are directly involved in service development and delivery. In education, this has been led by pressure and advocacy groups who are dissatisfied with services located in a system that is paternalistic, oppressive and perpetuates dependency.

These groups wish to promote self-advocacy – for example, in the field of learning disability (Williams and Shoultz 1982) with groups such as 'People First', a co-operative of people with learning difficulties offering training about disability awareness (Mitchell 1992). Groups have also evolved in the field of mental health, such as Survivors Speak Out and Mindlink. They argue that user groups should be involved in the education of professionals in order to change and enhance the care that is provided and as an antidote to the overwhelming power of health professionals (Ramon and Sayce 1993; Croft and Beresford 1990). They also suggest that to have true partnership there needs to be a removal of the power imbalance (Newnes 2001).

Croft and Beresford (1990) argue that the politics of the supermarket does not sit happily with the politics of liberation. It detracts from rights-based collective agendas, and can be used to perpetuate existing power structures and mask inequalities by claiming a user perspective and thus discouraging dissent.

The hospice and palliative care movement is not exempt from this critique. Despite having developed as a protest and advocacy movement for people at the most painful and vulnerable time of their lives (Small and Rhodes 2000), it is accused of having being overtaken by a managerial agenda, shifting from 'vision to system' (James 1994). It is now driven by the goal of developing a medical specialism in its own right and with its own paternalistic practice (Clark 1993). It has, over time, become more reliant on health service funding and the proposed move to payment by results could enable the culture and practices of the managerial and efficiency agenda to further permeate hospices, so further removing the user voice from the care provided.

As educators, we need to be critical of social policy changes and the user agenda. We need to question our own motivations and value base and to explore whether we involve users as true partners or whether our own practice in involving users is at present rhetoric (Maslin-Prothero 2000) or tokenistic (Forrest *et al.* 2000).

When developing user initiatives, we must take care not to create a homogenous user/carer which hides the reality of inequity, inequalities, differences and cultures. We must be aware that the user agenda can provide a smokescreen detracting from a rights-based agenda and true user involvement and empowerment. However, we also need to keep a foot in the consumerist camp and be mindful of priorities identified from users' feedback and interweave these into our education (O'Neill 2005).

While there is evidence to suggest that the public now has a much higher expectation of the quality of service provided, is better educated and 'consumerist', and requires more information and greater involvement in decisions about treatments, in everyday practice this rarely happens (Towle 2000).

Recent research in primary care suggests that the power imbalance remains, with fewer than 10% of encounters meeting basic criteria for informed decision-making, such as discussion of the nature of the decision and asking patients for their preferences (Braddock *et al.* 1999; Craig and Umscheid 2009). Involvement in end-of-life decision-making is paramount. We need to consider our role in educating students and practitioners to enable greater involvement of patients and their families, particularly those who are unable to speak for themselves. We must identify ways in which to educate professionals to be aware of paternalistic practices, to unpick professional and institutional power in palliative care and be skilled enough to enable the user to be an equal partner in everyday end-of-life clinical encounters. In summary, we need to learn to 'care with' rather than 'care for'. Students need opportunities to learn with users rather than learning about and from professionally driven agendas and practices.

USER INVOLVEMENT IN EDUCATION: IS IT OF VALUE?

'It is important to use 'users' in training health professionals to help them better understand the issues and emotions of the patients they serve and care for. The invaluable

information through education, that patients can impart, is necessary to ensure better understanding, better communication and thus better care, which will surely lead to less misunderstanding, less mistakes, better patient management and quality of care, and ultimately less stress for health professionals. Health professionals need to be better supported in their work and that means better education about the needs of patients they care for, to enhance their relationship, both medical and empathic.

Health professionals cannot address the needs of their patients if they do not have a dialogue with the people they serve. This information and ultimate understanding is empowering; ignorance only leaves a gap open to misunderstandings, mistakes and bad experiences. Health professionals will continue to struggle, and patients will continue to feel dissatisfied, if this gap is not crossed. The experience of illness is not just medical but also emotional.

No one can communicate the experience like the 'users' themselves, and this can be imputed through many forms, art and literature or even the direct impact of appropriate patients attending, presenting or even leading seminars and workshops.' (Petrone 2006)

Regrettably, there is a dearth of literature and research on user involvement in education, with little systematic evaluation of the impact of user involvement in the classroom (Flanagan 1999).

Literature and research demonstrates that user involvement remains a marginal and passive endeavour and that patients have been largely underutilised as active participants (Wykurz 1999). A literature search for an article in the *British Medical Journal* in 2002 identified 1848 references involving patients in medical education from 1970 to 2001, with only 23 articles on active involvement. The latter is predominantly used only in a small part of the undergraduate curriculum and is rarely used in post-registration learning (Wykurz and Kelly 2002). The value of involving patients as *teachers* for the student can be seen in the following list:

➤ provides insight into the experience of the journey of the patient
➤ enhances understanding
➤ can provide useful feedback
➤ minimises anxiety
➤ develops confidence and self-awareness
➤ impacts on future attitudes and behaviour
➤ increases respect for patients
➤ contextualises learning.

For the educator it provides extra valuable alternative teaching resources, and in doing so improves the quality of the teaching (Wykurz and Kelly 2002).

BENEFITS FOR PATIENTS
Research on patients involved with medical education suggests that they benefit through talking about their problems, are able to learn more about their condition, and feel useful by being able to give something back. Furthermore, involvement gives

patients an opportunity to demonstrate their expertise (Stacy and Spencer 1999).

Patients, in a study of user involvement in medical student training with socially deprived communities, described the value of being listened to:

> 'Yes, yes, I felt relieved that someone's listening to me, you know someone's going to do something different you know, going to alter the system.' (Jackson et al. 2003)

A key factor therefore was the ability to influence and improve care provision and practice by improving students' understanding of their experience, thus helping to bridge to the theory and practice gap:

> 'I think the thing that I enjoy is that you can actually tell them the little things that would make your life easier.' (Jackson et al. 2003)

It can also be valuable as a cathartic (McMahon 1986) and therapeutic experience and helps users to feel valued (Costello and Horne 2001).

As a patient with multiple sclerosis who worked with nursing students shared:

> 'It made me feel good to be involved in something I felt confident about and it was satisfying to receive positive feedback, as lacking of self confidence comes with the patient's role.' (Costello and Horne 2001)

BENEFITS FOR STUDENTS

Involving users supports holistic care, as students are able to focus on the whole person and gain a deeper emotional, cultural and social understanding and to challenge stereotypes and attitudes (Jackson et al. 2003).

Research with nursing students suggests that they found 'It was beneficial to listen to a patient telling you about their actual experiences rather than a teacher telling you about hypothetical ones.'

It also helps to raise students' awareness of patients' expectations, and patients' perceptions of nursing care and for students to identify issues that were important to a carer/user, resulting in better understanding and empathy (McGarry and Thom 2004).

Involvement of real patients in problem-based learning enhanced communication skills and feelings (Sen Gupta 1997), and involvement in communication workshops showed real changes in behaviour.

Students also recognise that it helps to 'redress the power imbalance', resulting in users being viewed as experts:

> 'Yes, I think it's about the difference. In clinical practice, we're the experts but when they come into class, they're the experts – it's for them to have their say, it changes your perception.' (McGarry and Thom 2004)

Meeting users outside of practice, especially if they are in the role of spokesperson for a group of users rather than as a patient, can assist in students developing a critical consciousness (Ramon and Sayce 1993). It can even have emancipatory effect on students (Evans and Hughes 1993), in that it can bring core values and conflicts into the open.

BARRIERS TO LEARNING FROM USERS

It would appear that to be the most effective, user involvement needs to be embedded within the curriculum with students meeting users throughout their undergraduate experience (Jackson 2003).

However, the culture of learning in the NHS doesn't promote involvement, far less participation (Ingham 2001). The theory–practice gap is well documented (Smith 1992).

Professional education socialises students into a particular set of values, which distance them from their original motivation and reduce their ability to identify with users. In research undertaken by Smith, it was found that in the beginning of their training students felt that nursing was about people and caring, but after six months they talked instead about the need to know different techniques and investigations. The emphasis was more on the technical and cognitive aspects of healthcare. By their third year, knowledge was evaluated almost exclusively in relation to medical and technical content (Smith 1992).

The dominance of technical and cognitive knowledge over emotional and people-centred aspects of nursing resulted in nursing students minimising emotional learning. The gap between what is formally taught and the reality of everyday emotional challenges in practice left them feeling inadequate, unsure and defensive (Smith 1992).

Menzies' seminal study in 1970 demonstrated the numerous ways in which nurses learn to defend and protect themselves from individually identifying with patients, resulting in denial of feelings and avoidance of excessive involvement (Menzies 1970).

This is true to an even greater extent in medical education, where 'we first teach science and then we teach detachment' (Spiro 1993). Fourth-year medical students in the Patients as Partners Project had already learnt to distance themselves and felt angry and threatened when asked to reflect on their experiences about self-exposure (Newbury 1996).

User involvement in education could provide a bridge between user and student, and theory and practice, thereby countering the damaging effects of socialisation and preventing students from disconnecting both from themselves and their patients.

User involvement in education requires a paradigm shift (Warne and McAndrew 2005) and needs to challenge traditional power relationships. Professionals are in a power relationship with each other and over service users and relationships are created and maintained as forms of power (Hugman 1991). Educators play their part in this hierarchical system and create and reinforce the theory–practice gap, by prioritising technical and cognitive knowledge over 'user' knowledge and maintaining themselves in power relationships with students. Students need to question their own position as disempowered users of higher education. If empowerment and participation are given to users, then students need to also become experts in their own empowerment (Henderson 1994; Newbury 1996).

Partnership rather than passive involvement or consultation requires a redistribution of power between educational professionals and users (Beresford 1994) Using users as teachers reverses power relationship and challenges the traditional role of users as objects of study (Kelly 1995). Educators need to commit to users but also give up their own power struggle (Hopton 1994).

Given that user involvement is still a marginal endeavour, those educators committed enough to develop partnerships are often marginalised by colleagues and experience indifference, opposition and resistance (Newbury 1996).

To be effective, the involvement of users requires a strategic approach with organisational commitment, and a climate and culture that actively promotes and incorporates user involvement (O'Neill 2005). Educators need support and training to develop their understanding of the issues involved (Beresford 1994).

INVOLVING USERS: HAZARDS, BARRIERS, PITFALLS AND RISKS

Opponents of involving users often argue that users have a biased and unrepresentative view (McHaffie 1993). It is important to recognise that there is a double standard operating, as the representativeness of professionals, teachers and policy makers is not challenged in the same way (Beresford 1994).

While it is necessary to try to recruit users with a variety of experiences and backgrounds, it is important to remember that it is the individual's subjective experience which is of unique value regardless of their being representative (Newbury 1996).

While it is essential to avoid coercion and explore motivation for involvement, it is equally important to cause no harm, so confidentiality and consent are crucial (Bindless 1998). Being involved as a user can be traumatic and physically and emotionally draining when repeated sessions are undertaken (Ramon and Sayce 1993).

Both students and users can feel vulnerable. In one study, some students found patients' presence inhibiting and felt embarrassed about asking questions about terminal aspects of their illness (Costello and Horne 2001). In another study, students were worried about being blamed for everything that is wrong with the NHS and were concerned that users may have their own agendas and use the sessions as forums to vent unresolved experiences. Students may also feel guilty, ignorant and deskilled (Ramon and Sayce 1993).

Students' own background and experience may resonate with that of the user (Ramon and Sayce 1993). Students who have been users need to be seen as a resource, although they may be uncomfortable at disclosing their experiences for fear of discrimination or prejudice. Yet sharing their experiences needs to be encouraged and acknowledged as valuable in order that other students gain further understanding of professional practice and power relations (Rooke-Mathews 1993).

Some educators also question whether user involvement is a manipulative exercise to play on people's emotions to bring about attitude change (McHaffie 1993).

PALLIATIVE CARE EDUCATION: AN EXEMPLAR OR NOT?

Palliative care requires practitioners to be aware of and to learn the art and science of care as it involves connecting within a therapeutic relationship rather than just fixing patients' problems. Understanding the experience of patient and carer is therefore paramount if healthcare practitioners are to approach the situation from a patient's perspective rather than their own agenda. Given the espoused patient- and family-centred philosophy of palliative care, what better specialism is there to fully involve users in educating others about their needs and experiences? Multi-disciplinary working is fundamental to palliative care, and user involvement has been shown to be of immense value in interprofessional learning. It can help to overcome barriers to interprofessional working, conflicts of power, values and language (Barr 1994). Newbury argues that shared learning, reflective practice and user involvement challenge power differentials and help to overcome professional rivalries and attests that users can become both equal and expert (Newbury 1996).

Involving users may therefore help to redress the power imbalance and contribute to shifting the culture, values and practice of palliative care away from paternalism and back to 'partnership'. We need to consider our approach carefully and identify the knowledge, skills and attitudes needed for this cultural shift. Furthermore we need to be mindful of heightened emotional distress and the potential for distancing and detachment when educating and learning about death.

The premise of user involvement is that people need to be able to commit and contribute to and make recommendations for changes and developments in practice. This is particularly difficult when people are at the end of their lives or have been recently bereaved. Partnership and active involvement is demanding when people are fragile and vulnerable.

The challenge for us is how to involve patients and carers as 'active' agents in the process at such a difficult time. Ethical questions need to be raised about their vulnerability and the appropriateness of student practitioners being voyeurs of people's sadness and distress. We need to be even more mindful of the need to avoid tokenism and exploitation. While recognising that partnership is the ideal, users may well be too ill or even dead before this can take place. We need therefore to be strategic, creative and flexible, developing both direct and indirect approaches to enable the voice of the user to be heard and understood.

FRAMEWORK/GUIDELINES FOR USER INVOLVEMENT IN PALLIATIVE CARE

The majority of current practice in palliative care education, sadly but understandably, is focused around one-off involvement with users. However, the one-off encounter can still be set up as a partnership.

Four key areas need to be considered in this: preparation, communication, support and debriefing. The key areas for user involvement in palliative care according to Gordon *et al.* (2004) are preparation, communication, support and debriefing. These are useful headings to assist in the planning of educational activities to maximise learning. A framework for involving users in education, developed by Hamilton-Gurney

(1993), provides a useful starting point for the reader to consider examples of ways in which users are engaged in palliative care education. From among the options provided, the reader can then consider ways in which they personally could engage with users as partners in palliative care and end-of-life education.

A model for user involvement in palliative care education could be developed by adapting a framework from Hamilton-Gurney.

LEVELS OF USER INVOLVEMENT IN PALLIATIVE CARE EDUCATION

Material in this section has been adapted from Hamilton-Gurney (1993). Four levels of user involvement will be considered: one-off passive involvement; consultation; active involvement; participation/a partnership approach.

One-off passive involvement

The majority of user involvement in palliative care education will be of this type. Some of the opportunities and ways in which one-off passive patient involvement can take place are:

➤ during inpatient stays, when patients might meet with students on clinical placements, undergo physical examinations, present their histories, provide feedback and become involved in decision-making
➤ by patients agreeing to take part in multi-disciplinary case conferences, meetings and significant events
➤ by patients agreeing to take part in the classroom, in one-off sessions to multi-disciplinary or uni-disciplinary groups, to present their experiences
➤ by using elements of actual patient cases in simulated, problem-based learning
➤ by using narratives, journals, mass media, literature and art that represents patients' perspectives
➤ by using videos and recordings of patients and their families
➤ by using websites with patient/user experiences, such as Rosetta Life, MAP Foundation and Health Talk (*see* Further information section).

The following section provides a brief illustration of how a few of these techniques are used.

Passive involvement case studies

North Devon Hospice
Sessions involving users are built into university programmes and one-off workshops. Users volunteer or are invited to share their stories and provide feedback about their care, and have contributed to sessions on: understanding the emotional impact of illness; understanding the impact of caring; sharing the impact of chemotherapy; communication skills; breaking bad news; patients as active communicators with health professionals; and young people's experiences of bereavement. The aim is to support and empower the user to share whatever they wish in a way that they feel most comfortable with.

Process of setting up a session with a user
- The education facilitator meets the user two weeks before the session and listens to the user's story.
- Together they explore key points and ways in which they wish to share/discuss with the group.
- Options range from an open-ended discussion, a session with key headings, an interview with the facilitator or open questions from the floor. The option used will be whichever the user feels most comfortable with.
- The facilitator negotiates their role in supporting the user, including what support the user wishes to have if they get upset.
- The facilitator phones the user the day before to address any last-minute concerns.
- The students/group are briefed about the user and the possible impact on themselves of hearing a user's story.
- The role of the facilitator in the session is to introduce the user and the group, to establish a group agreement and to hold the space and boundaries of the session.
- The facilitator debriefs with user, ensures that they have the user's contact details and arranges to phone a week later to reflect on the experience or to debrief if required.
- The facilitator debriefs and reflects on the session with the group.

Countess Mountbatten House Hospice, Southampton
Half-day interprofessional workshops are offered to medical, nursing, physiotherapy, occupational health and social work students working together in small groups. Carers are selected at random to talk to a small group of students. The aim of these sessions is twofold: for students to understand the feelings and experience of carers as well as their own professional role within the multidisciplinary team. The workshop facilitator debriefs the carer and the group (Wee *et al.* 2007).

Saint Francis Hospice, Essex
Patients in education: telling your story
Patients from the day hospice are recruited to participate in 'goldfish bowl' sessions with medical students via an information leaflet and the day hospice staff. The participating patients are prepared and supported by the education team and then have the opportunity for further debriefing by staff within the day hospice.

Consultation case study

St Christopher's Education Advisory Group
A small group of service users and carers attend selected workshops and courses to monitor them and ensure that 'the patient is always present in the classroom'. The group then meets with the Director of Education on a quarterly basis to provide feedback and evaluation and to bring ideas and contribute to future planning for new programmes.

Active involvement

Some of the opportunities and ways in which active patient involvement can take place are:

➤ by developing ongoing reflective practice groups with equal numbers of learners and users, with shared ownership and input and co-facilitation

➤ by involving patients and carers in curriculum development as paid, trained and accredited teachers.

Active involvement case study

St Wilfrid's Hospice, Chichester

A patient who was an English lecturer and also a member of the local cancer network forum approached her local hospice education department to explore ways in which she could be involved in educating health professionals and others about the 'patient experience'.

She co-facilitated 'Learning to Live with Cancer' programmes with the Head of Education.

She then developed and co-facilitated three-day courses for health professionals, 'Tales from the other side'. These involved her sharing monologues of patients' stories obtained from the Learning to Live with Cancer programmes, and the Head of Education providing a theoretical input on the lived experience of illness, as well as partnership working and role-play.

The patient further recruited other members of the network user forum to share their stories. This bears some similarities to the work of the playwright Nell Dunn and her experiences, and the subsequent development of *Cancer Tales* as described in Chapter 2 of this book.

Participation: a partnership approach

Some of the opportunities and ways in which patient participation can take place are:

➤ via advocacy groups or individuals proactively leading education in their own right – i.e. local self-help groups

➤ by employing patients as lecturers, accredited teachers and facilitators. Develop sustained involvement via meaningful relationships rather than just one-off guest appearances: involve existing groups, network user groups, and bereaved people, and utilise the experience of professionals and educators as users.

A partnership case study

Michele Petrone, artist and cancer patient, was a pioneer as a user educator. A professional artist, following his diagnosis of Hodgkin's disease in 1994 he painted and wrote *The Emotional Cancer Journey*. This work was widely used by health organisations and medical institutions in education, and toured hospitals and public centres, including the Chelsea and Westminster Hospitals and extensive tours across East Sussex and Surrey. In 1998 Michele's first residency, at St Peter and St James Hospice in Sussex, helped patients and carers to 'colour' their feelings through paint. This work, *Touching the Rainbow*, was published in 1999.

Moving Pictures, in 2000, extended this work to health professionals. He has exhibited at The Royal Academy and The South Bank Centre in London. Michele was also an honorary lecturer at the Royal Free and University College of London Medical School, as well as at the University of Northumbria, and contributed regularly to the King's Fund NHS Chief Executives and Top Managers Programmes.

Michele gave workshops and presentations, around the emotional issues of illness, nationally and internationally. In 2000 he co-founded the MAP Foundation, to promote expression, education and understanding of the complex issues of serious illness and dying.

> 'Michele's teaching inspired medical and nursing students and hospice staff. Through his art and his words Michele offered students and colleagues a unique insight into the lived experience of illness. He helped people understand how important it is for doctors and nurses to bring their humanity, as well as their knowledge and skills, to all their interactions with patients. He gave them the courage to believe in themselves and renewed their sense of purpose and vocation. To be taught by Michele, or to encounter his work was to be, quite simply, changed.' (D Kirklin, Senior Lecturer in Ethics and Humanities, Royal Free and University College Medical School) (Kirklin 2007)

While the passive approach is valuable, it maintains the power imbalance. Involving users as partners requires creativity, courage and a critical awareness of complex structural and personal challenges.

There needs to be organisational ownership and a strategic approach, and practitioners, students, educators and users need to be educated and supported.

There needs to be careful planning, preparation, partnership, resourcing and evaluation at every stage. We as educators need to be effective communicators and group facilitators. We need to be able to deal with unresolved issues and support students and users who feel emotional or find the experience too intrusive. Both users and students need the opportunity to challenge, feed back and be debriefed and educators require regular supervision.

KEY POINTS

- User involvement in palliative care education is a double-edged sword. While it must be considered and valued as an important and integral part of professional development, equally it must not be invoked in a merely tokenistic way.
- Truly involving users requires a cultural and paradigm shift, and the questioning of paternalistic attitudes and values and of our own fears and concerns.
- Involving users requires organisational ownership and resourcing; it is not a

cheap option. It requires champions who are passionate about the 'user voice' and who are prepared to think creatively and develop innovation.

■ The current government agenda could support people in this. The guidelines and framework provided will go some way to assist you in developing user involvement in your programmes and in your workplace.

CONCLUSION

Despite the long history of learning from patients in medicine and healthcare, involving users as visible partners in the educational process remains in its infancy. Over decades the rhetoric of government initiatives has been to enhance involvement and the user voice. However, we must not be fooled into thinking this goal has been already achieved but must instead learn to gain a critical understanding of the processes of politics, power and organisational culture.

Involving users in palliative care education is challenging. There are now a number of examples of good practice to build upon. However, there are real ethical and practical barriers and challenges in involving people who are very ill or emotionally distressed in education. It is a struggle to fully integrate the user voice and we need to be creative and imaginative in developing approaches which fully capture the user experience.

The development of user involvement and cancer network partnership groups, user and self-help groups and user conferences could enable cancer sufferers and survivors to develop a more sustained involvement in education. Palliative care educators need also to consider ways of encouraging bereaved people as well as patients and carers to become more involved as active partners in the education process. Long-term partnerships may enable users to share their experiences along the illness carer journey, utilising innovative ways of telling their stories.

User involvement in education needs to become embedded in institutional, organisational and everyday practices. Professionals require education on the challenges of involving users as 'partners in care' through initial education and training through to professional development. All of us have been or are potential patients and carers, and this rich experience or potential needs to be revealed and explored in education. This and involving users in education will have an impact on end-of-life care and enhance relationships between professionals, patients and families.

IMPLICATIONS FOR THE READER'S OWN PRACTICE

1 Are you interested in developing true partnership and being a user champion?
2 Reflect upon the last time you were a patient and consider the imbalance of power you may have experienced. Identify what you would like to have fed back to those caring for you.
3 Reflect upon your workplace over a week. Look for examples of imbalance in power within your organisation, teams/departments and between professionals and patients. What small step could you take to challenge/change this?
4 Reflect upon a dying patient with whom you have worked. Consider what may have

been important for them to have shared about their experience of being ill. What do you think the ethical implications may have been if you were to have supported them in this?

5 Identify as many different ways as you can think of to enable users to be involved in your education programmes. Who else will need to be involved? How will you be able to recruit/involve users as partners in your programmes? Do you know any who may wish to develop their own programmes?

REFERENCES

Barr H (1994) *Perspectives on Shared Learning*. London: CAIPE.

Beresford P (1994) *Changing the Culture: involving service users in social work education*. Paper 32.2. London: CCETSW.

Bindless L (1998) The use of patients in health care education: the need for ethical justification. *J Med Ethics*. **24** (5): 314–19.

Blair T (2000) Needs of patients top the new NHS agenda. *National Health Service News*. Summer. Leeds: NHS Executive and DoH.

Braddock CH *et al*. (1999) Informed decision making in outpatient practice. *J Am Med Assoc*. **282**: 2313–20.

Chipp E, Stoneley S, Cooper K (2004) The clinical teacher: clinical placements for medical students: factors affecting patients' involvement in medical education. *Med Teach*. **26** (2): 114–19.

Clark D (1993) Whither the hospices? In: Clark D, editor. *The Future for Palliative Care: issues of policy and practice*. Buckingham: Open University Press: 167–77.

Costello J, Horne M (2001) Patients as teachers? An evaluative study of patients' involvement in classroom teaching. *Nurse Educ Pract*. **1** (2): 94–102.

Craig A, Umscheid MD (2009) Should guidelines incorporate evidence on patient preferences? *J Gen Intern Med*. **4** (8): 988–90.

Croft S, Beresford P (1990) *From Paternalism to Participation: involving people in social services*. London: Open Services Project and Joseph Rowntree Foundation.

Department of Health (1997) *The New NHS: modern, dependable*. London: DoH.

Department of Health (1998) *A First Class Service: quality in the new NHS*. Health Service Circular. London: DoH.

Department of Health (1999a) *Saving Lives. Our Healthier Nation*. London: HMSO.

Department of Health (1999b) *Patient and Public Involvement in the New NHS*. London: HMSO.

Department of Health (1999c) *Making a Difference: strengthening the nursing, midwifery and health visiting contribution to health and health care*. London: HMSO.

Department of Health (2004) *Getting over the Wall: how the NHS is improving the patient experience*. London: HMSO.

Department of Health (2006) *Our Health, Our Care, Our Say*. London: HMSO.

Department of Health (1995) *Calman-Hine Report. Policy Framework for Commissioning Cancer Services: a report by the Expert Advisory Group on cancer to the chief medical officers of England and Wales*. London: HMSO.

Department of Health (2000) *The NHS Cancer Plan: a plan for investment, a plan for reform*. London: DoH.

English National Board for Nursing, Midwifery and Health Visiting (1995) Involving service users and carers in education and training development and evaluation. *ENB News.* **17**.

English National Board for Nursing, Midwifery and Health Visiting (1996) *Learning from Each Other.* London: ENB.

Evans C, Hughes M (1993) *Tall Oaks from Little Acorns: the Wiltshire experience of involving users in the training of professionals in care management.* Devizes: Wiltshire Community Care User Involvement Network and Wiltshire Social Services Department.

Evans T, Seabrook M (1994) Patient involvement in medical education. *Br J Gen Pract.* **44**: 479–80.

Farrell C, Gilbert H (1996) *Health Care Partnerships.* London: King's Fund.

Flanagan J (1999) Public participation in the design of educational programmes for cancer nurses: a case report. *Eur J Cancer Care.* **8** (2): 107–12.

Forrest S, Risk I, Masters H, Brown N (2000) Mental health service user involvement in nurse education: exploring the issues. *J Psychiatr Ment Health.* **7** (1): 51–7.

Gordon F *et al.* (2004) Involving patients and users in student learning: developing practice and principles. *Int J Integr Care.* **12**: 28–35.

Grayley R, Nettle M, Wallcroft J (1994) *Building on Experience: a training pack for mental health service users working as trainers, speakers and workshop facilitators.* London: NHS Executive.

Gupta K (1995) Medical education. *Lancet.* **345**: 1440.

Hak T, Champion P (1999) Achieving a patient centred consultation by giving feedback in its early phases. *Postgrad Med J.* **75** (885): 405–9.

Hamilton-Gurney B (1993) *Public Participation in Health Care Decision Making.* University of Cambridge: Health Services Research Group.

Harrison C, Beresford P (1993) Using users. *Community Care.* **1009**: 26–7.

Henderson J (1994) Reflecting oppression: symmetrical experiences of social work students and service users. *Soc Work Educ.* **13** (1): 16–25.

Hendry GD, Scheiber L, Bryce D (1999) Patients teach students: partners in arthritis education. *Med Educ.* **33**: 674–7.

Hogg C (1994) *Beyond the Patient's Charter: working with users.* London: Health Rights.

Hopton J (1995) User involvement in the education of mental health nurses: an evaluation of possibilities. *Crit Soc Pol.* **42**: 47–60.

Hoyes L *et al.* (1993) *User Empowerment and the Reform of Community Care.* Bristol: School for Advanced Urban Studies.

Hugman R (1991) *Power in Caring Professions.* Basingstoke: MacMillan Educational.

Illich I (1976) *Limits to Medicine.* Harmondsworth: Penguin.

Ingham M (2001) How patients can contribute to nurses' education. *Nurs Times.* **97** (24): 42–3.

Jackson A, Blaxter L, Lewando-Hundt G (2003) Participating in medical education: views of patients and carers living in deprived communities. *Med Educ.* **37**: 532–8.

James N (1994) From vision to system: the maturing of the hospice movement. In: Lee R, Morgan D, editors. *Death Rites: law and ethics at the end of life.* London: Routledge: 102–30.

Kelly D, Wykurz G (1998) Patients as teachers: a new perspective in medical education. *Educ Health.* **11**: 369–77.

King's College, London, and Worthing and Southlands Hospitals NHS Trust (2004) *Formative Evaluation of Cancer Partnership Project, Final Report.*

Kirklin D (2007) Tribute to Michele Petrone. Available at: www.mapfoundation.org/ (accessed 12 November 2008).

Maslin-Prothero S (2000) The rhetoric of user participation in health care [guest editorial]. *Nurs Educ Today.* **20** (8): 597–9.

Masters H *et al.* (2002) Involving mental health users and carers in curriculum development: moving beyond 'classroom' involvement. *J Psychiatr and Ment Health Nurs.* **9** (3): 309–16.

McGarry J, Thom N (2004) Users and carers view their involvement in nurse education. *Nurs Times.* **100** (18).

McHaffie HE (1993) *The Care of Patients with HIV and AIDS: a survey of nurse education in the UK.* Edinburgh: Institute of Medical Ethics, Department of Medicine, University of Edinburgh.

McMahon RA (1986) *Nursing as Therapy.* King's Fund: London.

Menzies IEP (1970) *The Functioning of Social Systems as a Defense Against Anxiety.* London: Tavistock Institute of Human Relations.

Mitchell D (1992) Running out of excuses. *Community Care.* **946**: 22–3.

National Council for Hospice and Palliative Care (2008) *Listening to the Experts. A summary of 'User involvement in palliative care: a scoping study'.* London. National Council for Hospice and Palliative Care.

National Institute for Clinical Excellence (2004) *Guidance on Cancer Services: improving supportive and palliative care for adults with cancer.* London: NICE.

Navarro V (1976) *Medicine Under Capitalism.* New York: Prodist.

Newnes C (2001) Clinical psychology, user involvement and advocacy. *Clin Psychol Forum.* **150**: 18–23.

O'Neill F (2005) Beyond the tick box: strategic direction to patient involvement in education. In: Warne T, McAndrew S, editors. *Using Patient Experience in Nurse Education.* Palgrave: Basingstoke.

Osler W (1905) The hospital as college. In: *Aequanimatus, to medical students, nurses and practitioners of medicine and other addressees.* London: HK Lewis.

Petrone MA (1999) *Touching the Rainbow: pictures and words by people affected by cancer.* Sussex: England Health Promotion Department.

Petrone M (2006) Notes prepared by Michele for the author (unpublished).

Ramon S, Sayce L (1993) Collective user participation in mental health: implications for social work education and training. *Issues Soc Work Educ.* **13** (2): 53–70.

Rixon W-Y (1995) Patients as partners. *Users Alliance for Health.* **3**: 4–5.

Rooke-Mathews S (1993) Working users. *Comm Care.* **980**: 14–15.

Salter R (1996) Learning from patients: unfashionable but effective. *Postgrad Med.* **72**: 385.

Sen Gupta TK, Hays RB, Jacobs HJ (1997) Problem based learning using ambulatory patients. *Res Dev Problem Based Learning.* **4**: 574–8.

Small N, Rhodes P 92000) *Too Ill to Talk? User involvement and palliative care.* London: Routledge.

Small N (2003) The changing National Health Service, user involvement and palliative care. In: Monroe B, Oliviere D, editors. *Patient Participation in Palliative Care: a voice for the voiceless.* Oxford: Oxford University Press.

Smith P (1992) *The Emotional Labour of Nursing: how nurses care.* Basingstoke: MacMillan.

Spencer J *et al.* (2000) Patient-orientated learning: a review of the role of the patient in the education of medical students. *Med Educ.* **34**: 851–7.

Spiro HM (1993) What is empathy, and can it be taught? In: Spiro HM *et al.*, editors. *Empathy and Practice of Medicine: beyond pills and the scalpel.* New Haven, CT: Yale University Press.

Stacey R, Spencer J (1999) Patients as teachers: a qualitative study of patients' views of the role in a community based undergraduate programme. *Med Educ.* **33** (9): 688–94.

Taylor M, Hoyes L, Lart R, Means R (1992) *User Empowerment in Community Care: unravelling the issues.* Bristol: School for Urban Studies.

Towle A, editor (2000) *Community-based Teaching: change in medical education.* London: King's Fund.

Tritter J, Daykin N, Evans S, Sanidas M (2003) *Improving Cancer Services Through Patient Involvement.* Oxford: Radcliffe Publishing.

Twinn SF (1995) Creating reality or contributing to confusion? An exploratory study of client participation in student learning. *Nurse Educ Today.* **15** (4): 291–7.

United Kingdom Central Council (1999) *Fitness for Practice: the UKCC Commission for Nursing and Midwifery Practice (the Peach Commission Report).* UKCC: London.

Wardle J (2002) Physician heal thyself. *Observer Review.* 17 March.

Warmsley J (1995) Helping ourselves. *Community Care.* 1–7 June: 26–7.

Warne T, McAndrew S (2005) *Using Patient Experience in Nurse Education.* Basingstoke: Palgrave.

Wee B (2007) Teaching large groups. In: Wee B, Hughes N, editors. *Education in Palliative Care.* Oxford: Oxford University Press.

Williams B, Grant G (1998) Defining 'people centredness': making the implicit explicit. *Health Soc Care Community.* **6** (2): 84–94.

Williams P, Shoultz B (1982) *We Can Speak for Ourselves.* London: Souvenir Press.

Wykurz G (1999) Patients in medical education: from passive participants to active partners. *Med Educ.* **33**: 634–6.

Wykurz G, Kelly D (2002) Learning in practice. Developing the role of patients as teachers: literature review. *Br Med J.* **325**; 818–21.

FURTHER INFORMATION

- Monroe B, Oliviere D, editors (2003) *Patient Participation in Palliative Care: a voice for the voiceless.* Oxford: Oxford University Press.
- Small N, Rhodes P (2000) *Too Ill to Talk? User involvement and palliative care.* London: Routledge.
- MAP Foundation: www.mapfoundation.org
- healthtalkonline (website of DIPEx): www.healthtalkonline.org
- Rosetta Life: www.rosettalife.org

ACKNOWLEDGEMENT

I would particularly like to thank my old colleague and friend Jenny Newbury for her contribution to this chapter via her 2006 Masters dissertation.

16

A patient and carer course: 'I have friends in the same boat'

Janis Hostad and Sally-Ann Spencer Grey

'The mere imparting of information is not education. Above all things, the effort must result in making a man think and do for himself.'

Carter G Woodson

AIM

The aim of the chapter is to illustrate the importance of patient and carer education in cancer and palliative care, and to demonstrate the benefits of a patient and carer course.

LEARNING OUTCOMES

By the end of this chapter, the reader should be able to:
- discuss the importance of patient and carer education in cancer and palliative care
- explore the benefits of running such patient and carer courses
- discuss different approaches, and illustrate one working model for patient and carer course delivery to this client group
- share an educational methodology, and present teaching approaches for a cancer and palliative care patient and carer course.

INTRODUCTION

This chapter is designed to allow the reader to peruse the history, drivers, educational theory and background to one method of patient and carer education for cancer and palliative care patients. This strategy is easily transferable and would be useful as a framework to develop a unique course to fit the reader's requirements.

Education allows vulnerable patients to adapt more effectively, so that positive outcomes for themselves, their families and society may be more widely achieved (Walker *et al.* 2005).

The National Health Service has provided healthcare professionals with the opportunity to deliver patient and informal carer health education. In the past this has generally been related to a specific disease, for example, arthritis and diabetes. The patient was usually the primary beneficiary of this education, with informal carers as incidental recipients. This education was designed to inform the individual about their disease and its treatment. Its intention was to inform and educate regarding health promotion and self-management activities. It may have involved some specific skills training, for example, stoma care. Informal carers were rarely identified as needing information and education about the patient's disease, illness and treatment, in their own right. This only became the primary focus of education and training when there were care tasks to undertake for the patient which required specific skills training, such as care-giving, lifting and handling. The impact of education was rarely assessed or evaluated.

Has this changed: is it any different today?

It is now recognised that written information should be provided to patients to support any verbal information and education, and must be tailored to their needs. However, within the NHS, information is rarely made available to informal carers which is uniquely tailored to their specific needs. It is even rarer that carer information and education needs are identified in their own right. Information to what the caring role may require, such as changes to lifestyle, to relationships, to their health, are uncommon. Though patient information may address how their disease might progress, the impact of disease progression on carers is rarely addressed. Information specifically designed for carers, usually highlights welfare benefits and finance, or access to practical and sometimes emotional support.

The information needs of informal carers, while still limited, are often better addressed by the voluntary sector by disease-specific groups, associations and charities. Some of these organisations are performing this function very efficiently (the Alzheimer's Association, for example). General carer resources do also have a wealth of information and advice, but sometimes it can be difficult for an individual to access these resources. Consequently there is little help to facilitate access, and there is little which is specific to cancer and palliative care.

SO WHAT DOES THE PATIENT CARER COURSE DELIVER THAT ISN'T ALREADY AVAILABLE?

Patient and carer education is a combination of information provision, learning and support. It aims to contextualise and support patients' and carers' adaptation and coping, by giving them understanding of their situation and of themselves. It also aims to reduce uncertainty, and to enhance quality of life for both, encouraging a sense of togetherness, and hopefully enhancing their relationship as a result. In addition, it encourages communication and sharing with, and between, health and social care professionals and participants. It is therefore essential that patient and carer education is an integral part of the service that is offered.

'Information is an important part of the patient journey, and a key element in the overall quality of patient experience' (DoH, accessed 2003). Regarding cancer, information, alongside support and specialist care, helps patients and their families to cope with the cancer and the cancer journey (Calman–Hine Report 1995; DoH 2000a; DoH 2000b; DoH National Patient and Cancer Patient Surveys 1998–2003; NICE Guidance for Supportive and Palliative Care 2004).

Information promotes autonomy

The capacity to exercise control over one's own functioning and events which affect one's life is the essence of humanness (Bandura 2001); it is autonomy. According to Williamson:

> 'The principles most important regarding patient autonomy are information, access, equity, respect, choice, shared decision making, safety, support, redress, and representation (Williamson 2001). Of these, information is the keystone' (Williamson 2003: 73).

Information is supportive

Patients initially are more likely to be attracted to support opportunities which focus on technical knowledge, information-giving and anticipating patient needs, and consider these more important than those opportunities which are marketed as providing emotional support (Larson 1986; von Essen and Sjoden 1991, Larsson et al. 1998).

However, patients report that they gained unanticipated emotional support from information-focused opportunities, which challenges assumptions that professionals may have about the nature of emotional support for patients (Skilbeck and Payne 2003).

Similarly, informal carers need information too, education and support during the patient's illness (Ramirez et al. 1998). In some research (Eriksson and Lauri 2000), informational needs are rated at a higher level than support needs.

Education is supportive

It has been known for some time that educating patients can reduce anxiety and increase patient satisfaction (Poroch 1995), and also that provision of an appropriate social environment for patients may be as important as one-to-one counselling (Langley-Evans and Payne 1997). There is much written, however, about the lack of education opportunities available to address these patient and carer needs (Hostad et al. 2004), but there is still little being done to remedy the problem.

It is interesting that 'students' in learning communities provide social, emotional and intellectual support for each other (Kuh et al. 1991), with the students in this instance being patients and carers. The result is 'social capital', in that the relationships between people enhance those people's abilities (Spencer Grey 2004). This social capital has been recognised in self-help groups for cancer patients (Adamsen and Rasmussen 2003), and in this qualitative research study, the role of the nurse as a social networker who encourages relationships between fellow patients has been highlighted. This corresponds well with the facilitator roles required to deliver patient and carer education.

It is recognized that learning is facilitated or hampered by emotions (Boekaerts 1993; Goleman 1995), and that emotions drive learning and memory (Sylvester 1994). This literature clearly indicates the usefulness of such education, including the social support of this vulnerable group.

WHAT ARE THE BENEFITS?

The authors of this chapter have surveyed patients and carers and healthcare professionals involved in each course, and the following illustrates the main themes identified. This includes the benefits that each stakeholder group feels it has gained from its involvement in a patient and carer course.

For patients and carers, a course can:
➤ improve adaptation and coping, by teaching how to manage stress, enable self-regulation and examine power issues, and by extending knowledge, understanding and self-development, thereby reducing the unknown
➤ improve personal relationships, by increasing understanding and communication and helping participants to get 'over the hump' or 'barrier' of putting on a 'brave face', being in control, not showing vulnerability, etc.
➤ improve interpersonal communication – between family members, between patient and informal carers (as well as formal carers), with the GP and with other health and social care professionals
➤ improve knowledge of how to access and understand conventional treatment, by increasing understanding of past, present and future events
➤ increase understanding of how to access complementary therapies, by examining the pros and cons, and preferences, how to be safe, what might work, and healthcare professionals' attitudes (such as reluctance, or support)
➤ provide peer support, assisting with empathy, normalisations, sharing and listening
➤ encourage greater autonomy, as outlined below:
  — by examining concepts of 'self-management', where health and healthcare are based on sharing knowledge, and encouraging users to take control
  — by promoting informed, shared decision-making, which ensures that patients and carers are part of the healthcare process, and that they can have their say, negotiate care levels and come to decisions together with health and social care professionals.

For health and social care professionals, a course of this type can:
➤ improve knowledge and understanding of patients' and carers' issues
➤ improve professional relationships, both with patients and carers and with colleagues
➤ improve interpersonal communication, both with patients and carers, and with colleagues

> ➤ improve practice, by their being more informed and aware
> ➤ promote advocacy, by their being better informed regarding patient and carer concerns and wishes, and thus better able to advocate on the users' behalf
> ➤ promote informed, shared decision-making, encourage self-management and autonomy
> ➤ promote user involvement – including improved understanding of the benefits of user involvement, better communication with users, and greater trust in patients' and carers' capacity for autonomy. User involvement is concerned with the meaningful and active participation and consultation of service users (patients, clients and carers) according to ability 'from their unique perspective' (Munroe and Oliviere 2003). User involvement is discussed in much greater detail in the next chapter.

Interestingly there were no negatives, other than that many participants wanted more time spent on all subjects – however, they did not want a longer course.

COURSE DELIVERY MODELS

At present, there is a wide range of different approaches employed to provide patients and carers with information and support. For example, there are support groups, self-help groups, and a variety of information and education sessions. The authors have, over the years, been involved in, and worked with, many of these approaches, and with different groups. Commonly, the groups were patients or carers, but sometimes combined groups were held. Having evaluated all these different models, the current patient and carer course is the only one to have had universally good evaluations by all the attendees, and by the facilitators.

THIS APPROACH
Course delivery timeframe

The course is delivered over five or six consecutive weeks.

The use of gap weeks can be introduced, to accommodate bank holidays or times of poor attendance, for example at peak holiday times.

The course should be kept short and focused, in order to promote independence and empowerment, and to reduce the possibility of any unhelpful dependency developing.

The course runs for one day per week.
> ➤ It can be run as a half-day, which might be easier for some patients and carers to attend. However, this can compromise the aims and outcomes, by not covering all the course content.

The daily schedule runs from 9.30 a.m. to 12 noon, followed by lunch, then 1.00 p.m. to 3.30 p.m. (approximately).

> For the first half-hour and last half-hour of the day, and lunchtime, everyone is together.
> Between 10 a.m. and 12 noon, and 1.00 p.m. and 3.00 p.m., family members/carers and the people with cancer are in separate groups.

The first half-hour in the morning session enables socialising, and time for housekeeping, any questions or general reporting back on homework from the previous week, which can then be developed as necessary in the two groups.

Lunch is a social occasion, a time to compare notes, to be reassured that your loved one is alright, and to touch base with the real world again. Facilitators (and maybe other volunteers) are also present. Conversation is kept light and simple. Participants reported valuing this time to share their experiences and to socialise.

The closing half-hour brings people back together with a brief sharing of issues produced by each group (agreed in advance), setting any homework, and evaluating the learning for this week. It seems to reduce emotional intensity, and brings people back to each other, making them feel emotionally safe before leaving. This section of the day, the authors feel, is one of the key elements which contribute to the success of the course. The sharing of issues between the groups as a collective seems to validate the issues, while to an extent ensuring that they remain anonymous. It is important to have these issues raised in such a way that no one person is singled out. Equally, such issue-sharing engenders a feeling for each individual that their issues and emotions are legitimate. The reason for this is that they have agreed, and are happy to have this brought out into the open; there is a bit of a 'see, it isn't only me' feeling, too.

A result of this sharing seems to be a bringing together of patient and carer, in a deeper level of understanding of each other's experiences and feelings. It also seems to negate any collusion between them about not saying how each is really feeling, for fear of hurting the other, and so in a gentle and supportive way it helps to restore honesty and trust. Repression can lead to uncontrolled and unpredictable emotional outbursts, emotional lability, or a lack of emotional expression, which can affect closeness. It takes much more energy to maintain secrets, collusion and repressing true feelings and emotions. However, being able to share, to be honest, yet sensitive, to communicate openly, is much less stressful, according to the participants. Energy levels are often already impaired due to illness, or side-effects of treatment, and stress. Mechanisms which can help to conserve, or make best use of, internal resources can only be of benefit.

Facilitation

Two facilitators are needed. These can be two healthcare professionals, or a healthcare and social care professional, or a healthcare professional and an educator, complementary therapist, counsellor or spiritual care advisor. It could also be run by two educators who have a background in cancer care and have a high level of communications skills.

Both facilitators are needed because they will have complementary professional skills. One needs to have expertise in the disease(s) of the patients attending (for example, cancer) and to be knowledgeable about healthcare systems.

Both facilitators need to be skilled communicators and facilitators. This not just about having good communication skills, though these are needed, too. They need a deeper dimension as well, encompassing linguistic, intellectual and experiential resources, in order to be able to reflect on the context and the relationships involved, and to gauge the effects of different ways of interacting by all participants (Hostad 2004).

Good communication skills will include being able to communicate empathy, genuineness and unconditional positive regard.

Some counselling, or therapeutic communication skills, and experience in facilitating groups, are needed, together with some life experience.

Having two facilitators enables the course to continue if individual support is needed by a participant. There are times when individuals need time out from the group, with a facilitator.

These facilitator skills are essential to ensure the smooth running of the group, as sometimes tensions do develop. This can be between different personalities, between patient and carer, or when topics are raised by one person which another feels uncomfortable about, or not quite ready to discuss at that point. In the main these issues can be successfully dealt with in the group, but occasionally one of the facilitators needs to spend time with the individual(s) in order to help them with their problems.

Attendance

Participants can attend as many, or as few, sessions as they wish. However, attendance at the first session is mandatory. It is hoped that they will come to all the sessions, but it is recognised that ill-health, treatment and family issues may affect attendance.

The patient, or their family member or carer or friend, can attend on their own or with each other (this may vary over the duration of the course). It is suggested that only one family member or carer attends, and that the same person comes along each time, because:

➤ having the same person attend each time enhances group cohesiveness and development
➤ introducing new members to an established group can be disrupting and uncomfortable for all parties.

If the same carer, family member or friend cannot attend each week, then another person can be introduced, but with prior agreement from the group. Though this sounds a formal process, it is really just involves a brief question. The group is usually very understanding and accepting. In fact, no issues have arisen from this in the past, and often the person coming new into the group is already 'known' to the group, because the patient or other carer or friend will have mentioned them to the group before.

Whole families cannot be accommodated within the course, but separate arrangements may be made if necessary.

Target audience: who is it for?

➤ Within the oncology department, this will be for adults with a cancer diagnosis, regardless of stage.
➤ Within the wider supportive and end-of-life care setting (supportive, palliative

and terminal care), it can be any adult with a life-limiting or progressive degenerative disease, regardless of diagnosis and stage (for example, cancer, neurological disease or organ failure).

➤ Adult family members, carers, or those significant to the patient, such as friends, can attend also.

➤ On occasion, with prior agreement with the facilitators and the group, children or young people significant to the patient can attend, but they must be accompanied by the patient, or a known family member or carer, who has been attending the course.

The presence of children and young people can affect the nature and quality of interactions. Some participants may feel inhibited by the presence of children. Attendance of children is not common, but is always negotiated with the group. If it is agreed that they will attend, then this will be for part of the day only. Children must be accompanied to ensure appropriate support and safety, and to adhere to child-protection recommendations. The content of that session may be altered to accommodate a child's presence, depending upon the topic or their age. Further support may be required.

In addition, a special session can be introduced, orientated around the children and young people. This, too, is negotiated with the group, and additional facilitation is essential, involving a person with particular expertise and experience of working with young people.

The latest development in the process is to hold one specific session during the course, where children and young people are targeted and invited to attend. This is facilitated completely separately from the main group. This approach seems to be the least disruptive to the main group, and provides the best feedback from the children.

How and why does it work?
Information

Information (at the right time, and which is consistent) supports communication, understanding, involvement, dignity and respect (DoH 2002; Swain *et al.* 2003).

Information is the key methodology in improving adaptation and coping. The more information received and processed on a topic, the less the uncertainty regarding that topic. Uncertainty can create and exacerbate anxiety and fear (Corney *et al.* 1992). Informed patients (for instance, those who have a good knowledge of their disease, procedure or treatment), have less anxiety, increased satisfaction and better outcomes than those less well informed (Poroch 1995).

Information has intrinsic worth, but is also a medium for learning, although merely providing access to information will not help people to learn. People often want information, without making the connection to learning, and many would, if asked, say that they did not want to learn. People will only engage with information, and learn from it, if it is relevant, timely and understandable (Hostad *et al.* 2004).

Learning has the potential to effect a permanent change in behaviour, or capability, or knowledge base. Learning can create change in thinking and understanding, even if it is not manifest in behaviour. Individuals often want learning, in the hope that it will increase understanding and knowledge, so that they have some choice in how they react and behave, and thus they are able to adapt and cope better than before. These courses are embedded with educational theory, which has underpinned the facilitators' approach, developing a user-friendly and effective course.

Education theory

A constructivist approach to adult learning is taken, because it is what adults need.

As adults, we have accumulated a foundation of life experiences and knowledge, and the wealth of our experiences must be recognised. Participants should all be treated as equals in experience and knowledge, and allowed to voice their opinions freely (Spencer Grey 2007).

Adaptation of Knowles' nine key principles of adult learning (Knowles 1980) to include information could be used in information development education (Spencer Grey 2007).

TABLE 16.1 Key principles of adult learning

1 Adults need to control the information they receive, and their learning
2 Adults need to feel that the information and learning has immediate utility
3 Adults need to feel that the information and learning focuses on issues which directly affect them
4 Adults need to be able to use this information and learning as they go along, rather than receive background theory and general information
5 Adults need to anticipate how they will use this information and learning
6 Adults need to expect better coping and adaptation to result from this information
7 Adult learning is greatest when it maximises available resources
8 Adult learning requires a climate that is collaborative, respectful, mutual and informal, and information must be provided under similar conditions
9 Adult learning relies on information which is appropriate to what is known at a given time

Source: adapted from Knowles 1980.

By using the adult learning criteria in Table 16.1, and by listening to patients and carers, we can tailor the 'teaching' to maximise effect. It can be assumed that what someone learns over and above what is taught when in a safe, well-intentioned learning environment will be valuable, however, it is difficult to measure this. Figure 16.1 illustrates the complexities of teaching and of the learners retaining knowledge.

As well as an understanding of adult education, the facilitators need to be aware of the stressors. Margaret Dimond talked about coping with stress by successfully adapting to chronic illness. She suggested that perhaps adaptation is ultimately measured by how a person finds a way of living, which takes account of the illness but is not controlled by it. Hence, quality of life is protected by maintaining hope, and lessening fear. Dimond further suggests that such a life may even rise above the limitations of the illness (Dimond and Jones 1983).

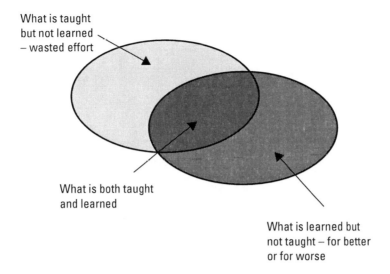

What is taught
but not learned
– wasted effort

What is both taught
and learned

What is learned but
not taught – for better
or for worse

FIGURE 16.1 What is taught and what is learned: a representation of one learner's learning

Source: Atherton (2005).

Stress management and coping theory

The main points made by stress management and coping theory (Spencer Grey 2004) are as follows.

➤ People tend not to resist outside disturbances, but instead react in significant ways to them; they do not 'shrug off' external influences, but are partly driven by them (for example, events and relationships). In the same vein, it is also suggested that internal influences (for example, biological, psychological or emotional disturbances) are not 'shrugged off'.

➤ Stress is the environmental condition under which homeostasis (balance) is interrupted. Stress equals pressure, or tension, exerted on someone, or a demand on physical or mental energy. Stressors are the external situations which lead to stress. Stress can be a constant, steady tension, or small daily hassles, or major life events.

➤ Two main healthcare outcomes for chronic, life-threatening or progressive degenerative diseases are adaptation and coping. The ideal is: coming to terms with the situation (adapt), while being able to live with the limitations of the situation (cope), while maintaining or improving quality of life (adapt), while being able to accommodate constant change (cope and adapt).

➤ Adaptation and coping are also appropriate health outcomes for carers and will include bereavement.

➤ The ability to achieve stability through adaptation is a possibility.

With this in mind, it is most important to ensure that the environment and the venue for the course are as comfortable, safe and stress-free as they can be. Much thought needs to be put in to how best this might be achieved, for minimum cost. Sometimes there are pleasant, quiet rooms in hospitals or health centres, or there might be an alternative venue which is more suitable and easily accessible to most patients.

Facilitation process

At all stages of the course, it is important to continue providing an environment conducive to comfort, safety and learning, for the participants. With this in mind (after the initial discussions), the group is divided into two. The first group is 'The Patients' and the other is 'The Carers'. Both groups receive the same information. Separating the groups in this way enables the safe expression of fears, needs and concerns, without patients or carers hurting and upsetting each other.

This is the first step in exposing vulnerability, in a safe environment, and having this accepted helps participants to find the confidence to take their issues back to the larger group, and/or to their partner or carer. There are common issues in the information and education needs of both patients and carers, and it was felt important by patients and carers that they receive the same information. This engenders trust and valuing each other equally. Participants also acknowledged that their information needs may differ, and the significance of information and issues could vary between them, so they would value further information which is tailored to their specific needs, and the opportunity to explore issues in order to meet these needs (Spencer Grey 2005).

Content

Education topics and information are useful in their own right, but can also serve as a vehicle for discussion, with open and sensitive communication.

The main topics are defined in advance by facilitators, but some negotiation is possible. Other topics are selected by the group, but these needs are usually met in the complementary session, not in the main teaching session. It is important to set the ground rules and expectations at the start of the course. These include suggestions which are discussed and negotiated with all attendees. There may be some additional individual group rules negotiated, particularly regarding the sharing of information and insights with the other group, and the anonymity of this sharing.

The main topics are as follows:
➤ 'Health and illness' – this looks at what these are in relation to having a disease (cancer, for instance); what this disease is; how it develops and spreads; taboos and myths surrounding it.
➤ 'Investigations and treatments' – this looks at the 'what' and 'why' aspects, such as how treatments work, their side-effects and exploring how to cope with them.
➤ 'One step at a time' – this includes loss of confidence and self-esteem, acknowledging changing circumstances, sexuality issues, body image, spirituality, quality-of-life issues, and forward planning.
➤ 'What is out there to help?' – this takes in who does what, and why; how to get the best out of the healthcare system; which charities can help; hospices and palliative care.
➤ 'A little bit of what you fancy does you good' – this focuses on diet and nutrition, and getting the most out of your life.

➤ 'Complementary therapies' – looks at what they are, how they work, and how to make safe choices.
➤ 'Stress management' – this covers what stress is, how it shows itself, how to manage it and how to cope with loss and change. This is usually looked at from a more individual and practical aspect, in the separate patient agenda session.

These seven topics are delivered using a variety of teaching methods. PowerPoint presentations and handouts are utilised, in an informal delivery style which stimulates many questions, much discussion, and lots of sharing and support. It is useful to record key issues on a flip-chart.

There is commonality in the general information and education needs of patients and carers, and it was felt important by both these groups that they receive the same information (Spencer Grey 2005). They also acknowledged that their specific information needs may differ, and so they would also value information which is tailored to their specific needs, and the opportunity to explore this in the separate groups. Patients, in particular, are very aware of the efforts, strains and problems that their illness creates for their carers and family, and they often feel a great need to help reduce this stress. There is weekly re-negotiation regarding what can be shared, in recognition that this may vary from week to week, because of the topic, regardless of ground rules.

Why these topics?

These topics have evolved from conversation and feedback from patients and carers. Even during bereavement support, some individuals reported that some of the very basic issues regarding the disease, investigations and treatment had not been fully explained or understood. At late stages of the disease, the patients still wanted to know why it develops, how it grows, spreads and progresses. Questions such as 'Why am I having these investigations?' and 'How does the treatment work' were also asked.

Concrete information, even regarding some of the unpleasant issues, helps people to cope better, as fear of the unknown is diminished. Facilitators should try to anticipate needs and suggest alternatives which can help people to gain control, have choice and self-manage, thereby maintaining independence.

Essential integral themes running throughout the course are communication, autonomy, self-esteem, and valuing the patient and carer experience and expertise.

The separate session, away from the main teaching session, offers other topics. These may include introductory talks on complementary, alternative medicines (CAMs), or specific topics selected by the group to meet their specific needs. This session may show more variation between groups than the taught session. Each course has a different agenda, which meets the specific group's requirements.

Why this approach?

This is one very useful way of running a course, but one size does not fit all, and therefore there needs to be variation. This is one choice which may be good for some people but not for all. However, this approach does allow people with illness, and carers, to be treated as equals, with the same information, the same amount of individual time and attention, and both can negotiate what is shared with the other.

Having time apart, and together, provides the opportunity for the patient and carer to value each other as individuals, equally respecting of their relationship, as this is the basic tenet of holistic practice. They often talk in these separate groups in a way that they would not if they were together. However, this initial discussion of many topics is often the catalyst which gets them talking together with their loved one.

CONCERNS AND QUESTIONS

These are the main questions asked by other professionals:

➤ *What happens if some people in the groups are newly diagnosed, and others are close to death?*
While the facilitators had some concerns around this issue, it was found that these anxieties were unnecessary, as the patients and carers supported one another. Those who are in early diagnosis comment on how well the others are coping. Perhaps this is due in part to the type of person who comes to this type of course – they tend to be individuals who are keen to find ways to cope. This approach by people who are at the end of their lives seems to encourage and allay the anxieties of those at the beginning of their journey.

➤ *Is it possible to mix patients with different diseases?*
Yes, it is possible, and many of the issues would be the same. However, some disease-specific sessions would need to be included as well. It would definitely require the help or partnership of the appropriate clinical nurse specialists. As the number of individuals wanting this type of education grows, then some disease-specific sessions can be considered.

➤ *Does this format work for other specific palliative type illness or disease, for instance multiple sclerosis, or advanced heart disease?*
Yes, it does. The format can easily be adapted to a particular illness, as mentioned above. However, there may be some exceptions, as the patient is expected to participate as an equal, and this might not always be possible with advanced dementia, or Parkinson's disease.

➤ *Does separating the patient and carer really work?*
Yes, it does. However, patients and carers are always a little apprehensive on the first week about separating, and understandably so. Interestingly, the feedback says that this is the most beneficial aspect of the course. They begin together, and are then separated into different groups, then come back together for lunch. After lunch, they go back into separate groups, and come back together again for the final session. This seems to be the winning format, and, as already mentioned, allows for much discussion by the 'couple', and completing of 'homework' ready for the next week's meeting.

➤ *What about the gender mix? Is it mainly women?*
There seems to be a greater number of women in the patient group, but in the carer groups, there are usually more men. Thus, when they are all together in the main session, it is fairly evenly distributed.

➤ *Can you run these courses on your own?*
No. As previously mentioned, these courses always need at least two facilitators

to run them, due to the two groups being separate most of the time. In fact, it is useful if you can have a third facilitator to help with the main group and provide support where needed. While it appears to be expensive with regard to facilitated hours, feedback has shown quite the opposite. The course prevents much time being spent by many health professionals with each one of the participants with regard to problems and issues that are sorted out as a result of the course.

The success of these courses has been evaluated by written, or verbal, feedback.

Some of the effects of this course on different individuals are perhaps better illustrated in three 'example' vignettes.

Example 16.1 Latent learning and group support

One patient (Mary) who had attended the whole course was at the complementary session regarding pain and pain management, although she was not in pain at the time. As the weeks progressed, Mary began to develop some pain, and immediately started to keep a pain diary, as had been discussed in the pain session. At the next session, she discussed her diary with one of the other patients (Brian) and his carer (Brenda). Brenda showed Mary how she had helped her husband Brian to keep his diary and monitor his pain with forms she had devised. Brenda gave Mary a copy, on a computer memory stick, of the diary sheet and a form which he used, and Mary set this up on her own computer at home. Armed with her diary, she said she felt that she was in a better position to describe and monitor her pain, and felt her pain would be better controlled as a result. Mary also reported that it made discussion with her doctor less stressful and more productive, and that she felt more in control.

Before the end of the course, all participants had received a copy of the tools which Brenda had devised, just in case they might need them in the future.

Example 16.2 Group autonomy, camaraderie and peer support
(all encouraged throughout the course)

A lady with advanced lung cancer (Susan) developed a spinal cord compression while attending the course. She was immediately admitted to hospital for radiotherapy. Even though she was unwell, she wanted to ask the group, via the facilitators, whether they would be happy for her to attend the next session, given that her condition had altered so drastically. She said she would accept the group's decision. (They unanimously agreed to allow Susan to attend.)

Susan was brought, on her bed, for the next three weeks while she was in hospital.

She said, 'I really enjoy the company, and have so much fun. I always gain lots of support, and who knows, I might still learn something useful!'

The other patients and carers were very supportive, and though they found the situation distressing, they were very glad Susan wanted to come.

Her situation provoked many discussions regarding the fears which people have about bone metastases, and other signs of advancing disease.

One of the other patients, with advanced breast cancer (Carol), took it upon herself to visit Susan every day while she was in hospital. Carol knew that Susan's husband couldn't be there as much as he would have liked, because of the long travelling distance and having to look after their two young children.

Susan felt comfortable enough to share her feelings with the staff on the ward, and with Carol, which she said was a direct result of attending the course. While it was very traumatic, she used her time in hospital and when attending the classes most effectively. Together with her husband, she completed the end-of-life work that she wanted and needed to do. This included preparing presents, cards and letters for her children's eighteenth and twenty-first birthdays, engagements, marriages, and other life events when she thought they might need her or a message from her.

The facilitators also supported Carol, who, while initially upset by all the emotional and emotive work by Susan, went away impressed by her new friend's courage and tenacity. It prompted Carol to ensure that her own affairs were in order, and to adapt some of Susan's ideas to her own circumstances.

Example 16.3 Sexuality session

The two facilitators have found this session most interesting, particularly conversations which have developed as a result of input on this topic. Sarah, who had problems with her body image and refused to have a breast prosthesis, started to share her concerns and misgivings. As she did so, five of the other ladies popped their prosthetic breasts on to the table for everyone to see. There was much frivolity and discussion, and Rob and Trevor (the only males) joined in.

The reassurance of the women, and their openness to share all aspects of each of their issues relating to body image, helped to address many of Sarah's concerns and worries. However, it was the men's reactions which she said really helped. They initially joked about never seeing (or feeling) so many breasts in one go. Then they talked, in a very matter-of-fact way, about how little the loss of a partner's breast would mean to them. They encouraged her to talk to her husband about it (he was in the other group). 'He can't be that bothered, or why is he here!' This good, commonsense comment by Trevor really helped Sarah to turn the corner in coping with her body image. Issues like this are very seldom dealt with effectively, and certainly not in a group (Hostad 2007).

There are many other examples which the authors would have liked to share, but unfortunately space constraints do not allow. However, it does begin to give a flavour of how this course runs, and the benefits it may have.

As such courses continue to be developed and are updated, further consideration should incorporate the difference and diversity between individuals and client groups.

Some demographics will have cultural groups for whom English is not a first language. This situation has not had to be accommodated as yet, but it may arise in the future. It could suggest that this sector of the target audience is not yet being reached. This issue will need to be investigated further.

English as an additional language can be accommodated with prior warning, but family members should not be used as interpreters. It may be that language-specific courses need to be established with facilitators proficient in that language, or that facilitators may need to be bilingual or multilingual, or that interpreters are appointed to the facilitators and not to an individual participant.

Regarding those from minority ethnic groups, the effectiveness of this model of delivery, and the suggested topics, would need to be evaluated and reviewed in light of cultural sensitivity and cultural needs.

Similarly, the success of the model, and the suggested topics, with adults with learning difficulties, or adults with cognitive difficulties, has not yet been evaluated.

This model has been most successful, and the reader may wish to take some, or all, of this approach to utilise in their clinical or education setting.

KEY POINTS

- Nationally, public education related to cancer and palliative care is neglected, especially patient and carer education.
- There is no specific national initiative, or support from government, regarding cancer and palliative care education for patients and carers.
- Professionals who facilitate patient and carer education may require further training.
- Relatively few resources are allocated to intervention of this type.
- Consideration should be given to incorporating this important aspect of care into different health professionals' job descriptions.
- Further investigation into the different approaches, methodology, settings and good practice would be beneficial.
- There is need to consider specific research into these interventions.

CONCLUSION

This chapter has considered the many aspects of patient and carer education, and has focused on stress, information giving, support and learning. It has looked at how intrinsically they are linked, and how all of these elements need to be incorporated into such educational programmes.

The authors have endeavoured to provide readers with much food for thought, so that they might look again at the patient and carer education which they provide.

One size does not fit all, and different individuals, groups and settings require their own unique approach. However, the process outlined is very flexible, and may be adapted to the reader's locality and needs. It has certainly produced unexpectedly and overwhelmingly excellent evaluations, so it is hoped that there will be something useful for readers to take away.

This is an important, but sadly neglected area of education within cancer and palliative care.

'We suggest that public information should be "formalised" and that it should be given the credence it deserves. Public education implemented appropriately will ensure that *it achieves its overall aim of empowering the public, so that they are able to adapt to their new situation, in whatever form this takes.'* (Hostad *et al.* 2004: 50)

It is imperative that this aspect of public and patient information is given the focus it requires, so that ultimately there will be more support, information and education on offer. The more of this type of education that is available (for example, the Macmillan Cancer Care or the Caring with Confidence carers' course – *see* Further reading), the more choices the patient, carer and general public will have as to what, how and when to receive it. This is ultimately so that patient and carer education becomes an essential and integral dimension of cancer and palliative care provision, so that the patient and carer receive the best quality holistic care they so richly deserve.

IMPLICATIONS FOR THE READER'S OWN PRACTICE

1   Is this method of patient and carer education used in your clinical area?
2   Do you see any potential problems for the implementation of patient and carer education at your workplace? How might these be overcome?
3   Who else could you work with in order to ensure the success of such an initiative?
4   How could you evaluate whether the course has been of benefit to your patients and their carers?
5   What other innovative ways might you deliver patient and carer education?

REFERENCES

Adamsen L, Rasmussen JM (2003) Exploring and encouraging through social interactions: a qualitative study of nurses' participation in self-help groups for cancer patients. *Cancer Nurs.* **26** (1): 28–36.

Atherton JS (2005) Learning and teaching: what is learning? Available at: www.learningandteaching. info/learning/whatlearn.htm (accessed 13 April 2009).

Bandura A. (2001) Social cognitive theory: an agentic perspective. *Annu Rev Psychol.* **52**: 1–26.

Boekaerts M (1993) Being concerned with well being and learning. *Educ Psychol.* **28**: 148–67.

Calman K, Hine D (1995) *A Policy Framework for Commissioning Cancer Services: a report by the Expert Advisory Group on Cancer (EAGC) to the chief medical officers of England and Wales. Guidance for purchasers and providers of cancer services.* London: HMSO.

Caring with Confidence (2009) Available at: www.caringwithconfidence.net (accessed 13 April 2009).

Corney R, Everett H, Howells A, Crowther M (1992) The care of patients undergoing surgery for gynaecological cancer: the need for information, emotional support and counselling. *J Adv Nurs.* **17** (6): 667–71.

Department of Health (2000a) *The NHS Plan.* London: DoH.

Department of Health (2000b) *The NHS Cancer Plan: a plan for investment, a plan for reform.* London: DoH.

Department of Health (1998–2003) *National Surveys of NHS Patients.* London: DoH.

Department of Health (2002) *Delivering the NHS Plan: next steps on investment, next steps on reform.* London: DoH.

Dimond M, Jones SL (1983) *Chronic Illness Across the Life Span.* Norwalk, CT: Appleton-Century-Crofts.

Eriksson E, Lauri S (2000) Information and support for cancer patients' relatives. *Eur J Cancer Care.* **9**: 8–15.

Goleman D (1995) *Emotional Intelligence: why it can matter more than IQ.* London: Bantam Press.

Hostad J (2004) An overview of hospice education. In: Foyle L, Hostad J, editors. *Delivering Cancer and Palliative Care Education.* Oxford: Radcliffe Publishing: 203–23.

Hostad J, Macmanus D, Foyle L (2004) Public information and education in palliative care. In: Foyle L, Hostad J, editors. *Delivering Cancer and Palliative Care Education.* Oxford: Radcliffe Publishing: 37–51.

Hostad J (2007) 'Let's talk about it, we never do' – Sexual health in cancer and palliative care: an educational dilemma. In: Foyle L, Hostad J, editors. *Innovations in Cancer and Palliative Care Education.* Oxford: Radcliffe Publishing: 197–219.

Knowles M (1980) *The Modern Practice of Adult Education: from pedagogy to androgogy.* Chicago, IL: Pollett.

Kuh G, Schuh J, Whitt E and Associates (1991) *Involving Colleges: successful approaches to fostering student learning and development outside the classroom.* San Francisco, CA: Jossey-Bass.

Langley-Evans A, Payne S (1997) Light-hearted death talk in a palliative day care context. *J Adv Nurs.* **26**: 1086 90.

Larson PJ (1986) Cancer nurses' perceptions of caring. *Cancer Nurs.* **9**: 86–91.

Larsson G *et al.* (1998) Cancer patient and staff ratings of the importance of caring behaviours and their relations to patient anxiety and depression. *J Adv Nurs.* **27**: 855–64.

Macmillan (2009a) *Get Support: living with cancer course.* Available at: www.macmillan.org.uk/Get_Support/Who_to_turn_to/Living_with_cancer_course.aspx (accessed 13 April 2009).

Macmillan (2009b) *New Perspectives: course overview.* Available at: http://learnzone.macmillan.org.uk/file.php/86/living-with-cancer/New_Perspectives_-_course_overview_V6.0.pdf (accessed 13 April 2009).

Munroe B, Oliviere D (2003) *Patient Participation in Palliative Care: a voice for the voiceless.* Oxford: Oxford University Press.

National Institute for Clinical Excellence (2004) *Guidance on Cancer Services: improving supportive and palliative care for adults with cancer.* London: NICE.

Picardie R (2000) *Before I Say Goodbye: recollections and observations from one woman's final year.* New York: Henry Holt.

Poroch D (1995) The effect of preparatory patient education on the anxiety and satisfaction of cancer patients receiving radiation therapy. *Cancer Nurs.* **18** (3): 206–14.

Ramirez A, Addington-Hall J, Richards M (1998) ABC of palliative care: the carers. *BMJ.* **316**: 208–11.

Rogers C (1980) *A Way of Being.* Boston, MA: Houghton Mifflin.

Skilbeck J, Payne S (2003) Emotional support and the role of Clinical Nurse Specialists in palliative care. *J Adv Nurs.* **45** (3): 521–30.

Spencer Grey SA (2004) Psychoneuroimmunology and its role in cancer and palliative care education. (Chapter 9.) In: Foyle L, Hostad J, editors. *Delivering Cancer and Palliative Care Education.* Oxford: Radcliffe Publishing.

Spencer Grey SA (2005) *Cancer Services Users Information Project Report.* Hull, Humber and Yorkshire Coast Cancer Network.

Spencer Grey SA (2007) Information for service users: educational implications. (Chapter 10.)

In: Foyle L, Hostad J, editors. *Innovations in Cancer and Palliative Care Education*. Oxford: Radcliffe Publishing.

Swain J, French S, Cameron C (2003) *Controversial Issues in a Disabling Society.* Buckingham: Open University Press.

Sylvester R (1994) How emotions affect learning. *Educl Leader.* **52** (2): 60–85.

von Essen L, Sjoden PO (1991) The importance of nurse caring behaviours as perceived by Swedish hospital patients and nursing staff. *Int J Nurs Stud.* **28**: 267–81.

Walker L, Walker M, Sharp D (2003) Current provision of psychosocial care within palliative care. In: Lloyd-Williams M, editor. *Psychosocial Issues in Palliative Care*. Oxford: Oxford University Press.

Williamson C (2003) Principles and theoretical background. (Section 3.) In: *Raising the Standard: information for patients*. London: Royal College of Anaesthetists.

Yaniv H (1992) Sexuality of cancer patients: a palliative approach. *Int J Gynecol Canc.* **2**: 282–90.

FURTHER READING AND USEFUL CONTACTS

As well as setting up a course similar to that of the authors of this chapter, you might like to also consider being involved in developing one of the following, or checking to see if there is one of these types running in your area.

- **Macmillan (Macmillan Cancer Care)**. Macmillan provide a course for people living with cancer, facilitated by people living with cancer. The New Perspectives course is free, and runs over six weeks. Attendees meet weekly for two and a half hours, to learn new skills and techniques which help them to 'identify ways of managing symptoms and side effects of treatment' (Macmillan 2009a). A wide range of topics is covered (Macmillan 2009b). The latter also available at: http://learnzone.macmillan.org.uk/file.php/86/living-with-cancer/ New_Perspectives_-_course_overview_V6.0.pdf) Macmillan in Northern Ireland have designed a self-management course for carers, and in London a course is available which is specifically designed to meet the needs of South Asian people living with cancer (Macmillan 2009a). The latter also available at: www.macmillan.org.uk/Get_Support/Who_to_turn_to/ Living_with_cancer_course.aspx

- **Caring with Confidence**. This is a government initiative, and part of their 'New deal for carers' which aims to improve support for carers. It is 'a knowledge and skills based programme' for carers, and can be accessed free through local group sessions, self-study workbooks, or through online sessions. Carers can chose to access some, or all, of the sessions. There are six in total: Caring and Coping, Caring and Me, Caring Day-to-Day, Caring and Resources, Caring and Life, and Caring and Communicating. If attending a local group, each session will last three hours (Caring with Confidence 2009). www.caringwithconfidence.net

- Patient and Carer Education 'I now have friends in the same boat' Facilitators Guide.

  This facilitator's guide will be published by Radcliffe in 2010, by the authors of this chapter. It will cover all aspects of the course, with examples of step-by-step teaching sessions and including ground rules, handouts, PowerPoint presentations, key learning points, alternative exercises, sessions and much more. It is designed to be used as it is, or adapted to suit the needs of the facilitator and the group.

17

Climbing the mountain to self-awareness and self-care in cancer and palliative care education

Eileen Mullard

'The miracle of self-healing occurs when the inner patient yields to the inner physician.'

Vernon Howard

AIM

The aim of this chapter is to explore the issues in and around the area of self-care and its relationship to cancer and palliative care education.

LEARNING OUTCOMES

By the end of this chapter, the reader should be able to:

- improve students' knowledge of how self-awareness can lead to self-care and prevent burnout
- empower teachers to assist students to recognise the importance of self-care and the associated educational aspects
- facilitate the development of insight into how self-awareness assists in caring for others
- understand that incorporating a model of self-care within their lives is equally as important for educators as for students.

INTRODUCTION

Our global society is currently facing major issues related to human performance and wellness. One of these issues relates to the quest to obtain optimum performance, health and wellness and a better quality of life for all concerned in the provision of cancer and palliative care. This objective is not unique to cancer and palliative care; it is also relevant to all aspects of healthcare delivery and affects everyone including patients, carers and healthcare professionals. In order to meet the challenge of achieving well-being, we need to understand and embrace the concept of self-awareness. Education in this topic is vital.

As healthcare professionals, our focus tends to be on what is best for the patient. It is tempting to place patients' needs first. Our attention is focused on meeting those needs, then subsequently those of our families, friends and colleagues. It is all too easy to forget to care for ourselves. Educators are caregivers and not only should we care for ourselves but by doing so we act as role models for our students.

It is in these changing times that we need to be extremely aware of self so as to give the best of care to others. Looking after oneself benefits not only one's patients, family and friends but, importantly, ourselves. In looking after ourselves, we become the model of self-care.

IMPLICATIONS OF A LACK OF SELF-CARE

Not taking care of oneself can create a multitude of effects. These effects may begin with the healthcare professional not being aware that he or she needs self-care. The knock-on effect leads to poor delivery of patient care and generates more work for other team members. This then impacts on patients, causing them to stay in hospital longer, and inhibits their ability to heal. The additional stress of increased workload affects other healthcare professionals, which can result in a variety of negative responses – such as ringing in 'sick' due to 'physical or psychological' reasons. These then create more stress for the staff and the patients and so the cyclical process continues.

As has been outlined, this has implications not only at the patient level but for ward staff and at an organisational level. There are also financial and efficiency consequences. Inevitably, there are long-term effects in both morale and staff retention (Cordes and Dougherty 1993). This chapter seeks to explore this phenomenon and deepen understanding that climbing the mountain to self-care can sometimes be a difficult path to self-awareness. It is therefore essential that self-care is taught. This may be as a stand-alone topic or integral to the various aspects of cancer and palliative care education.

DEFINING SELF-CARE

Self-care is a universal requirement for sustaining and enhancing life and health. In the NHS document *Self Care: a real choice* (DoH 2005), self-care is defined as 'a part of daily living taken by individuals towards their own health and well-being and includes care extended to their children, family, friends and others in neighbourhoods and local communities'.

Self-care is a lifelong habit. It is the action that individuals take for themselves and their families to stay healthy and to manage minor and chronic conditions, based on their knowledge and the available information. Orem (1991), a nursing scholar and theorist, defines the self-care process as 'activities that individuals personally initiate and perform on their own behalf in maintaining life, health, and well-being. Self care is an adult's personal, continuous contribution to his or her own well-being.'

Self-care is the creation and maintenance of a healthy relationship with oneself. Although this may sound like a simple statement, it is a practice that is not often fully embraced in healthcare. It is easy to become so immersed in the medical model that self-care is often neglected (Lachman 1996). Yet focusing care and attention on what causes one's stress and one's response to it will assist in understanding oneself better. This process assists individuals to become familiar with themselves and in return to have the capability to help others fully. As already stated, self-care is about self-awareness. Self-awareness is very much linked to the concept of self-care. How can one take care of self if there is no insight into being 'aware' of the concept of 'self awareness'?

Words such as 'alertness', 'watchfulness' and 'knowingness' are attributes of self-awareness (Wakefield 2000; Lachman 1996). Another word to describe self-care is self-reflection. It is merely a process of turning one's awareness or watchfulness towards one's own inward feelings, beliefs and behaviours (Dossey *et al.* 2000). It is a structured, deliberate process with the outcome of learning new information of the self. This process of reflection is taught and learned in basic health educational training for patient care.

Kolb and Fry (1975) and Schon (1983) describe reflection as a way of learning – for example, using reflection after a task. What is needed for self-care is deliberately to utilise reflection appropriate for the quality care of patients on one's own thoughts and behaviours. In this way what is provided for others will be provided for the health care practitioner. This is explored in greater detail by Chris Johns (*see* Chapter 6), who outlines several approaches to teaching reflection.

THE WOUNDED HEALER

> 'The doctor is effective only when he himself is affected. Only the wounded physician heals. But when the doctor wears his personality like a coat of armour, he has no effect.'
> (Carl Jung, quoted in Dunne 2000)

The 'wounded healer' that Carl Jung was referring to can be anyone involved in healthcare provision. This includes teachers who facilitate others. They must gain students' trust in order that students are prompted to give themselves permission to feel that which has previously been too painful for the emotional psyche to cope with and express.

There is not a healer archetype and a patient archetype; the healer and the patient together constitute the whole archetype. Within the wounded one is a healer and within the healer is a wounded one.

In healthcare, there are many who are wounded healers and do not realise it. This is because they are caught up in the chaos of caring and not tending to their own self-care. When individuals acknowledge that they are wounded healers – that is, when they embrace their own accumulated grief and 'woundedness' – they are far more effective as healthcare providers.

In the education of healthcare professionals, the wounded healer concept is important to achieve the ultimate outcome of improved patient care. This is achieved by raising the self-awareness of healthcare providers (Turkel 2004). What sort of exercise would you undertake in the classroom to achieve this?

Exercise 17.1

One approach might be to prepare a detailed story relating to a nurse working in palliative care and how she becomes increasingly involved with certain patients to the detriment of other patients, but fails to recognise this. Her behaviour and attitude to other members of her team is changed and distant, and she even starts phoning the patients' relatives from home when she is off duty!

The participants could be asked to answer a number of questions at various stages during the exercise, such as these examples.

1 When do you know that this individual is wounded?
2 At what point does great compassion and care become over connection?
3 Is it better to be too connected than not connected enough?
4 How can you facilitate and listen to patients repeatedly, sharing their inner most soul pain, without becoming wounded or over connected?
5 What symptoms did you pick up which illustrated her difficulties?
6 What could you do to help and support this individual?
7 How could this nurse build her self-awareness and self-care?

A number of different scenarios could be used to illustrate specific points, in particular emphasising the value of being non-judgemental and offering support to the individual.

BURNOUT

In the absence of self-awareness and self-care, the accumulation of stress over a period of time can cause burnout to occur. Burnout has been identified with stress and workload. Burnout can be interpreted as the individual's ignoring their own well-being. A metaphor that can be applied to this is that healthcare practitioners are like batteries and, when not charged properly, they cease to work.

The individual delivering care to others often forgets to care for self. The individual continues to care for the client. Caring can be conscious but the effects of caring can be absorbed unconsciously and re-emerge, giving cause to various levels of pain, sorrow and joy, on physical, mental, emotional and spiritual levels.

The carer can either become a victim or choose to transform themselves and their wounds into a source of healing. In this healing process, the ability to heal others can be maximised through learning and can empower others through this positive experience.

However, if the carer's self-care and own 'woundedness' is ignored, the signs of burnout can manifest. It is important therefore to use methods such as those described above to teach students this concept.

Burnout is a state of exhaustion that has been much written and researched about in the literature (Cordes and Dougherty 1993; Maslach and Leiter 1997). It is a psychological term for the experience of long-term exhaustion and diminished interest, usually coming immediately after an extended period of overwork (Lee and Ashforth 1990). It was originally identified with social workers. However, the literature reveals that it affects all healthcare professionals. The *Western Journal of Medicine* devoted its entire January 2001 issue to offering guidance in living positive and healthy lives. This might be useful pre-session reading, which could then be discussed and analysed in the classroom.

While burnout is an extreme, it happens because of the lack of self-care. Maslach and Jackson (1981) defined burnout as a three-dimensional syndrome of emotional exhaustion. The three themes that emerged in this research were emotional exhaustion, depersonalisation and diminished personal accomplishment. To avoid burnout, the carer needs to be self-aware and vigilant in this area.

An exercise which could be utilised in the classroom might be to provide different case studies in which students could identify the above themes.

The concept of holistic nursing suggests that nurses have well-being at the core of their practice – more specifically, self-care (Dossey *et al.* 2000). The holistic nurse needs to be able to define and integrate this concept of self-care, not only as a professional but as an individual. Self-care is critical in preventing burnout.

It could perhaps be said that the education system is at fault for not incorporating self-care within the curriculum. The seeds of self-reliance, fatigue and emotional exhaustion often germinate at the beginning of training for nurses and other healthcare professionals. By the time these healthcare professional are midway into their career, this attitude is reinforced and acknowledged by peers. Subsequently the reputation for being a 'hard worker' is ingrained, as is the concept of ignoring self. Maslach and Leiter (1997) write of burnout as an 'erosion of the soul'. It spreads gradually and continuously over time, allowing the individual to be in a challenging and downward spiralling place from which it is hard to recover ground.

This risk pervades right from the beginning of the healthcare educational pathway. Burnout then encroaches as practitioners' workloads expand with extra demands and the individual experiences a sense of losing control. Education provided early on and repeatedly on self-care can avert this from happening.

Signs and symptoms of burnout

Since burnout is not an overnight occurrence, it is important to be alert to its early signs. Knowledge of these early signs can help to avert the complete meltdown that can occur if signs are not heeded.

Therefore it is critical that students in healthcare are educated on signs and symptoms of burnout, including a rationale for self-care management.

Often, healthcare practitioners begin a new job feeling 'energised and optimistic'. Then disillusion and disappointment occur when self-appointed targets are not met, which can be normal. The individual then continues to strive harder and better and they can be lulled into a false sense of security and ignore the prevailing signs of burnout.

Exercise 17.2 The signs of burnout

The students might be encouraged to identify the different effects of burnout by discussing them in groups. They might also signal whether they have experienced them or witnessed them in colleagues.

Physically, the individual may feel that they experience:
- digestive problems
- headaches
- high blood pressure
- heart attack
- strokes
- teeth grinding
- fatigue.

When the individual is on the *verge* of burnout, they may feel:
- powerless
- hopeless
- drained
- frustrated
- detached from people and things around them
- little satisfaction from work
- bored
- resentment for having too much to do
- a failure
- stuck in a situation from which they cannot extricate themselves
- unsure of their job or career
- withdrawn, isolated from co-workers and friends
- insecure about their competence and abilities
- cynical
- irritable
- anxious.

In literature reviews, both Maslach and Leiter (1997) as well as Cordes and Dougherty (1993) agree that burnout results in both physical and psychological symptoms as noted above. As the symptoms continue, the individual feels tired and sometimes jealous of others who are happy with their jobs. Ironically, when experiencing burnout individuals often push themselves harder. They will try to balance numerous roles, multitask and respond to a variety of challenging and changing situations, often at the expense of their own well-being. They feel like they are running on a treadmill that will not stop.

These symptoms of burnout are often sown in healthcare when change is a constant and is the norm. It is expected. The individual's physical and psychological well-being is ignored. The individual begins the spiral downwards.

Exercise 17.3 Identifying individuals suffering from burnout

The student groups can be given the task of producing sentences which they might utilise when trying to broach a conversation with a stressed individual.

Then ask them to respond to these questions about the early signs of burnout.
- Do work activities that you once found enjoyable now feel like drudgery?
- Have you become more cynical or bitter about your job, your boss or the company?
- Are non-work relationships (marital, family, friendships) affected by your feelings about work?
- Do you find yourself:
  - dreading going to work in the morning?
  - easily annoyed or irritated by your co-workers?
  - envious of individuals who are happy in their work?
  - caring less now than you used to about doing a 'good job' at work?
- Are you:
  - regularly experiencing fatigue and low energy levels at your job?
  - easily bored with your job?
  - depressed on Sunday afternoons thinking about Monday and the coming week?

If you answered 'yes' to five or more of the above, you may be suffering from job burnout (Canaff 2006).

Exercise 17.3 usually generates a discussion about how the above signs have been felt by the students or observed in colleagues. This can be followed up by giving them the case study outlined in the next exercise.

Exercise 17.4 Case study

The students are asked to discuss the case study outlined below and to identify the negative and positive aspects of it.

Recently a university student who was post-registration and a new graduate in her early twenties verbalised how she was working night shifts and for long periods. During a short-staffed night duty shift, she hurt her back and now finds it difficult to do her work. She feels guilty because statements are made to her that she is not doing her job and it is *only* a back injury. Her GP provided her with a prescription for analgesics so she could go back to work and yet no one is supportive. No referrals have been made to occupational health. The student is now beginning to exhibit the signs and symptoms of burnout: insomnia, feeling tired all the time, depressed, having no joy for the job that she was thrilled about initially, wishing that she did not have to go back and work the night shift. This student has now been counselled by her general practitioner and referred to occupational health for guidance. As of this time, she is in counselling and relocating to a different job. She is feeling better.

This case study demonstrates that this is a very real situation, occurring right now in clinical areas of NHS.

Can burnout be prevented?

Little emphasis has been placed on the potential health consequences for nurses providing care. The issue of self-care is never more important than now globally for all healthcare professionals. To prevent burnout, the individual needs to become familiar with the symptoms. What better time to educate students about the early signs and symptoms of burnout and about self-care strategies for prevention of burnout, early in their training. Hill Jones (2005) speaks of a self-care plan as a way of being proactive with self. These self-care strategies will not only improve the individual, but also facilitate the individual's having a productive life with family and friends, providing better patient care and outcomes, and preventing patient and medical errors as well. Burnout or lack of self-care – or the other term 'compassion fatigue' – can be prevented. It will take support of management and educational institutions to begin the work of educating students from the start of their 'caring' careers.

Lack of self-care affects the individual at physical, mental, social and spiritual levels.

So what can the educator do to address these symptoms? Also, what techniques can the educator bring into the student's life to improve self-awareness and self-care? All the previous exercises and the one outlined below are some of the tool range available to bring individuals' attention to the importance of self-awareness.

Exercise 17.5 Self-management to prevent burnout

Have the students discuss in groups what these symptoms are, and the techniques and technique points for self-management which they can use to improve self-awareness and their self-care. When they have reported back, they can compare their feedback to the list below.

Self-management checklist

If you feel that you are experiencing burnout, you might find it useful to consider the following.

1 See your GP to schedule a complete physical check-up and discuss any signs or symptoms that you are currently experiencing.
2 Make certain that you are getting more than four hours of sleep and preferably seven to eight hours.
3 Eat healthy foods and focus on treating your body with high-quality fuel of high-protein breakfasts and snacks to help with your energy levels.
4 Drink eight glasses of water a day and not eight cups of coffee.
5 Increase exercise by walking up the stairs at work and parking your car further away to walk, doing stretches at your desk, and walking at breaks and lunch. Taking up hobbies such as yoga and pilates can help as well.
6 Find an individual with whom you can share your problems in confidence, e.g. a trusted colleague, manager or counsellor.
7 Investigate the possibility of clinical supervision at work.
8 Complete a time analysis of an average week to see how much satisfaction you receive and how that could be improved.

---

9   Look at ways in which you can improve your self-esteem and become a much more positive person.
10 Use education to learn new ways to cope better.

This is not meant to be an exhaustive list, but it does offer a few ideas for helping to prevent burnout. The latter two methods could be achieved effectively through NLP (*see* Chapter 4 for more details).

As carers, students are always giving and sometimes this activity seems endless. To assist them in developing self-care, one can encourage them to self-manage by taking several proactive measures.

It is suggested that they improve their coping skills by using other techniques from neuro-linguistic programming (NLP), such as positive self-talk, mental imagery, muscle relaxation techniques and meditation. Where possible they should access a counsellor or life coach to improve skills. Alongside improving coping skills, individuals should develop self-awareness – that is, the ability to know and understand self. Get them to recognise whether they are perfectionists, or have a low level of assertiveness or a strong need for approval. If they admit to any of these traits, they may be more prone to burnout than someone who is authoritarian or task-focused. It is essential that they recognise their strengths and weaknesses in order to help them deal with life stressors. They can also use journalling and reflective practice, as outlined in Chapter 6 by Johns.

Depression can be an outcome of stress. Stressed individuals need to be aware of depression, particularly if they have a history of it, as burnout can re-activate depression. Ensure that they are aware of the signs and symptoms of depression.

In the everyday tumult of balancing personal and professional lives, it is important that students learn – or re-learn – time management skills to inject some control into their jobs and life. A time management strategy is a crucial source of stability. Therefore, it is important begin to say 'no' more often, to schedule more time off and to delegate more tasks.

Insist that students set realistic goals for clarity and direction in their lives. Make them set meaningful goals for the short and long term so that they can feel a sense of accomplishment when they achieve them.

Finally and perhaps 'firstly' try to get them to put themselves first. Ask them to allocate 'me' time regularly to do something they enjoy. Tell them to schedule 'me' time into every day or week and to keep to it as if they were keeping a GP's appointment (Ricardo 2007). 'Me time' should allow them to put balance back into their personal lives. It can assist in creating new relationships and in reconnecting them with family and friends. This is all about creating a sensible lifestyle.

Encourage students to work on nurturing their relationships with partners, children, pets and friends. It is equally important for them to develop these personal relationships as much as the relationships they develop at work. Similarly, by following a 'looking after themselves' programme they may create a community of new friends which may offer another avenue for support with like-minded individuals.

In the work context, you can recommend that they speak with their supervisors and address the issues at work by exploring ways to alleviate stress. Sometimes it may be necessary to consider the possibility of job change if this is warranted.

Some of the above strategies may help to prevent individuals from reaching complete burnout. The students can learn from these and so be helped to regain life–work balance.

The ideal solution to address stress management would be to deliver a specific module on the topic in a cancer and palliative care pathway. However, if circumstances are against the development of such a module, then dedicated sessions can be created in core curricula. These sessions might include the following exercise.

Exercise 17.6 Increasing self-awareness

The students first identify their strengths and weaknesses.

They should then identify the ways in which they cope with life's stressors – for example, do they overeat or not eat?

The key to this exercise is to get them to become aware of themselves. This can be done by getting them to identify, over a designated time period, repeated patterns that demonstrate high levels of stress. In this regard, writing a journal during the allotted timeframe would be most useful.

Through these patterns, the student will be able to identify a proactive self-care plan. This plan could be a compulsory element of the curriculum. It is meant to be changeable and fluid so that it can be adapted as the individual changes their perspectives over time.

The teacher can motivate students to incorporate small changes at first. Class members should stick with the changes for a six-week period. Change takes time to become habit and this usually occurs after about six weeks. Get them to make a date with themselves and reflect on these changes. They should ask themselves whether the changes are working and whether they have improved their quality of life.

The individual can verbalise the importance of the concept of self-care and understand the theories associated with self-care. It is the modelling of the self-care that effects change. The lived experience is very powerful and moving.

KEY POINTS

- Self-care is a universal requirement for sustaining and enhancing life and health.
- In multidisciplinary healthcare education, self-care is not addressed specifically as a core area.
- A pattern has emerged over time for students, which challenges healthcare students, managers and teachers.
- Not being self-aware leads ultimately to poor patient care and burnout of individuals.

■ Self-care is a basic for all individuals, although it can be a forgotten topic.
■ Burnout is a real type of stress and preventable through diligent self-care. It can be avoided by utilising some creative teaching methods.

CONCLUSION

It appears that stress and burnout are still prevalent among healthcare professionals. Therefore educational strategies that raise self-awareness and provide stress management should be an integral part of healthcare training. As healthcare professionals become increasingly involved with the care of others, they can become paralysed and lose their sense of self. This situation can be avoided if self-care is taught early in their training. To reach the pinnacle of self-care, one has to scale the heights of self-awareness. The mountain might seem difficult to climb, but the view is worth the effort. Seeing and feeling the achievement of self-care and well-being is an outcome worthy of all healthcare educators' efforts.

'You cannot teach a man anything; you can only help him find it within himself.'

Galileo

IMPLICATIONS FOR THE READER'S OWN PRACTICE

1 How do you, as an educator and carer of students, incorporate self-care into your life? Give an example relating to each of the physical, emotional, mental and spiritual areas of your life.
2 What innovative strategies could you use to mark the importance of the concept of self-care?
3 How would you as a healthcare educator motivate other healthcare professionals to incorporate self-care into their teaching?

REFERENCES

Cordes CL, Dougherty TW (1993) A review and an integration of research on job burnout. *Acad Manag Rev.* **18** (4): 621–56.
Department of Health (2005) *Self Care: a real choice.* London: DoH.
Dossey B, Keegan L, Guzzetta C (2000) *Holistic Nursing: a handbook for practice.* 3rd ed. New York: Aspen Publishers.
Dunne C (2000) *Carl Jung: wounded healer of the soul – an illustrated biography.* London: Continuum Publishing.
Hill Jones S (2005) A self care plan for hospice workers. *Am J Hosp Palliat Care.* **22** (2): 125–8.
Howard V (2006) www.ThinkExist.com, Quotations
Kolb DA, Fry R (1975) Toward an applied theory of experiential learning. In: Cooper C, editor. *Theories of Group Process.* London: John Wiley.
Lachman VD (1996) Stress and self care revisited: a literature review. *Holist Nurs Pract.* **10** (2): 1–12.

Lee RT, Ashforth BE (1990) On the meaning of Maslach's three dimensions of burnout. *J Appl Psychol.* **75** (6): 743–7.

Leiter MP, Maslach C (1988) The impact of interpersonal environment on burnout and organizational commitment. *J Organ Behav.* **9** (4): 297–308.

Maslach C, Jackson S (1981) The measurement of burnout. *J Occup Behav.* **2**: 99–113.

Maslach C, Leiter MP (1997) *The Truth about Burnout: how organizations cause personal stress and what to do about it.* San Francisco, CA: Jossey-Bass Publishers: 13–15.

Orem DE (1991) *Nursing Concepts of Practice.* 3rd ed. New York: McGraw-Hill.

Ricardo C (2007) The importance of valuing yourself through the practice of self care. Available at: www.therapist-psychologist.com

Schon D (1983) *The Reflective Practitioner.* New York: Basic Books.

Turkel M (2004) Creating a caring environment through self renewal. *Nurs Admin Q.* **28** (4): 249–54.

Wakefield A (2000) Nurse's responses to death and dying: a need for relentless self care. *Int J Palliat Nurs.* **6** (5): 245–51.

West J Med (2001) January edition.

18

Promoting leadership by education

Ian Grigor

'Life is change. Growth is optional. Choose wisely.'

Karen Kaiser Clark

AIM

The aim of this chapter is to review approaches to leadership, and behavioural leadership in particular.

LEARNING OUTCOMES

By the end of this chapter, the reader should be able to:
- understand the basis of the leadership topic area
- analyse the sub-aspects that comprise behavioural leadership
- evaluate the elements of effective leadership
- use and adapt the leadership knowledge gained from this chapter, transferring all relevant aspects to cancer and palliative care education and practice.

HOW DID LEADERSHIP IN HEALTHCARE EVOLVE?

Management has played a significant role in healthcare, though arguably less so in health education, since the inception of the National Health Service in 1948. Strictly speaking, it was administration rather than management that was prevalent in the first 30 years of the NHS, until the report from the Merrison Commission (1979) which identified weak management and too many management (administrative) tiers, leading to an inability to make concise judgements. In the same way that administration and management were considered as one and the same, up until the early 1980s, the words 'leadership' and 'management' are often used synonymously, today – a source of not inconsiderable confusion and debate.

In essence, it was really the advent of the current ten-year strategy, *The NHS Plan:*

a plan for investment, a plan for reform (DoH 2000a), which truly opened the door to leadership in the NHS. Specifically, the Department of Health (2000a) demanded the development of:

> 'Leaders who can establish direction and purpose, inspire, motivate and empower teams around common goals and produce real improvements in clinical practice, quality and services. We need leaders who are motivated, self aware, socially skilled and able to work together with others across professional and organisational boundaries.'

The call for leaders has been reinforced in subsequent White Papers, *The NHS Improvement Plan: putting people at the heart of public services* (DoH 2004) and *Our Health, Our Care, Our Say: a new direction for community services* (DoH 2006). Taken literally, the Department of Health appears to be calling for superheroes who can fit the somewhat demanding person specification for leaders.

So who are these wonderful souls, where do they come from and how do they behave if they are to achieve the desired effects?

In the last century, when it began to be studied by academics, leadership was considered to be a trait of 'great men', an innate ability to demonstrate charisma, out-standing strategic ability and, at the same time, great humility and sensitivity to those being led, i.e. the followers (Roe 1957). Hewison (2004), however, has suggested that too many traits were identified in that era and that not many of these are actually pos-sessed by all 'natural born' leaders.

Swansburg and Swansburg (2002), on the other hand, argued that certain back-ground variables do have strong links to the abilities of various leaders: these are, educational experience, previous and current career experience, and age. Therefore, there are elements of academic, sociological and psychological development. This fits well with the alternative perspective of Reitman (1961) and Storey *et al.* (2002) on the trait theory: that it may be based on a socialisation phenomenon whereby children of well-organised, assertive, resilient parents grow up showing these skills and attributes, probably because they rubbed off on youngsters brought up in such households.

Over a period of academic scrutiny, the trait theory gradually fell out of favour and was replaced by a series of other theories of leadership, including the behavioural styles, previously favoured by Lewin (1935). However, the trait theory is currently enjoying a resurgence, not so much in the sense of congenital aptitudes but, rather, as an acceptance of the types of skills that can be acquired at an early age and honed due to life experiences.

In this brief chapter, it would be impossible to do justice to the many theories and philosophies of leadership, so the focus will be exclusively on the more commonly debated behavioural styles.

LEADERSHIP: WHAT IS IT?

To set the ball rolling, there is a need to define 'leadership', in general terms. Leadership may be defined as *'a process whereby an individual influences a group of individuals to achieve a common goal'* (Northouse 2004: 3). Leadership, however, is a powerful word, worthy of conveying much more than can be contained within a concise definition and capable of meaning many different things, to different people, in different contexts. Despite the multitude of ways that leadership can be conceptualised, the following components can be identified as being central to the phenomenon. First, it is a process or an activity; second, it involves influence, and this means that a relationship between people is not always passive (Daft 1999); third, it occurs within a group context involving people who are both leaders and followers; and finally, leadership involves the attainment of goals, but also the commitment of individuals to such goals (Sadler 1997).

However, there are as many definitions of leadership as there are books on the topic, demonstrating the contentious nature of this area, but some of the less controversial definitions come from Milner and Joyce (2005), Sullivan and Decker (2005) and van Knippenberg and Hogg (2003), who all agree with Northouse (2004) that leadership is a process of influencing people towards the attainment of goals. This identifies that the players in a leadership scenario are the leader and those who are led, the followers. Their joint role is to achieve goals and it appears to be the leader's skills and aptitudes that orchestrate the achievement of these goals.

In healthcare, it is implicit that nursing goals, either directly or indirectly, impact on the quality of care afforded to patients. However, with regard to the care environment, Rigolosi (2005) related leadership to contemporary healthcare by claiming that all healthcare professionals are, in fact, leaders in some form, relating closely to the concept of self-leadership, particularly relevant to those autonomous practitioners that work in primary or intermediate care, for example.

What is a leader and what do they do?

A leader's role, as has been established, is to galvanise the team to achieve the required goals which, in turn, are aligned to the organisation's aims. Of key importance is that the leader always wants the team to be successful and thrive. The leader may have been formally appointed to the leadership role and, thereby, given the necessary authority to lead. Another way in which a leader can assume authority is when the team, usually informally, appoints an individual to take the lead, recognising that person's competence to achieve (Chemers and Ayman 1993). However, in certain situations, a leader may arise from the background, as it were, in times of need. For example, in a crisis, there may be an expectation that the appointed leader will take charge in resolving the situation but, on occasion, someone else, often totally unexpectedly, will assume authority, perhaps by dint of their experience of a previous, similar incident. On reflection, after the event, team members may express surprise at the identity of the individual who assumed leadership authority. Whatever the situation, whether formal authority has been given or a leader has arisen to take on that position, due to circumstances, the leader needs to exhibit leadership characteristics, if the team is to follow.

In clinical areas, the followers, according to Swansburg and Swansburg (2002), are groups composed of members who are interdependent, who have shared goals and must successfully cooperate to complete these goals. Therefore, the role of the leader is of paramount importance in conducting their orchestra of followers and facilitating efficient and effective attainment of their goals.

Characteristics of a successful leader

Arguably, the most important asset that a leader requires is excellent communication and negotiation skills. By definition, therefore, such an individual needs to be highly visible and cannot spend their working days secreted in their office. Effective communication and negotiation occurs only if the receiver understands exactly the information or idea that the sender wants to give, and successful clinical leaders tend to be skilled at listening and taking time to hear the suggestions and concerns of those they seek to lead. Stone *et al.* (2004) stressed that communication is a process of coaching, counselling, coordinating, supervising and evaluating. To that list may well be added questioning, because insightful questioning can often illuminate areas of potential miscommunication. This series of skills includes not only the ability to talk convincingly but to listen convincingly, too: to be able to pick up signals and cues from followers. One issue that is often overlooked, in terms of listening skills, is that team members invariably have different communication preferences and styles (Huczynski 2004). Without knowing what these preferences are, it is easy to miscommunicate without realising it, so it is invaluable for the leader to understand the communication preferences of their staff, as well as to be aware of the respective competences of these staff. Body language, of course, also plays a significant part in communication.

In order to understand the communication process fully, a leader needs to have self-awareness and awareness of the needs of individuals in their team, particularly at the ward or department level (Weiner 1995). Learning about this can help to identify one's own strengths and weaknesses and give an insight as to where development is required. It is apparent from the research by van Knippenberg and Hogg (2003) that a leader should set an example for a team, and, therefore, if the leader's own standards are beneath those they expect themselves, team members are likely to practise only to their leader's standards.

The successful leader uses skills associated with recognising the potential of their staff, including sensitivity to the current challenges and their likely demands on colleagues. This would include, for example, knowing when to stop piling work on already stressed staff. This talent, emotional intelligence, is considered to be the skill of observing and assessing one's own and others' emotions while using that information to plan and guide action (Taylor-Moss 2005). Goleman (1996) previously stated that emotional intelligence enables a leader to manage team relationships more effectively and sense the impact of their own actions on others' emotions. Therefore, leaders need to be aware of the needs and objectives of their staff, and to be conscious of the social and physical conditions that might affect their working environments. It is imperative that a positive philosophy of leadership is established which values the need for such an approach (Milner and Joyce 2005).

If a leader is going to successfully guide a team to achieve their set aims, then that leader needs to have the capability to recognise the resources and assets at their disposal and match these to the demands of the tasks. Almost invariably, the prime assets will be the staff and their skills, so, having identified resources, the successful leader needs to influence the team to complete the challenges ahead (Haslam 2001). The process of influencing the team to commit to achieving the set aims includes a subset of influential leadership skills such as delegating, decision-making and, occasionally, conflict management (Hewison and Griffiths 2004). Cook and Leathard (2004) identi-fied additional attributes required for an effective clinical leader: these were creativity, highlighting, influencing, respecting and supporting.

In return for their commitment, however, followers need to be motivated to achieve the stated goals by, for example, pay, personal development opportunities or, simply, job satisfaction (Deci and Ryan 1991). The need for motivation may seem to be somewhat surprising, especially in healthcare, a setting wherein most people tend to work because it is considered to be vocational: literally 'a calling' to give care and help to other people. However, how many healthcare workers would be happy to do their jobs, often giving up considerable personal time and effort, without pay? Pay is considered to function as an extrinsic motivator – that is, it is a tangible reward that people can see, feel and weigh in their hands, so to speak. Personal development, such as the acquisition of new skills, or job satisfaction, are motivators too but these are classed as intrinsic, basically feelgood factors that make an individual glow inside but without any immediate, tangible benefit (Carson and Carson 1997).

A closer look at behavioural leadership

Behavioural leadership focuses, literally, on the ways in which leaders and their fol-lowers behave and can be broadly categorised as below.

Autocratic leadership

The autocratic style places heavy emphasis on the task and job requirements, with less emphasis on people and the aforementioned interpersonal relationships (Northouse 2004). Arguably, this style might be seen as having more of an association with man-agement than leadership, since the common consensus of leadership is that, ultimately, it promotes success for the group. The autocratic style of leadership is results driven and the leader is often seen as controlling, demanding, hard-driving and overpower-ing (Margerison 2002). Northouse (2004) believes that an autocratic leader is one who uses threats, punishments and negative reward schedules. Communication from the leader, in such an environment, tends to be loud, hostile and with an air of superiority. Whitehead *et al.* (2007) argue that authoritarian leaders more commonly criticise the work of their followers, a perspective that van Knippenberg and Hogg (2003) concur with. All of these authors agree that the criticism provided by an autocratic leader is both more frequent and more destructive, personal and hurtful in comparison to the more constructive appraisal seen in other behavioural leadership styles. Accordingly, continued use of autocratic leadership within a team has been linked to a rise in absent-eeism and sickness rates. Swansburg and Swansburg (2002) have identified that these behaviours suggest low morale within followers, that being apparent in team members who are fearful, devious, turbulent in their intra-team relationships and indifferent about job performance.

Although autocratic leadership can be viewed as being a form of bullying, it is sometimes necessary to adopt this style in clinical practice. However, an autocratic leader is primarily there to give direction; they do not necessarily have to use punish-ments or to be viewed as a bully.

In essence, autocratic leaders tell people exactly what they want done. Followers are expected to obey orders, often without receiving any explanations.

The authoritarian leadership style exists along a spectrum, with a more aggressive approach at one end, that has been criticised as invoking a bullying approach (Crail 2001), and a more gentle, leading mode at the other end, which may be referred to as 'benign dictatorship', identified in Figure 18.1.

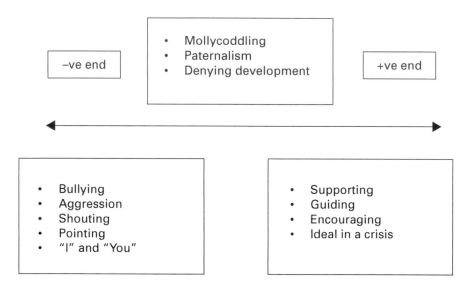

FIGURE 18.1 Autocratic leadership across the spectrum

The model in Figure 18.1 demonstrates a spectrum wherein, at the positive end, there is a gentle but firm leadership style that would suit new staff who do not know the ways in which the ward functions. Some subordinates may actually prefer a benign autocratic style and being told exactly what to do. Therefore, they need to be shown the expected ways of working in a non-threatening manner. However, the degree of support, at least initially, implies that there is little latitude for the new staff members to make suggestions or changes.

At the opposite end of the spectrum is the style that tends to be associated with autocratic leadership: commands are given in a unidirectional manner; there is no room for questioning or debate; the leader exerts authority, perhaps by shouting, and the atmosphere tends to be visibly hostile. Nonetheless, this is exactly the style of leadership that is required in an emergency, when there is no room for debate, e.g. if a patient has a cardiac arrest. Under such circumstances, the best outcome for the patient depends on a knowledgeable individual who can take charge. In the main, however, if the negative paradigm of autocratic behaviour is the norm, research suggests that autocratic leaders experience higher turnover among their staff.

Between the positive and negative variants of autocratic behaviour sits paternalistic leadership, wherein the leader becomes over-protective of their followers and does not allow them to make decisions in case they make the incorrect choices. While this approach may be laudable, in the short term, it can be damaging to development of staff, in the longer term, because as most are aware, it is by making mistakes that many people learn.

Democratic leadership

Martin (2006) stated that democratic leaders are more likely to consider the team as a whole and value each individual's skills within it. The democratic leader encourages participation and debate, relies on followers' knowledge for the completion of tasks, and depends on the team's respect for influence (Margerison 2004). This style of leadership is, therefore, a much more inclusive approach. Debate and free communication, in a bi-directional flow, is encouraged as the leader seeks the views of staff members who are held in high regard. The democratic leadership style is most effective when the leader wants to provide opportunities for employees to develop a high sense of personal growth and job satisfaction (Crail 2001). This, as widely reported in staff feedback, is regarded as being the preferred leadership style for nurses to work with as it leads to a sense of community and fulfillment for team members who are, for example, involved in planning and implementing strategies. Being involved in decision-making boosts staff morale, which in turn leads to a happier and more satisfied team. As such, this enhances the personal development of followers, a process which good leaders should encourage so that, if or when they leave their role, there is no detrimental effect on the team, the organisation or, in the healthcare scenario, patient care. Democratic styles are found to be at their most successful where there are few time constraints, and when the group is motivated and experienced.

While democratic leaders encourage the team to participate in decision-making, they remain in control of the final decision (Whitehead *et al.* 2007). Swansburg and Swansburg (2002) argue that democratic leaders place importance on valuing individuals and team work. Consequently, levels of job satisfaction and absenteeism rates are found to be improved under the democratic leader.

As is the case with autocratic leadership, the democratic leadership style also exists across a broad spectrum with strongly positive and negative elements. At the positive end, followers feel valued, involved and liable to enjoy personal development because

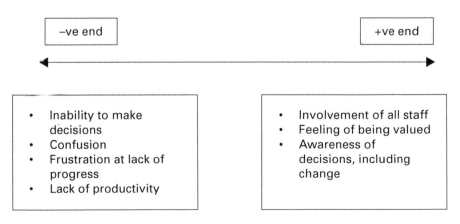

FIGURE 18.2 Democratic leadership across the spectrum

of either their involvement in making key decisions or, at least, their awareness of the issues under consideration. However, at the negative end, there could be a pervasive culture of indecision, even regarding the least important of judgements, including, for example, when colleagues should take their coffee breaks. This, in the fullness of time, would inevitably lead to a lack of productivity.

From practice it has been discovered that this style of leadership could fail to produce positive results if the group is unenthusiastic or inexperienced. Furthermore, Whitehead *et al.* (2007) identify that democratic leadership is not as efficient as autocratic leadership, although the work of a democratic-led team is more creative and self-motivated. However, this assertion may be open to question because evidence suggests that a happier team is more productive than a team characterised by fear of the leader. Figure 18.2 shows the spectrum of democratic leadership and its effects on followers.

Laissez-faire *leadership*

There is an absence of any obvious leadership in the *laissez-faire* style. This type of leader is, ostensibly, a very easy-going individual who will appear to allow everyone to do as they please. There are, however, two radically different interpretations of the *laissez-faire* leader: the individual who 'retires on the job' or the leader who knows that their followers are highly skilled and highly motivated individuals who do not require direct leadership. In the former case, this may be characterised by the leader who is not seen on the ward because they spend all their time in their office. If such a leader's intervention is required, they will be likely to turn a deaf ear, allowing their followers to flounder. In the latter case, the leader will consider that their experienced and able followers do not need interference with their daily routine which they all know so well. However, if direct intervention is required, such a leader will be quick to respond in a positive manner. As was seen in the cases of autocratic and democratic leadership styles, *laissez-faire* leadership also exists along a spectrum, as depicted in Figure 18.3.

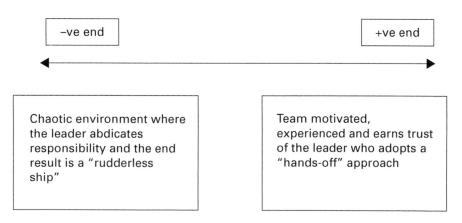

FIGURE 18.3 *Laissez-faire* leadership across the spectrum

The end result of *laissez-faire* leadership can be two entirely different groups of followers. On the positive side, there arc those in a *bona fide* team who know that their leader trusts them to do an excellent job, without the need for checking up on them. However, members within this group of followers know that, if they require help, it will readily be available. On the negative side, the worst scenario is a disparate bunch of individuals, who are definitely not able to function as a team, but who find themselves in a hopeless situation because neither they, nor apparently their leader, know in which direction they should be heading.

Situational leadership

While the three main aspects of behavioural leadership styles have been identified above, the successful leader should be able to move seamlessly between each, dependent upon the situation (Whitehead *et al.* 2007). The philosophy of being able to react to all situations that arise is known as the contingency or situational theory of leadership. As above, there is an argument that behavioural leadership can be explained as a mega-spectrum with autocratic leadership at one end and *laissez-faire* leadership at the other. In the middle lies democratic leadership and its close relatives, such as the paternalistic aspect of autocratic leadership, seen in Figure 18.4A.

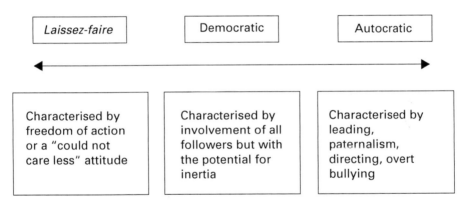

FIGURE 18.4A Behavioural leadership across the spectrum
Source: Tannenbaum and Schmidt 1973.

Tannenbaum and Schmidt (1973) created a simple but powerful model (Figure 18.4B) to demonstrate the range of leadership styles that can be experienced under the global banner of behavioural leadership.

Situated at the lower left corner is the novice nurse who is joining the ward. Ideally, the leader adopts a directive, benign autocratic stance in guiding the novice nurse in the ways of the ward. Note that there is no need for 100% direction from the leader because, for example, the novice nurse is aware of how a professional should act and how he or she should present for work. Progressively, there is less direction from the leader as the novice becomes more experienced and eventually, when the nurse has attained expertise and a thorough understanding of the ways in which the ward is run, there is minimal direction from the leader. Note, again, that there is never a situation of

100% freedom being exercised towards the expert nurse and this, of course, is because there will always be policies and protocols that guide practice.

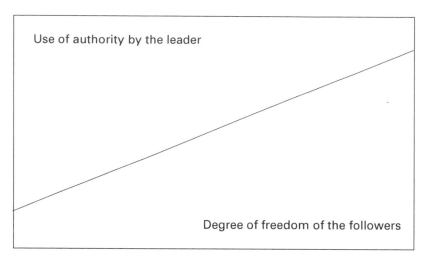

Use of authority by the leader

Degree of freedom of the followers

FIGURE 18.4B Leadership across the spectrum

WHY IS LEADERSHIP IMPORTANT?

Leadership is important to ensure not only that goals are achieved by the healthcare team but also that scarce resources, including staff, are used most cost-effectively. This takes into account the advanced skills and knowledge of practitioners who have bene-fited from studying in higher education. In contemporary society, the aim is not just to achieve goals but to make team members feel valued for their contributions.

Applications to cancer and palliative care education

The Nursing Contribution to Cancer Care (DoH 2000b) specifically recognised the need for leadership skills in those who would be responsible for delivering the National Cancer Plan. In particular, there was the acknowledgment that funding needed to be identified to facilitate leadership training and development for nurses, in the cancer care community, in order to meet the goals of the contemporary NHS. Part of the funding was ring-fenced for establishing the Leadership Centre for Health, closely allied to the Modernisation Agency, that was to be charged with supporting leadership development of clinicians and managers, to prepare them for the changes required in the twenty-first-century NHS.

EVIDENCE OF GOOD EDUCATION PRACTICE

For more than 30 years, the King's Fund has run leadership programmes for a spectrum of individuals from nurses to board members. The Department of Health-sponsored programme 'Leading an Empowered Organisation' (LEO), arguably the best known leadership programme, has been delivered to some 60 000 health workers in the past ten years. However, research into the effectiveness of LEO in enhancing patient care is, at best, equivocal (Cooper 2003; Hancock and Campbell 2006; Werrett *et al.* 2002; Woolnough and Faugier 2002).

In 2005, the Department of Health developed 'Improvement Leaders' Guides' which offered leaders the chance to develop their skills and knowledge to become competent leaders. This placed a great deal of emphasis on creating an environment in which individuals are constantly encouraged and supported to enable them to think for themselves. There appears to have been no evaluation of the effectiveness of these guides, as yet.

The Royal College of Nursing (2007) runs a clinical leadership programme to help practitioners develop patient-centred leadership strategies to cope with day-to-day management. It claims that clinical leaders who have attended the course have been converted to adapt their leadership styles, with improvements in patient care and working relationships, which suggests that leadership style and emotional intelligence can be taught.

ISSUES SALIENT TO LEADERSHIP

Adopting leadership behaviours was reported to hold significant implications in the 'Agenda for Change' (DoH 2004) role evaluations. Workers who demonstrated leadership behaviours and skills, in the views of team members and patients, were reputedly progressing through gateways faster and rising up the pay scale quicker (DoH 2004).

KEY POINTS

- The need for leadership in the care environment has been driven by contemporary policy direction from the Department of Health.
- Analysis of leadership behaviours demonstrates that there are multiple variants of behavioural leadership.
- The effective leader must be able to adopt the leadership style appropriate to the context.

CONCLUSION

Effective leadership is essential to the optimal functioning of clinical practice. There is no single, overriding, best style of leadership but, ideally, a leader should have a mixture of skills to use in supporting their team (DoH 2005). A good leader must be able to know their followers in terms of ability, knowledge, desire and willingness. The author leaves the reader to use this material to make their own connections to cancer and palliative care. An effective leader must be able to balance tasks and relationships within their team and be ready to move from one style to another, depending on the situation, using appropriate behaviour for any given situation (Storey 2003; Yoder-Wise 2003). In conclusion, each style has its role in the workplace and can be used for different situations and tasks, and for the maturity and level of professionalism of employees.

IMPLICATIONS FOR THE READER'S OWN PRACTICE

1   How can you incorporate leadership training into the field of cancer and palliative care?
2   In what ways will the theories of leadership impact and contribute to your teaching?
3   What creative teaching activities could you employ to illustrate the different styles of leadership?

REFERENCES

Carson KD, Carson P (1997) Career entrenchment: a quiet march toward occupational death. *Acad Manag Exec.* **11** (1): 62–75.

Chemers MM, Ayman R, editors (1993) *Leadership Theory and Research: perspectives and directions.* London: Academic Press.

Cook M, Leathard H (2004) Learning for clinical leadership. *J Nurs Manag.* **12** (6): 436–44.

Cooper SJ (2003) An evaluation of the 'Leading an Empowered Organisation' programme. *Nurs Stand.* **17** (24): 33–9.

Crail M (2001) *Leadership in the NHS.* London: Emap.

Daft RL (1999) *Leadership: theory and practice.* Fort Worth, TX: Dryden Press.

Deci EL, Ryan RM (1991) A motivational approach to self: integration in personality. In: Dienstbier RA, editor. *Nebraska Symposium on Motivation.* Lincoln, NE: University of Nebraska Press: 237–88.

Department of Health (2000a) *The NHS Plan: a plan for investment, a plan for reform.* London: DoH.

Department of Health (2000b) *The Nursing Contribution to Cancer Care.* London: DoH.

Department of Health (2004) *The NHS Improvement Plan: putting people at the heart of public services.* London: DoH.

Department of Health (2005) *Developing Excellence in Leadership with Urgent Care.* London: DoH.

Department of Health. (2006) *Our Health, Our Care, Our Say: a new direction for community services.* London: DoH.

Goleman D (1996) *Emotional Intelligence.* London: Bloomsbury.

Hancock H, Campbell S (2006) Impact of the 'Leading an Empowered Organisation' programme. *Nurs Stand.* **20** (19): 41–8.

Haslam SA (2001) *Psychology in Organizations: the social identity approach.* London: Sage.

Hewison A, Griffiths MM (2004) Leadership development in health care: a word of caution. *J Health Organ Manag.* **18** (6): 464–73.

Huczynski A (2004) *Influencing Within Organizations.* London: Routledge.

Lewin K (1935) *A Dynamic Theory of Personality.* New York: McGraw-Hill.

Margerison CJ (2002) *Team Leadership.* London: Thomson.

Martin V (2006) Leading in teams: part one. *Nurs Manag.* **13** (1): 33–6.

Merrison A (1979) *Report of the Royal Commission on the National Health Service.* London: HMSO.

Milner E, Joyce P (2005) Lessons in leadership, meeting the challenges of public service management. *Pub Admin.* **84** (4): 1104–8.

Northouse PG (2004) *Leadership: theory and practice.* 3rd ed. London: Sage Publications.

Reitman WR (1961) Need achievement, fear of failure, and selective recall. *J Abnorm Soc Psychol.* **62**: 142–4.

Rigolosi ELM (2005) *Management and Leadership in Nursing and Healthcare: an experimental approach.* 2nd ed. New York: Springer.

Roe A (1957) Early determinants of vocational choice. *J Couns Psychol.* **4**: 212–17.

Royal College of Nursing (2007) Clinical Leadership Programme. Available at: www.rcn.org.uk/resources/clinicalleadership/

Sadler P (1997) *Leadership.* London: Kogan Page.

Stone AG, Russell RF, Patterson K (2004) Transformational *versus* servant leadership: a difference in leader focus. *Leader Organ Dev J.* **25** (4): 349–61.

Storey L, Howard J, Gillies A (2002) *Competency in Healthcare: a practical guide to competency frameworks.* Oxford: Radcliffe Medical Press.

Storey J (2003) *Leadership in Organisations: current issues and key trends.* Abingdon: Routledge.

Sullivan EJ, Decker PJ (2005) Leading and managing. In: Connor M, editor. *Effective Leadership and Management in Nursing.* 6th ed. Upper Saddle River, NJ: Pearson Prentice Hall: 43–66.

Swansburg RC, Swansburg RJ (2002) *Introduction to Management and Leadership for Nurse Managers.* Sudbury, MA: Jones and Bartlett.

Tannenbaum R, Schmidt WH (1973) How to choose a leadership pattern. *Harv Bus Rev.* **51**: 162–80.

Taylor-Moss M (2005) *The Emotionally Intelligent Nurse Leader.* San Francisco, CA: Wiley.

van Knippenberg D, Hogg MA (2003) *Leadership and Power: identity processes in groups and organizations.* London: Sage Publications.

Weiner B (1995) *Judgments of Responsibility: a foundation for a theory of social conduct.* New York: Guilford Press.

Werrett J, Griffiths M, Clifford C (2002) A regional evaluation of the impact of the 'Leading an Empowered Organisation' programme. *Nurs Times.* **7** (6): 459–70.

Whitehead DK, Weiss SA, Tappen RM (2007) *Essentials of Nursing Leadership and Management.* Philadelphia, PA: FA Davis Co.

Woolnough H, Faugier J (2002) An evaluative study assessing the impact of the 'Leading an Empowered Organisation' programme. *Nurs Times.* **7** (6): 412–17.

Yoder-Wise P (2003) *Leading and Managing in Nursing.* 3rd ed. London: Mosby.

19

The ultimate challenge: a successful, productive, cohesive and dynamic team?

Lorna Foyle and Janis Hostad

'Snowflakes are one of nature's most fragile things, but just look what they can do when they stick together.'

Vesta Kelly

AIM

This chapter aims to look at the multi-layered, complex issues which health-care professionals encounter within their work teams. The teacher's role in developing methods to tailor training to each unique individual team will be explored.

LEARNING OUTCOMES

By the end of this chapter, the reader should be able to:
- examine current team theory and models
- identify policy drivers which determine that interdisciplinary team-working is core to clinical practice
- celebrate the work of highly effective teams in these specialities
- equip teachers and facilitators with the ability to distinguish between effective and dysfunctional teams
- explore different methods of team-building in the speciality of cancer and palliative care
- identify appropriate teaching methods to enhance team-working.

INTRODUCTION

Team-working is now part of the everyday language of all healthcare professionals, yet few of these professionals would be able to describe what team-working is, or how team-working impacts on patient and carer outcomes. Although this could be deemed a criticism, it is hardly surprising considering the amount of training that professionals receive on team-working during their training and subsequent continuing professional development. Most training is generally on an *ad hoc* basis. Formal training which links team-working to organisational structural issues and policy development and implementation is minimal. The trend for interdisciplinary working has arisen from a raft of government policies, and most of the literature in the first decade of the twenty-first century tends to focus on the impact of interdisciplinary and multidisciplinary meetings. In stark contrast, the literature on effective uni-disciplinary team-working has diminished, and yet this, too, is an essential component of delivering effective care in the specialities of oncology and palliative care.

Nursing teams are responsible for 24-hour care of patients when they are treated in the acute hospital setting or as an inpatient in hospice care. It is not in the scope of this chapter to compare and contrast the benefits and limitations of uni-disciplinary and multidisciplinary team-working. However, it is crucial to grasp that any disharmony within single discipline teams, such as nursing, must inevitably impact on the relationships with other professional groups. The first part of this chapter is more theoretical, and questions and debates some of the literature in the context of cancer and palliative care. The second part of the chapter is more practical in nature, and seeks to provide the reader with useful ways to team build and teach the topic.

BACKGROUND

Payne (2004) traces the history of teamwork, which originated in the 1930s in response to the rational science movement, which later became known as the human relationship school. The concept of team-working developed in other industrial organisations until the mid-1960s, when the notion of teamwork finally migrated to the health services. Teamwork in various healthcare settings is based on three assumptions.

The first assumption is that teams, whether they are multidisciplinary or uni-disciplinary, are more effective than individuals working in isolation.

West (1994) points out that this is not necessarily a correct assumption, and researches experiments which social psychologists refer to as 'social loafing' (Fuller and Tulle-Winton 1996). Social loafing describes the fact that individuals work less hard when their efforts are combined with those of other team members, compared to the effort that individuals can make when working in isolation on the same task. This challenges the notion that teams are more effective than the sum of the contributions of individual members. Team decision-making can often fall short of the quality of decisions made by their most capable individual team members (Rogelberg *et al.* 1992).

The second assumption about team-working is that integrated and cohesive teams are more effective than fragmented, dysfunctional teams. Comparative studies on functional teams and dysfunctional teams are virtually non-existent. Dysfunctional teams rarely declare their frailties, and therefore it is difficult to enrol them into comparative studies. It is important therefore to have a clear definition of what a dysfunctional team is. Lencioni (2002) discusses team failure, and postulates that the five dysfunctions of a team are:

➤ absence of trust
➤ fear of conflict
➤ lack of commitment
➤ avoidance of accountability
➤ inattention to results.

Research is still needed to define clearly what is meant by a 'functional team' and a 'dysfunctional team'.

Assumption three is based on the belief that team-working is an inherent skill, and does not require developing or training (West 1994: 97).

Despite these thought-provoking assumptions, a range of policies has determined the current status of cancer and palliative care teams in healthcare provision in the UK. Throughout the NHS, the old hierarchal ways of working have given way to more flexible team-working between different clinical professions (DoH 2000). Teamwork is seen as a central feature of current NHS healthcare (DoH, NHS Executive 2000).

The NICE Guidance on Cancer Services (2004), *Improving Supportive and Palliative Care for Adults with Cancer*, defines the multidisciplinary team as:

> 'a group of health and social care professionals from a range of disciplines, who meet regularly to discuss and agree plans of treatment and care for people with a particular type of cancer or problem, or in a particular location. This includes primary care teams, site specific cancer teams and specialist palliative care teams.'

Multidisciplinary teams tend to be the favoured model of team-working in cancer care. In this setting, multidisciplinary team meetings may happen once or twice a week, have a very structured process, and are generally led by a doctor. Contrast this with the interdisciplinary model that is favoured in palliative care, where there appears to be a closer connection between the various members of the team, and meetings will also be scheduled on a regular basis. In this model, the leadership role may be adopted by a different team member, as the necessity arises. Different disciplines will take on the leadership role, depending on the requirements of the task. Multidisciplinary teams are often perceived as having a well-defined hierarchical management structure, compared to palliative care teams which appear to have a flat management team structure, although there is no strong evidence to support either viewpoint.

Team types

Healthcare professionals do not just work in one team. They are members in a variety of teams. For example, nurses who work on a cancer ward will be members of the nursing team, the multidisciplinary team, the organisation that they work for and even any specialist projects in which they are involved. They may also be affiliated to local, regional and national policy groups or professional associations. These teams may often require the same level of commitment from members, whether it is a short-term or long-term team commitment. Replicate this level of team membership to all professionals providing healthcare, and the number of different healthcare teams that exist at any one time in a healthcare system is almost boundless. Effective team-working is well documented in the literature, particularly in the multidisciplinary team-working arena. Yet minimal evidence is available on the type of team-building educational strategies for educationalists and facilitators, to improve team dynamics and functioning.

The authors of this chapter have been involved in team-building across acute trusts, primary care trusts, hospices, and the voluntary and independent sectors in healthcare provision. Team-building activities were designed with uni-disciplinary and multidisciplinary teams in mind when the authors were commissioned. Some activities are a regular feature on all team-building sessions, while others were employed to meet specific team needs in the diagnostic phase. Many of these teaching endeavours will be detailed later in the chapter.

One discipline which regularly commissions team-building from the authors is nursing. The Nursing and Midwifery Council Code of Conduct for the UK emphasises that *'registered nurses must co-operate with others in teams and work effectively as part of a team'* (NMC 2008). Likewise, multidisciplinary teams will request team-building activities to enhance team dynamics and interactions.

Qualities of effective team functioning

The aim of every high-quality team, whatever its composition, is to optimise the use of information, people and resources to achieve the best clinical outcomes for patients.

In order to meet this aim, teams will have key characteristics in place: effective leadership, positive attitudes, successful collaboration and efficient communication. Teams possessing these key components create an atmosphere of mutual trust and expertise (Firth-Cozens 1992; Driskell *et al.* 2006). A cohesive team will have effective communication and successful collaboration, and will provide mutual support for each member. Any team, regardless of the care setting, should have a competent leader.

Leadership has become associated with the qualities of being inspirational and promoting team cohesion. The leadership role can often be compromised by the incumbent's managerial role in the employing organisation.

Leadership involves the ability to coordinate the activities of team members by ensuring that team actions are understood, changes in information are shared, and team members have the necessary resources to deliver quality patient care. Leaders can assume one of the many models of leadership to develop their personal leadership style. This is discussed in greater detail by Ian Grigor in Chapter 18.

A dynamic leader has confidence, awareness of personal strengths and weaknesses, and motivation and enthusiasm to attain standards of care. An effective leader will foster a positive environment that will encourage all team members to learn and contribute. A positive environment in turn will develop cohesion and collaboration, and will ultimately help to create an excellent team. A well-functioning healthcare team is additionally made up of team members who all exhibit a positive attitude, and contribute to the team effort, and trust and value their colleagues (Cashman *et al.* 2004; Molyneux 2001; Pethybridge 2004).

The terms 'teamwork' and 'collaboration' are often used interchangeably. Successful collaboration is a vital phenomenon to healthcare providers and patients. Collaboration within a healthcare team is a complex process which requires intentional knowledge-sharing and joint responsibility for patient care. The level of collaboration that takes place among healthcare team members can directly impact patient outcomes. Effective team-working relies on collaborative working, the sharing of goals, an understanding and respect for roles within the team, and key communication skills (Vanclay 1997).

The majority of chapters in this book focus on the importance of communications skills in our relationships with our patients and their carers, and with our colleagues. Most of the literature (Payne 2004; Borrill *et al.* 2001; West 2003; Maddocks 2006) that looks at effective team functioning emphasises the importance of communications within and outside the team. Despite this call to ensure effective communication skills within teams, other studies report that poor communication skills between professionals (Bliss *et al.* 2000; Street and Blackford 2001; Hansford and Barry 2002; Sasahara *et al.* 2003; O'Connor *et al.* 2006) remain in the majority of teams. The authors of this chapter would certainly agree that the work that they have undertaken with dysfunctional teams has discovered a lack of open communication between members (although often with the most noble of intentions). Some of the teams we have worked with have also had leadership and managerial issues that have caused conflict, in either a small or large degree. Roles and responsibilities have been a source of contention for team members who have attended our team-building courses. Sometimes the source of these tensions is not between disciplines, but between team members who have the same professional background. Responsibilities and expectations are typically blurred, so what one team member is 'supposed to do' (O'Connor *et al.* 2006) may overlap with activities undertaken by another team member. When roles become blurred, there is a need for clear demarcation of specific roles and responsibilities, while identifying activities that can be mutually accomplished by a combined effort. To summarise, team members are expected to communicate well, and to build up a sense of self-belief and affinity to the team. To achieve this, individuals need a certain level of self-knowledge and confidence in their own professional role and skills. Individuals also demand appropriate levels of respect, recognition and encouragement while working in teams (Molyneux 2001).

Teams cannot develop in organisations that do not recognise that the institutional structure and processes have the potential to create highly effective, functioning teams. Conversely, some organisations can stifle innovation and be the direct (or indirect) cause of dysfunctional teams. There needs to be flexible, respectful and responsive workforce development opportunities if teams are to maintain their effectiveness (Cashman *et al.* 2004).

BUILDING AN EFFECTIVE TEAM

Over time, the authors have been commissioned to provide team-building education in a variety of institutions, and they have become increasingly aware of contributing factors that made teams appear dysfunctional. These have been discussed in the first half of this chapter. It is important to stress here that not all teams are dysfunctional, but some teams feel the need to engage facilitators to enhance their estimable team-working processes, in the pursuit of excellence. Teams are frequently exhorted to indulge in team-building activities, and Payne and Olivierc (2006) suggest that 'everyday team-building' can happen on a daily basis through the use of case discussion in the speciality. However, embryonic teams may not have reached this stage in the development of the team, and may feel that they have not the capability to interact at this level. As far as the authors are concerned, every time a team member leaves or a new one arrives, the team dynamics shift and the team reverts back to being an embryonic team, which parallels the forming stage of Tuckman's (1965) model of the developmental sequence in small groups.

In order to assist in meeting the requirements of each team's unique needs, a process was developed which enabled identification of each team's individual requirements, and then specific activities could be matched to those needs.

The process has been refined, and this model can guide towards providing the appropriate level of team support and team-building activities. Other team-building research-based projects that have been undertaken at a national level in the NHS have financial implications for hard-pressed healthcare organisations, which they can ill-afford involvement at this level. Alternatives to this costly approach need to be sought in the future. The authors' well-formed model provides facilitators with a useful process, and it is economical, because it limits the time needed for extensive facilitation and time away from practice. The authors do always recommend at least two days (and depending on the team and its needs, possibly more). These are usually conducted separately, so that the identified work can be applied back into practice (in between each session), with the knowledge that change needs time, and is best completed in a step-by-step approach.

Figure 19.1 illustrates the model, which has six clear stages.

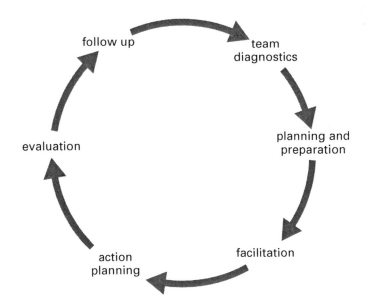

FIGURE 19.1 Model of the team-building process

The stages are detailed below, and are illustrated with activities which the authors use regularly. These explanations provide clarity regarding this approach, and useful exercises for facilitating team-building. Additionally, many of them will be helpful in the classroom when teaching. The authors believe that the phrase 'team-building' is applicable to any activity (or programme) that is designed to help a group of *interdependent* people to generate and create a lasting behaviour change, resulting in a more motivated, cohesive, efficient and productive culture.

To illustrate how this model might be used in practice, Stage 3 will be much longer than the others, to incorporate 'how to' exercises, which might be useful to the reader.

Stage 1: diagnostic phase

This is a crucial phase, and does require the facilitator to find out as much information as possible prior to setting a team-building date, and before the preparatory planning work is initiated. However, what the team or manager describes as the reason for requiring the team-building is usually a 'surface issue' rather than the 'deeper' major issue which has necessitated the team-building day. Often, the manager and the team provide different agendas, which make the planning and preparation interesting.

Possible reasons for team-building include:
- improving communication
- making the workplace more enjoyable
- motivating the team
- getting to know each other better, and increasing self-awareness
- planning new goals, or getting everyone to work towards the same goals
- teaching the team self-regulation strategies
- identifying and utilising the strengths of team members
- improving team productivity
- dealing with conflict inside and outside the team
- learning and practising effective collaboration with team members.

So, the 'diagnostics' start here at this point. However, this diagnostic stage is ongoing, being changed and refined depending on the results of questionnaires, visits and other exploratory investigative work prior to the event. On the day, group dynamics, individual participation, group activities and group interaction will further refine the initial diagnosis. Even prior to the follow-up meeting, the diagnostics will continue, possibly leading to further changes.

Occasionally questionnaires are completed prior to the event. However, the authors prefer not to do so. Anything which might pre-empt or affect what happens on the day is best avoided. It always works better if the group does not have the chance to discuss their answers together.

To start to gain a clear picture of what is required, it is useful to ask some pertinent questions, such as:
- What does your organisation want to get out of this exercise?
- What are the needs of the current team?
- What is the general age of the participants within this team?

This is followed by more specific questions, such as:
➤ What is happening within this group which illustrates that its members are not working efficiently as a team?
➤ What areas can team-building be useful in helping this team to improve?
➤ Are there areas of miscommunication, which slows down work activity?
➤ Are there conflicts, which bring down morale?
➤ Do members of this team focus on their own success at the expense of others?
➤ Would it be difficult for new members of staff to fit in with the existing team members?
➤ Are changes in strategy and policy resisted by team members?
➤ Do team members feel as though they have no influence in strategy and policy-making?

At the beginning, it is always useful to ask what their well-formed outcomes are for the day, which helps to initiate the diagnostic stage.

On one occasion, a questionnaire was sent out prior to the event in order to ascertain individuals' viewpoints and to focus the planning and preparation. This was on a ward where a member of their staff was being tried for manslaughter. This meant that all the staff had to be interviewed in depth, and their ward procedures and care were put under great scrutiny. It was a difficult time for everyone, and morale was very low. Many of the ward staff perceived that health professionals outside their ward were implicating all their ward team, suggesting that they had been covering up for their colleague. This caused much distress, but also brought about a special unity between them. However, they mistook their unity for everyone feeling the same. From contact with some of the staff prior to the event, it became clear that individuals were struggling to cope in many different ways. So, a pre-event questionnaire was sent out just prior to the event and the participants replied anonymously (with over 90% return). These results were presented to them at the beginning of the day. This proved not only to be an excellent diagnostic tool, but also very useful for raising 'self' and 'group' awareness. The group did much hard work that day, having found that while they *were* united, they were suffering in *many different* ways. They went on to successfully support each other as individuals, and with a renewed feeling of togetherness.

Stage 2: planning and preparation
Prior to any event of this nature, much planning and preparation needs to be completed in order to ensure the smooth running of the day(s). If this is a new team (brand new or including new team members), the activities will be different from those needed for a dysfunctional team. The plans for many team activities will have some commonality. For instance, there will always be ground rules, agenda-setting and action planning. During the planning stage, it is essential that two facilitators are present. It is impossible to do a really first-rate job of team-building as a lone worker. There are too many elements to consider, and too many individuals to observe, as well as the overall group dynamics. Another consideration should be that the facilitators are comfortable with and trust each other. This is vital to the success of the team-building exercise, as each of the facilitators has to have faith in the other's ability, and be able to rely on their

judgement. Conversely, the relationship has to be strong enough so that they can question each other's observations, ideas and plans. This means being confident and flexible enough to change the carefully prepared plans (at a moment's notice) to run with the group's agenda. So, in summary, this co-facilitation works best when each facilitator can be reliant on and have faith in their partner, and when this partnership remains interdependent at all times.

During this stage, the facilitator will actively work to produce a plan by assessing the team, making recommendations, and providing activities (exercises which comprise appropriate team-building interventions) for the team. These responsibilities usually require the facilitators to write a proposal (or possible plan) after their diagnosis of the team, indicating how they would go about improving the team's performance. The manager and the team usually follow the advice of the facilitator in determining which recommendations will be utilised.

The facilitator is then responsible for providing useful interventions which will transfer effectively back into the team and the organisational setting. This requires creating a detailed plan of events, while allowing for flexibility.

Stage 3: facilitation

To discover the underlying issues and problems of teams, assisting them to work towards finding their solutions, takes time. Therefore, at the beginning of any day, it is essential to start establishing rapport and gaining trust. Introductions are completed first, which starts to build familiarity. However, the ground rules are crucial for starting to establish trust.

Ground rules

This involves ensuring that the rules are generated by the group. They need to be written down and displayed visibly, so everyone can see them. There may be additions by the facilitators, but the rules must always be agreed to collectively by the group. Considerations include issues related to mobile phones, constructive comments, respect, and time-keeping, and many more. Confidentiality obviously needs to be addressed in the normal manner. In addition, with this type of teamwork, the team also needs to know what the facilitators will 'take away' or 'leave' in the room. Another important ground rule, which the authors insist on, is the use of 'I' language, so that the individual owns their thoughts (and does not presume to 'mind read' those of others). This does have a proviso in that, towards the end of the day, the facilitators will then, on occasion, encourage 'we' thinking and 'we' language.

The team's manager(s) may require a report on the day, so that they can see the time invested in this venture is being utilised effectively. If this is the case, the authors send the report to the team first, to ensure that the rules of confidentiality have not been broken, and to check the content, allowing them to veto anything which is not acceptable. Then, after the report has been accepted or adapted, it is sent to the managers. This report does not go into content detail, but only outlines the main agreed principles of action which the team plan to take. This is fully discussed as part of the ground rules.

Agenda-setting

The next routine item on team-building days is the agenda. This is gained in different ways, depending on the team and on whether the facilitators are familiar with them. Sometimes participants are asked to provide their ideas on 'post-its', anonymously in the first instance. If people are working in groups, they are asked to ensure that every-one's opinions are captured on paper. This is so that everyone's needs are heard equally. The facilitators are mindful that it might not be everyone's agenda, however, and will find ways of confirming this during the day. The agenda is written on a flip-chart, and agreement is sought. The flip-chart page is then pinned to the wall, for reference during the day.

On the first day, there are a few key sessions that will remain the same in 'essence', but will be adapted to take account of the team's agenda items. However, this is also the point when a number of the pre-planned sessions will be discarded, as the facilitators respond to the immediate needs of the group.

For example, one team which had new members wanted to be positive and proac-tive, moving on from previous difficult times, for themselves and also for their new colleagues. As this issue was clearly very important to several of the team, it was neces-sary to deal with it at the beginning of the day. This allowed the team to look forwards, rather than to dwell on the past. The previously planned activity was replaced, to deal with this more immediate issue. The participants were given 'post-its' and asked to write on separate pages what they wished to leave behind (from their previous team) in order to move on. They were also asked what they wished to take with them from the old team (to their new team) in order to move forward positively.

The rationale for this is the power of writing down issues and feelings, as the act of writing clarifies a situation, detaches the individual from it, reduces its hold, and often starts to show the way forward. Participants were then asked to get up and to cross 'the line' (this can be imaginary, or a line created using string). This is to help to symbolise a place where they are going to leave these things behind. They each tell the team what they are leaving behind, and why, and then drop the written issue into a rubbish bag. When they have done this, they walk back across the line, away from the troubles and back to where their new solutions will be created. The team is performing a ritual, and ritual can emphasise intent. This creates a symbol of what was previously troubling them – the 'post-its' detailing their problems – which were deposited over the line into a rubbish bag. Throwing them away in this way can absolve and release team members from their concerns. The state of despair and 'stuckness' which some team members can face is a solitary and isolating one. Ritual can take them away from their negative feelings and reconnect them with the positive team spirit. This part of the exercise can be very emotional, and there might well be tears. The second part of the exercise is for each person to stand up and place their positive 'post-its' on the flip-chart, explaining to the group what they are taking with them from the old team and why (staying on their side of the line). This sheet of paper is displayed where everyone can see it, for the rest of the day.

Never underestimate the importance of this type of exercise. Everyone is interested in what the new team members want to leave and to bring. However, it is even more important for the old team members to communicate that they want to leave these issues in the past. Also, if old team members are 'recovering' from past problems, it is very useful for the harmony of the group for the new members to be aware of this, while keeping it as content-free as possible.

Team activity

At this stage of the day, the team is usually asked to participate in 'team' exercises, which are designed to be challenging but non-threatening, and as much fun as possible. However, some exercises may, due to their function and nature, be a little more serious. The first exercise acts as an ice-breaker, and helps the team to start to relax. Many of the exercises (that the authors have invented themselves) tend to be multifunctional and match the outcomes for the day. However, some are designed to be very specific in assisting participants to work towards the team's goals. The authors usually use their own exercises, or ones which they have adapted (or ones recommended by colleagues). The components of a team-building exercise should be as follows.

Instructions

This part of a team-building exercise involves providing simple instructions for the exercise and ensuring that everyone has understood. It can be most useful to accompany this with written instructions if there is much to remember.

Activity

This is the exercise itself. The facilitators should observe the groups constantly, not only to check that they have understood what they are to do, but also to observe the group dynamics. The facilitators will be assessing how the group works together, who works with whom, who tends to get left out, who takes the lead, how they process the information and work towards their goal, and so on.

Feedback and debriefing

This is the most important part of a team-building exercise. When the facilitators have closed the exercise, it is crucial to review the purpose of the exercise, and how the team accomplished it. A debriefing is important to reiterate the purpose of the exercise, and to keep participants focused on the positive outcomes of the exercise. Feedback on specific body language, paralanguage, types of questions, approaches, time-keepers, behaviours, and many other components relevant to the exercise, is very effective. The authors have found video-recording the group to be useful. Often, the group members are surprised and enlightened by their behaviours. However, being aware of the video camera, the participants might not act in their normal manner.

Type of activity

Team-building exercises consist of a variety of tasks designed to develop group members, and their ability to work together, effectively. There are many types of team-building activities, including exercises involving unusual tasks (sometime simple, and sometimes more complex) and others designed for specific needs. The purpose of team-building exercises is to assist a team to become a more cohesive unit, so that they can work together effectively to complete a variety of tasks. (There are also team-building activities that are composed of multiple fitness exercises, such as ropes and assault courses. These types of activities will not be discussed as part of this chapter.)

The rationale for using each exercise needs to be clear and appropriate, depending on the desired outcome. For example, there are mainly four types of exercises: ones which are specific to communications, or problem-solving, or which are change orientated, or trust-building related.

➤ *Communications exercises* are ones which focus on improving communications via problem-solving activities. The issues which teams encounter in these exercises are solved by communicating effectively with each other. The goal, via this exercise, is to highlight the many potential problems with poor communication, and the importance of good communication to team performance. These communication-type exercises (and the next ones regarding problem-solving and decision-making) seem to be the ones most commonly used for cancer and palliative care professionals.

➤ *Decision-making and problem-solving exercises* are ones where the team is given a problem which requires a creative solution, or where the solution is not immediately apparent, or, as in real life where, just when the team thinks they have solved it, the problem gathers more dimensions (provided by the facilitators, depending on the way the exercise is progressing) and becomes rather more difficult to solve. The goal of these exercises is to focus specifically on groups working together to make difficult decisions, and to solve problems efficiently and in a timely manner. The feedback will be constructive and the endeavours of participants praised, but point out any methods which might have been quicker or more effective.

➤ *Change-orientated exercises* focus on aspects of planning, and being adaptable to change. There are many important problems for teams to be able to solve when they are assigned complex tasks, or in order to make difficult decisions. The main aim for this type of activity is to illustrate the importance of planning, as well as raising awareness, in terms of how each individual reacts when they choose to be involved in change. On the other hand, how do these same individuals react when change is imposed? The debriefing offers a chance to discuss how they react and how they might plan, cope and actually embrace all types of change in the future.

➤ *Trust exercises* involve engaging team members in a way that will induce trust between them. They are usually not difficult to implement, as long as they are not introduced too early in the day. Later is better, because by then the group has built trust in the facilitator and on account of this feels more comfortable in taking risks. The goal of this exercise is to increase (or in some instances, to create) trust between the team members. It is also important that, during the debrief, the team members relate this back into the context of their work. They can discuss how differing levels of trust between individuals, and different degrees of individual comfort in trusting others, always exist in the workplace. The session ends with the team exploring ways in which they might increase this trust in future.

The next section will detail two team tasks produced by the authors. These types of exercises have been used by multidisciplinary healthcare teams, hospice bedded-unit staff, Macmillan teams, cancer ward teams, administrative staff, and many more.

Examples of team activity

Exercise 19.1

In this activity, the team is asked to produce a magazine. They are divided into groups, and each group is given a 'feature' item, such as a problem page, a fashion article, news item, and so on. However, they are asked to liaise with the other groups in order to maintain their corporate identity, and have a theme running throughout.

They are given a deadline, which changes during production. Also, they asked to liaise with the other groups to collectively devise an acceptable publication title and front cover.

Each team has to elect a spokesperson, who will liaise with the magazine editors (the facilitators) when required to do so.

They are given a criteria sheet, which explains what they will be marked on.

The team are given coloured pens, old magazines, glue, scissors and sellotape, to assist in their task.

The debriefing

The groups always enjoy completing this exercise, and are usually very proud of their publication. Having praised the participants' masterpieces (for they often are), the facilitators then ensure that conclusions from this exercise are discussed.

- How did the groups work together?
- Did they accomplish the desired outcome?
- Did everyone take part?
- How did they liaise with the other groups to reach agreement?
- What happened when the deadlines changed?
- How would they have felt if they had not been praised?

All these aspects are discussed in relation to this specific exercise, even though the processes are very much the same in their clinical practice. Often, initially this is easier and more comfortable than discussing work directly. Later, the parallels to the work situation can be drawn out, and discussion encouraged by the facilitators.

This exercise can be adapted to reflect a specific team difficulty. For example, individuals from one particular feature-article group could be taken away to start up a new feature, leaving the original group short-staffed. Alternatively, there could be much more editorial interference.

These similarities to their own difficulties tend to provoke much discussion, and it is well worth including them.

This exercise is both a communication and a problem-solving type of exercise, and so questions need to reflect this, together with guidance of things which participants can do to improve aspects of these issues.

After performing these exercises in the past, the authors have made many interesting observations. For example, NHS staff seldom try to negotiate a later deadline. In many cases, they work through their coffee break in order to finish the task. When they suddenly find themselves short-staffed, they complain, but carry on nevertheless. These observations are very useful to feed back to the teams.

Another exercise which the authors use in a similar way involves the whole team working together. It calls for them to allocate roles appropriately, in order to complete an *Apprentice*-type project. They are required to 'invent' an exciting new health drink. They must explain what it is, and what it contains, and produce a creative name for it. They will report back on how the team will market it, and they have to come up with an advertising 'catch phrase', and make a formal presentation to the board. This is always a fun exercise, and it is very useful to see how the group divides into different tasks, whether they negotiate between themselves, and how, when they divided up the roles, they played to their strengths. On completion, they are asked to reflect on how they worked on the task. Are they normally so creative? Do they always play to their strengths? How might they do better?

Trust-building and 'getting to know you' activities

During the day, it might also be useful to incorporate 'getting to know you' exercises, and other 'bonding' or trust-building exercises.

A simple, but efficient, exercise is to ask everyone to describe something they are passionate about (away from work) and to tell the team all about it (preferably something others don't already know). This is safe because participants choose what they want to share, and it usually causes lots of interest and laughter.

Another exercise in this category is as follows.

Exercise 19.2 Messages behind your back

Each person is given a sheet of flip-chart paper. Each then draws another team member's name out of the hat. Each then has to design a wide border around the flip-chart sheet they have been given which is appropriate to the personality of the person whose name they have drawn.

On completion, everyone can go to all the flip-charts (but not to their own), in order to add anything which they think might have been overlooked. Finally, each person's flip-chart paper is pinned to their backs, and then the other team members write something positive about him (or her) in the centre.

Debriefing

Participants discuss how they felt about the comments on their flip-chart, and whether they agreed with other people's perceptions of them. This can be most enlightening. This is then developed into a discussion about why people talk 'behind the backs' of others. What is it that stops people from complimenting each other regularly? How difficult is it when people are saying negative things 'behind the backs' of others, and what can be done about it?

Another exercise, which is useful as the group starts to settle and become more trusting and willing to share, is as follows.

Exercise 19.3 The mask

Each member of the group is asked to produce a face mask. On one side of the mask, they will draw the 'side' of themselves that they think everyone sees, and on the other side, the 'side' of themselves that other people don't normally see.

They can use coloured pens, paper, sellotape, rubber-bands, and scissors to produce this mask. When it is complete, they each tell the group about the different sides of their masks.

The group can provide praise and constructive comments, and share how they think the individual appears, and whether the mask fits their personality or not.

Much discussion usually ensues regarding how personalities have so many facets, with some only being visible depending on the situation and the circumstances. Many team members ponder whether or not everyone wears different masks at different times, depending on their circumstances.

Another exercise, which the authors often use after this first mask exercise, involves knowing the group individuals well. The authors have several masks which have different facial expressions on them. A mask is chosen by the facilitator for a participant, which does not fit with his (or her) personality. For instance, a happy, smiling person is asked to wear a very sad mask, or an angry mask. The person does not know what expression is on the mask he (or she) is wearing. (Only a few participants wear masks, as there are only a few expressions which can be easily drawn.) They then mix and socialise with the rest of the group. The mask-wearers feed back first about how it felt, and generally report being surprised and startled at the difference in interactions. They are then asked to guess the type of expression on the mask. The other members of the group usually comment about how strange it is to interact with a person who appears different to their usual personality. Useful discussions often highlight that how a person is treated depends on their appearance. This has relevance in the clinical setting with cancer and palliative care patients.

Personality-type activities

Exercise 19.2 and Exercise 19.3 start to look at specific aspects of personality, and would link to other personality-type exercises. Readers who are trained to complete Myers Briggs (Briggs Myers and Myers 1995) personality profiles might find this useful as a component of team-building. Full profiling of this type is most helpful and revealing, but less useful on a single team-building day due to lack of time (but it could be more usefully addressed on a separate day). The authors often use a 'personality compass' activity. The personality compass is a simple identification model, and the 'personality compass type instrument' (PCTI) is specially designed to probe and identify the various fine distinctions of an individual's personality, using a reliable method which makes misidentification of type much less likely (Turner and Greco 1998). Unlike a number of other personality-typing systems, its simplicity and the visual impact of the compass imagery make it easy to see how the four fundamental natures (clusters of attributes of personality) all work together, and need to be developed together in order to create more well-rounded behaviours and thinking processes. It is a quick, easy and accurate instrument for measuring all the different dimensions of an individual's personality. The information can then be used to make significant improvements for the individual personally, and in the workplace. During the authors' team-building day, only a few questions are used and this cannot give a true profile. However, for anyone to ask their colleagues to suggest where they think he (or she) might come on the compass can be most enlightening. It is less important what type the individual actually is, and more important how their colleagues believe them to be, and so it is mostly an exercise of perceptions and the messages which might be given to others. If participants are interested, just a few hours of enjoyable training will provide them with the information they need, and can often lead to the method's providing the common vocabulary of a workplace, with interesting results.

The above section is about personality-typing, which contrasts with the 'team roles' approach made famous by Belbin (Belbin 1993), who described the team role as a tendency to behave, contribute and interrelate with others in a particular way. The team roles were designed to define and predict potential success of management teams, recognising that the strongest teams have a diversity of characters and personality types.

Belbin's work identified nine clusters of behaviour, termed 'team roles'. Each team role has its particular strengths and allowable weaknesses, and each has an important contribution to make to the team. Very few people display characteristics of just one team role. Most people have three or four preferred team roles, which can be adapted as the situation requires.

Exercise 19.4 Team role identification and implications

It should be noted that the self-perception inventory (SPI) is copyright to Belbin, and should not be reproduced in any form. Individuals may purchase the book and complete an SPI for their own personal development. Facilitators who propose to use SPIs in their training should contact Belbin Associates in Cambridge for permission and cost information.

The group completes Belbin's SPI questionnaire in order to gain insight into each individual's natural behavioural tendencies in a team context, which can be used to create and develop better-functioning teams.

The group members complete the questionnaire individually; meanwhile the facilitators prepare the flip-chart, dividing it into sections for each of Belbin's nine roles (which have been identified as being necessary for a successful team).

Then, each individual says which of the nine roles is their strongest and their initials are placed in the corresponding column. After they have all spoken, it is easy to see whether the team possesses all the different roles that it requires to succeed.

The second part of this exercise is to see if it is possible to fill in the gaps, by identifying participants' second-role strengths, and adding these to the flip-chart.

This should provide much better coverage of all the necessary team roles, and much discussion could follow about how individuals can adapt to their second (or even third) strength, for the sake of the team.

It could be useful to headline the strengths and allowable weaknesses of each role, which might create lively discussion and possible solutions. It has been reported that using Belbin's SPI can often have a dramatic effect on a team, as illustrated below.

A situation was reported to the authors where two facilitators were asked to assist in a team-building exercise. Their manager said that he had a really great team, but that they were very 'set in their ways', and never wanted to embrace change, or find new ways of working.

On the day, the facilitators reported that it was undoubtedly the Belbin SPI exercise which was the most enlightening. Every individual in the team had a very high team-worker role score, but the other eight scores were very low. They immediately diagnosed the team's problem. Their action plan therefore involved each person deciding which of their next highest scores they would focus on and develop, with the help of their colleagues. As team workers, they lived up to their profile, which was used to advantage. They were most cooperative, and wanted to help each other, so ways they might do this were built into the action plan. At the follow-up day, the team were much improved and they used the day mainly as a celebration of their success. Their manager decided, as a result of this, to re-examine the interview process to find the type of individual they would be seeking to attract in the future.

It is recommended that anyone new to team-building, who found this SPI information interesting and useful, might like to enrol on the two-day Belbin team role accreditation course (*see* Further reading).

Another exercise useful for bonding and increasing self-awareness is shown below. This exercise is most effective with larger groups. The authors have used it with cancer ward staff, and hospice bedded-unit staff.

Exercise 19.5 Values

The participants are asked to work in triads. To avoid simply working with their friends, they are asked to find two people who are wearing predominantly the same colours as themselves. Each triad's members find a place where they can talk together. They should be instructed to discuss an issue which is specified and clearly displayed on the flip-chart. The facilitator then gives them a new topic every few minutes. Start with the easiest, and then work towards the more difficult ones.

Here are some examples:

- What is one goal you have for next year?
- Talk about the most important thing you learned this year.
- What do you want to be doing in five years' time?
- What do you value in a friend?
- What do you value in a work colleague?
- What are the easiest and hardest emotions for you to express, and why?

- What is something that most work colleagues don't know about you?
- What is a motto you try to live by?
- What has been one of the greatest challenges?
- What is one of the greatest challenges you are facing at the moment?
- What do you like most about yourself?
- What do you value in a loving relationship?
- What do you value most in life?

These questions allow the team member to say as much, or as little, as they want. (Everyone should be reminded that confidentiality is part of the ground rules.) Obviously, not all these questions will be used. Some will be included which best fit the group's agenda. For instance, 'What is most challenging about working in a multidisciplinary team?' The group then discuss the exercise. What did team members learn, what was most difficult about it, in what small ways might it change their working relationship with the people with whom they worked in this exercise, and how does sharing in this way lead to improved team cohesiveness?

This exercise can easily be adapted for use in smaller groups, where this type of work might be of value.

Choosing the right activity

Before moving on to the 'action stage', it is important to address how imperative it is to ensure that the activity suits the team and their goals. Team-building exercises are useful for all types of team. Some exercises can be designed for smaller teams, and some for larger, some can be designed for new teams, others targeted to specific areas needing improvement in an established team. (Team-building exercises might also turn out to be for different age groups, so think about aspects such as the fitness of the group.) In addition, some team-building exercises that are found in books are intended primarily for children or teenager teams. Sadly though, because these are being mis-used with more mature groups, this has contributed to the negative stigma frequently associated with team-building exercises. This is often a reason why the facilitator has to spend much time gaining the group's trust at the beginning of the day.

When the different exercises are completed, the team will move on to the action stage of the team-building.

Stage 4: action planning

This is a key stage. All the hard work achieved will go to waste unless what has been diagnosed and learnt can be applied in the shape of a well-formed action plan. At intervals during the day, the individuals will be reminded of their agenda, to keep them focused on the final plan. Most exercises (as shown above) are designed to raise their 'self' and 'group' awareness, so they will often be prompted to find out what this will mean for them, and for the team, keeping them relating and converting their issues to problem-solving in future. Therefore, as an integral part of any team-building day, the group will address what they are going away to do, both individually and as a team, and then sign up to it. These resolutions should be recorded on paper if possible, and time should be set aside to do this either as a full team, or in subgroups. The facilitator should assist participants to merge their plans before the end of the day. This means that, as a final activity, it is useful to reinforce this commitment by asking every member verbally what they have found useful and what *they* are going to do to improve team-working.

Please note that people usually change their lives in small steps, one step at a time, and teams are no different.

Stage 5: evaluation

The evaluation is completed verbally at the end of the day, and also in a written evaluation form. The facilitators should accept the comments from the group, but remember that if there are any entrenched problems this might affect the evaluation, and it is useful to compare the verbal and written comments, because they are not always congruent. The facilitators, too, should reflect on and evaluate the day, focusing on what went really well, and what might have gone better. This is essential in order to translate the information into improvements for future training days elsewhere, and specifically for planning the next team-building event for this present group. If a report is required, it is produced at this point and sent to the team for ratification. After the discussions with the team, the facilitators will typically evaluate the team-building programme, produce a report, gain ratification from the team and communicate the results to the managers. The increased motivation resulting from a day of this type means increased productivity and, it is hoped, the investment in people will encourage them to remain with the team and the speciality in the future.

Stage 6: follow-up

The need for a mandatory follow-up day is discussed before any training commitments are entered into, and often the proposed dates for both the training day and follow-up day are settled at the same time. However, this follow-up day may need to be changed to an earlier or later date, depending on the conclusions from the team-building day. If the follow-up day has not been organised prior to the training day, it is always arranged before the participants leave. The authors will not undertake team-building with a group unless the managers and team are committed to having a follow-up session. The follow-up offers an opportunity to report back in a safe environment, where they can celebrate their successes with like-minded individuals who are genuinely interested and delighted in any progress which has been made.

It also provides an environment for discussing those opportunities which seemed more elusive, or planned actions which actually failed, for whatever reason. The follow-up is useful for keeping them on track, as well. Often, the authors will send a gentle reminder to the team halfway between the days in order to keep them focused.

Sometimes the training has been initiated because the participants are a 'new group', due to changes in membership. If, as the day progresses, the facilitators can see that this is a very productive and dynamic team in the making, they will have the group do short-term and long-term action plans. Then, in the final concluding session, these favourable facilitator observations should be shared with the group, and the suggestion made that they need not reconvene, unless they have unexpected problems which makes it necessary. Alternatively, many teams find it helpful to stay focused and remain cohesive by 'team-building' as a positive and fun activity once a year.

It must be acknowledged that team-building is never as easy as it might look, and it is the sign of a skilled team-builder who gives this impression. Therefore, it is wise, before embarking on this for the first time, to work alongside an accomplished facilitator, until skills and confidence reach the necessary level. It is also a good idea to always have different types of exercises available, because events seldom go to plan. Once those fairly new to this type of facilitation have become practised at it, it can become 'almost fun', with participants responding creatively to unexpected and immediate issues as they present themselves, with original solutions.

MOVING FORWARDS

The first section of this chapter focused on the history, research and underpinning models relating to teams. The second section was about team-building and how to facilitate productive sessions using a simple model.

The final section is designed to explore what should be taught pre-qualification and post-qualification about team-working. Team members can then identify their role and the part they play in their team's success. They can also be more proactive in working to their strengths, which will allow the team to flourish. Further, they can then recognise when their team is 'fatigued' or 'unwell' before it becomes completely dysfunctional and burnt out.

What health professionals should be taught about team-working

Teaching about teams is essential. How can anyone aspire to be an eloquent and effective team player if they don't know what constitutes an efficient 'team' and an effective 'team player'? Therefore it is both imperative and urgent that health professionals, both pre-qualification and post-qualification, are taught about group dynamics, efficient teams, effective team profiles, individual team roles and personality traits. They need to recognise when the team is becoming 'fatigued', 'unwell', or dysfunctional, and when there might be a 'saboteur' in their midst. This might be achieved by teaching the theory which is found at the beginning of the chapter, and by bringing it to life with some of the exercises which are found in the middle section. Teaching the subject with these types of exercises can be most helpful. Consider the exercise below.

Exercise 19.6 Developing a new team

Part One

Having discussed the theory, now work in a group to identify how you would put together a team to operate a new out-of-hours palliative team service.

To complete this, and aid your planning, utilise Topchik's (2007) steps, as detailed below, for building a new team.

Be prepared to illustrate how the theory and discussions in class have enlightened and informed your thinking.

> Topchik identifies ten steps for building a new project team.
> 1   Get upper-management support.
> 2   Define the purpose of your team.
> 3   Identify timeframes.
> 4   Select team members.
> 5   Classify team-member openings.
> 6   Share the overall purpose.
> 7   Decide team name.
> 8   Create team mission statement and goals.
> 9   Determine core team issues.
> 10   Establish team norms.
>
> **Part Two**
> Consider what type of induction programme you might develop, and what might need to be included within it.
>
> NB Ensure that subgroups are prepared to share the process, as well as the answers, back in the main group.

This is a long exercise which could be split into two. The exercise encourages the participants to consider the underpinning strategies, philosophies, guidelines and policies which need to be in place. This illustrates all the planning, preparation, time and effort which need to be carried out to ensure the success of a new team. Other teaching activities might include asking the participants to draw a picture or make a list of all the teams to which they belong, and note how some of them overlap, and what this means for confidentiality, trust and other significant issues. Another exercise would be to have the participants consider the characteristics of their *best* team experience, and look at the commonalities. The group usually identify the most common characteristics to be a clearly defined role and responsibilities, a supportive and knowledgeable leader, trust in one another, open communication, some degree of autonomy, and praise for a job well done. Another exercise might be to get them to identify what constitutes a good team spirit, and to identify ways to build one. Many of the exercises in the previous section can be used for teaching purposes, as mentioned earlier. Equally, some the exercises here would work well adapted for team-building.

Table 19.1 is not meant to be an exhaustive list, but rather to provide suggestions for some of the aspects of teams that it would be useful to teach to health professionals.

TABLE 19.1 Possible topics to teach on the subject of teams

• The theory of teams
• Definitions of a team
• Team types
• Team dynamics
• Role identification

- Personality types, and the effect on team-working
- An examination of the different types of teams and how they work
- What makes an effective team?
- What causes a team to become dysfunctional?
- Teamwork and its application to the cancer or palliative care setting
- What is 'social loafing' and how can it be minimised?
- Daily team-building, what is it, and how can it be accomplished?
- Building a new team
- Team member qualities
- Qualities of an effective team player
- Establishing a team spirit

Many of the items on Table 19.1 can be taught collectively, although the table does illustrate that there is a lot to teach, and it might act as a preliminary checklist.

The authors have found that many participants, when asked to identify the characteristics of an 'effective team', claim that they have never actually worked in one. This is a cause for grave concern. This clearly illustrates that there is a lot to be accomplished by both teachers and facilitators of team building.

The authors are passionate about team-working, and spend much time identifying ways to make teams succeed, and to help them reach their true potential. This chapter, in pursuit of this aim, has dedicated many of its pages to team-building exercises, which, it is hoped, the reader may be able to use or adapt. These are just a taster of many such exercises used by the authors, and, like them, the reader might like to develop a full portfolio of team activities in the future.

KEY POINTS

- Teams need to be considered as important commodities, bearing in mind that when they are not functioning efficiently, they will ultimately affect the overall performance of the organisation.
- Individuals working in the specialities of cancer and of palliative care do not always work in the same types of teams. Research could identify whether or not this is appropriate and effective.
- It is laudable that teams are an integral part of the national agenda, and are documented in so many policies and strategies. However, if there is no underpinning evidence or guidelines for researched good practice, could this be considered as paying only lip-service?
- If day-to-day team-building is considered important, then training must to be given to ensure that those who will be expected to facilitate it have the knowledge and skills to do so.
- The importance of communications to those working in cancer and palliative care is well appreciated, but because of the problems inherent in team-working, and the emphasis now placed upon the team, much more must be done to support these team workers.

■ Senior skilled staff working in cancer and palliative care could be trained to team-build. A regional (or national) programme of 'training the trainers' about team-building could be set up, to pass on these skills in a flexible and adaptable manner.

CONCLUSION

Much has been written by theorists about teams, most of it useful to those working in this speciality. However, little has been written about the effectiveness of uni-disciplinary or multidisciplinary working, as discussed in the first section of the chapter. Is one better than the other, or is it relative to the tasks and roles? Do all teams require a leader? Can leadership be successfully shared on a task, or project, or specialised knowledge basis? For example, some multidisciplinary palliative care teams have a medical consultant as the lead person on all pain and symptom issues, and a member of staff who takes the lead on education, another who takes the lead on implementing the Liverpool pathway, and so on. There are still many questions relating to the development of a highly effective and functional team, and the answers are, as yet, unclear.

This is still ground-breaking territory and, because of this, it needs further research and experimentation. Those who have the courage to try out new ways of working will most likely reap the benefits. So, maybe it is (as the catch phrase made popular in *Only Fools and Horses* says – and originally the SAS motto) 'He who dares, wins'!

In the title of this chapter, the authors asked whether 'the ultimate challenge' is developing a successful, productive, cohesive and dynamic team. To answer, yes, quite possibly it is, but undoubtedly it is worth it.

The final point to be made is that while this chapter has been about encouraging teams to work together cohesively and productively, and while the initial quotation was about 'togetherness', it is not about everyone being the same. Cancer and palliative care does not require a single role model to which all health professionals should acquiesce or aspire. There are some very different, but excellent, individuals in teams, who, each in their own way, is a prime example of what epitomises a ideal team player in cancer and palliative care. So, in the words of one inspirational coach:

'Strength lies in differences, not in similarities.'

Stephen Covey

IMPLICATIONS FOR THE READER'S OWN PRACTICE

1 How much do you know about group theory? How might improving your knowledge-base enhance your team-working?
2 Think about the different teams you have worked in. How effective were they, and what were the antecedents which produced the team's success, or its downfall?
3 Do you believe that 'social loafing' is a necessary evil to ensure the harmonious relationships between team members, or is it the product of a dysfunctional team?

4   How do you think you might facilitate team-building in the future?
5   How do the patients fit in as members of these teams?

REFERENCES

Amos MA, Hu J, Herrick CA (2005) The impact of team building on communication and job satisfaction of nursing staff. *J Nurs Staff Dev.* **21** (1): 10–16.

Belbin MR (1993) *Team Roles at Work.* Oxford: Butterworth Heinemann.

Bliss J, Cowley S, White A (2000) Inter-professional working in palliative care in the community: a review of the literature. *J Interprof Care.* **14** (3): 281–90.

Borrill CS *et al.* (2001) *The Effectiveness of Healthcare Teams in the National Health Service.* Birmingham: Aston University.

Briggs Myers I, Myers PB (1995) *Gifts Differing: understanding personality type.* Palo Alto, CA: Davies-Black Publishing.

Cashman SB *et al.* (2004) Developing and measuring progress toward collaborative, integrated, interdisciplinary health care teams. *J Interprof Care.* **18** (2): 183–96.

Department of Health (2000) *The NHS Cancer Plan: a plan for investment, a plan for reform.* London: DoH.

Department of Health, NHS Executive (2000) *Improving the Quality of Cancer Services.* HSC 2000/2001. London: DoH, NHS Executive

Driskell JE, Goodwin GF, Salas E, O'Shea PG (2006) What makes a good team player? Personality and team effectiveness. *Group Dyn.* **10**: 249–71.

Fewster-Thuente L, Velsor-Friedrich B (2008) Interdisciplinary collaboration for healthcare professionals. *Nurs Adm Q.* **32** (1): 40–8.

Firth-Cozens J (1992) Building teams for effective audit. *Qual Health Care.* **1**: 252–5.

Fuller R, Tulle-Winton E (1996) Specialism, genericism, and others: does it make a difference? A study of social worker services to elderly people. *Br J Soc Work.* **26** (3): 679–98.

Hansford P, Barry L (2002) Changing practise: overcoming resistance in a community palliative care. *Nurs Manage.* **9** (1): 18–21.

Lencioni P (2002) *The Five Dysfunctions of a Team.* San Francisco, CA: Jossey-Bass.

Maddocks I (2006) Communications: an essential tool for team hygiene. In: Speck P, editor. *Teamwork in Palliative Care: fulfilling or frustrating?* Oxford: Oxford University Press.

Mickan S, Rodger S (2000) Characteristics of effective teams: a literature review. *Aust Health Rev.* **23** (3): 201–8.

Molyneux J (2001) Inter-professional team working: what makes teams work well? *J Interprof Care.* **15** (1): 30–5.

National Institute for Clinical Excellence (2004) *Improving Supportive and Palliative Care for Adults with Cancer.* London: NICE.

Nursing and Midwifery Council (2008) *The Code: standards of conduct, performance and ethics for nurses and midwives.* London: NMC.

O'Conner M, Fisher C, Guilfoyle A (2006) Interdisciplinary teams in palliative care: a critical review. *Int J Palliat Nurs.* **12** (3): 132–7.

Payne M (2004) *Teamwork in Multi-professional Care.* 2nd ed. New York: Springer.

Payne M, Oliviere D (2006) The interdisciplinary team. In: Walsh D, editor. *Palliative Medicine.* New York: Elsevier.

Pethybridge J (2004) How teamworking influences discharge planning from hospital: a study of four multi-disciplinary teams in an acute hospital in England. *J Interprof Care.* **18** (1): 29–41.

Rogelberg SG, Barnes-Farell JL, Lower CA (1992) An alternative group structure facilitating effective group decision making. *J Appl Psychol.* **77**: 730–77.

Sasahara T, Miyashita M, Kawa M, Kazuma K (2003) Difficulties encountered by nurses in the care of terminally ill cancer patients in general hospitals in Japan. *Palliat Med.* **17** (6): 520–6.

Street A, Blackford J (2001) Communication issues for the interdisciplinary community palliative care team. *J Clin Nurs.* **10** (5): 643–50.

Topchik GS (2007) *First-Time Manager's Guide to Team Building.* New York: Silvestar Enterprises.

Tuckman BW (1965) Developmental sequence in small groups. *Psychological Bulletin.* **63**: 384–99. The article was reprinted in *Group Facilitation: A Research and Applications Journal.* No. 3.

Turner D, Greco T (1998) *The Personality Compass: a new way to understand people.* London: Thorsons Publications.

Vanclay L (1997) Team-working in primary care. *J R Soc Med.* **90**: 268–70.

West MA (1994) *Effective Teamwork.* Leicester: British Psychological Society Books.

West M (2003) *Teamwork: Practical Lessons from Organizational Research.* 2nd ed. Oxford: Wiley Blackwell.

FURTHER READING

For those readers who are unfamiliar with team-building, the authors would recommend three sources.

- Topchik GS (2007) *First-Time Manager's Guide to Team Building.* New York: Silvestar Enterprises.

  This covers the very basics of team-building. Its style is easy to read, due to its simple but engaging, conversational style. Topchik explains the five essential qualities of a high-performing team: goals and standards; decision-making; honest communication; clear roles and responsibilities; and celebrating success.

  It has activities and assessments useful for educators, managers and team members. This is a very helpful (but basic) guide for any 'would-be' team-builders or managers who strive for team-building success. (For managers, the book helps with discovering how their own leadership and management style influences the success of their teams.)

- Belbin Associates Cambridge. Website: www.belbin.com

  This address provides the reader with information on Belbin team role theory and application. It explains the easiest and most cost-effective ways for individuals and small teams to obtain a Belbin Team Role profile. It also provides useful information on the Belbin team role accreditation courses.

- Speck P (2006) *Teamwork in Palliative care: fulfilling or frustrating?* Oxford: Oxford University Press.

  This book places team-working in the context of palliative care, and addresses key issues regarding the importance of collaborative teamwork and enhancing understanding of team structures.

20

Managing death in a hospital context: creative approaches to teaching and learning about death and dying

John Costello

'My father is out on the frontier. He is going where he has never gone before – to his death. Each time I leave the ward, I leave him alone with that knowledge. Dad deserved dignity, not this.'

Paul Cable

The Times, 20 August 2007

AIM

This chapter aims to examine methods of helping practitioners to manage death in a positive way, in a hospital setting.

LEARNING OUTCOMES

By the end of this chapter, the reader should be able to:
- appreciate the various perspectives on good and bad deaths
- explore a number of different approaches to teaching methods related to managing death in a hospital setting
- focus on specific ways of improving communications through education
- consider how the more emotive aspects of death and dying may be taught in the most sensitive manner possible.

INTRODUCTION

Despite advances in medical science and healthcare, together with the push towards individualising approaches to patient care in the developed world, significant variation in the care of dying patients still exists. Healthcare professionals often find the subject of death and dying difficult. Encouraging them to discuss dying with patients who have a life-threatening medical illness is very daunting for some (Taylor 1993). This chapter examines a number of teaching methods designed to help healthcare professionals support patients and families at the end of life. The chapter focuses on improving communication with patients and families about diagnosis and prognosis to ensure that effective communication takes place and 'blocking behaviour' is avoided (Wilkinson and Mula 2003). There is an abundance of literature on palliative care and cancer highlighting how important it is for practitioners to have access to education about how to effectively manage end-of-life issues. This information aims to provide experiences likely to prevent complicated grief reactions and to leave families with memories of death that are as positive as they can be. Using research evidence and clinical case studies, the chapter will challenge practitioners to focus attention on death as a process and how to promote good death experiences. The chapter will outline why we find death and dying difficult and explain educational approaches for overcoming these fears, as well as developing greater self-awareness about a range of end-of-life issues. Moreover, it is important that practitioners feel confident about managing end-of-life experiences, in order to provide patients with quality care and to enable relatives to cope effectively with the loss of a loved one.

DIFFERENT TYPES OF DEATH

Many healthcare practitioners will recall experiences of caring for dying patients using terms such as 'good' and 'bad' types of death. As an ideology, good death has been sustained from traditional times to postmodern society, permeating many aspects of contemporary palliative care (Kristjanson 2001; Taylor 2001; Hopkinson *et al.* 2003). Notions of death as being good or bad are complex (Emanual and Emanual 1998), context dependent (McNamara *et al.* 1994; Lawton 2000) and involve a series of inter-relationships between patients' desires, the ability of others to meet their expectations and the extent to which social control is exerted over the dying process (Payne *et al.* 1996; Bradbury 2000). The literature on good and bad death reveals that such deaths are often sentimentally idealised as being personal and individualised. Good death evokes images of death as being peaceful, natural, dignified and not prolonged (Keizer 1996; Seymour 1999; Clark 2002). Good deaths are often characterised by families having control and a lack of patient distress. Conversely, bad death has the potential for causing trauma and a sense of crisis for dying people and others (Payne *et al.* 1996). Kellehear's (1990) conception of good death included an acknowledgement of the social life of the dying and the creation of an open climate about disclosure, with the patient's being aware of their impending death, whereas bad death experiences (also referred to as traumatic, chaotic or gruesome) raised conflict among ward nurses. A number of studies indicate that the fewer difficulties patients experience in their passage towards death, the greater the likelihood of the death being perceived positively by nurses (McNamara 2001; Hopkinson *et al.* 2003; Costello 2006). A recurring feature of the hospital-based literature is the association of 'poor death' experiences with organisational issues such as staff shortages and lack of resources (Rogers *et al.* 2000).

Exercise 20.1 Reflections on professional experience

Reflect for a few moments on your professional experiences of patients dying in hospital. Would you agree that some deaths might be described as good or bad experiences? Try to think back to your personal experiences and check out whether this dichotomy of good and bad death reflects your experience and, if so, try to think or make a list of why some deaths may be considered in this way.

TALKING ABOUT DEATH AND DYING

Discussion about death and dying can be awkward for certain people and it is often useful to introduce sensitive topics using group exercises. One particular exercise I use with clients and students to enable them to become more aware of the impact of loss is called 'loss lines'. This is an interesting way of helping people to reflect and consider personal experiences of loss, as well as enabling them to get in touch with their feelings about the experience. This exercise also aids reflection and promotes greater consideration of the impact of previous loss experiences, as well as offering a reminder of how they managed to cope with loss.

Exercise 20.2 Loss lines

The aim of this exercise is to raise awareness of the complexities involved when loss takes place and also to remind the group that loss is about *being deprived of something of value* and is not necessarily about human death. A loss line involves doing an inventory of the significant losses that have taken place in the person's life. The exercise can be carried out individually with one person or in a group with students agreeing to share their loss experiences. The facilitator can ask students to identify specific aspects of the loss, such as the type of support provided and the most helpful and unhelpful things that they can remember about the loss experience.

Each person is given a piece of paper and asked to make a note of the losses they have experienced, starting from as early as they can remember up to the present. The greater the intensity of the loss, the longer the horizontal line denoting the loss. The facilitator indicates that losses may be tangible, such as the death of a pet, or intangible, such as that relating to the loss of independence one can experience when being hospitalised. Below is an example of my own loss line. The most significant loss was my mother's death; interestingly, the loss of my pet dog Beauty, when I was 10, was more intense than the loss of my grandmother, who I hardly knew.

'Loss lines' is an interesting exercise because it enables facilitators to go as far as students wish to go with it. It can be used simply as a reminder of personal loss experiences, or it can be expanded to include focusing on how well or otherwise you coped with the loss. The group may decide to share loss experiences, or the exercise can be limited to non-disclosure. These conditions need to be discussed in advance and time allowed if the exercise is developed to include discussion of personal experiences. Certain losses

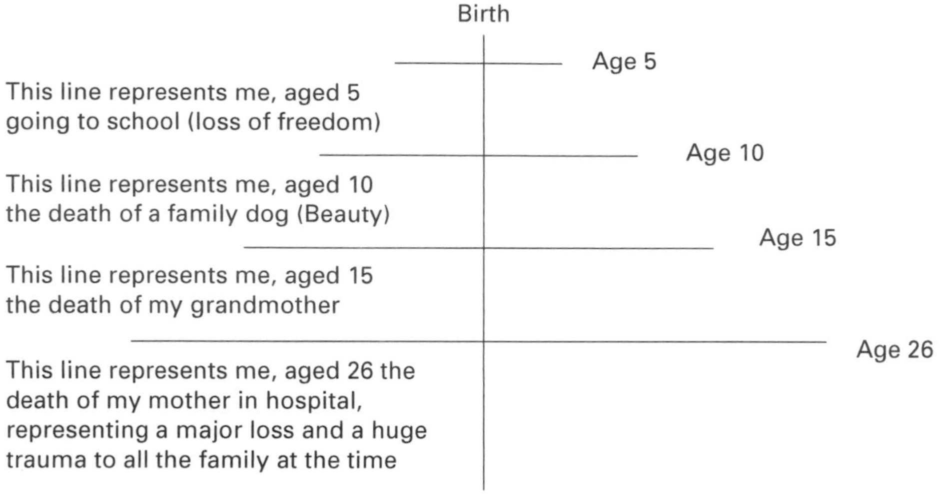

FIGURE 20.1 Loss lines

such as cot death, abuse or suicide can be particularly painful to recall and sensitivity in managing this type of loss is important.

There are many ways of enabling students in a group to discuss sensitive issues around death and dying, in a gentle and relatively non-threatening way. One particular exercise I often use with nurses to reveal anxieties or concerns about death and dying is a game called 'fear in a hat'. The exercise involves participants writing their anxieties about death and dying on a sheet of paper, then folding the paper and placing it in a box (or hat). Group participants then take a fear out of the hat offered around the group. Participants discuss their anonymous worries, fears and concerns (putting their own fear back, if picked out). This exercise, like many others, is relatively quick to do and can be adapted to promote discussion on a range of subjects, such as breaking bad news, talking about death or supporting specific groups such as children or older people. It is important to acknowledge fears, accepting the individuality and diversity of apprehensions, as well as their importance to the learning experience. At the end of the session, the facilitator may reflect on the general range of ideas, thoughts and concerns of the group through discussion, identifying specific concerns as well as strengths of group members that can be utilised in future group work exercises. Nurses often express concerns about truth-telling and informing relatives about a death, breaking bad news and the fear of sudden death. The facilitator needs to be sensitive about individual student needs and perhaps make clear before the exercise that students should feel free to take time out of the discussion if they feel particularly emotional about the topic. It is important to follow up students who become upset to 'check out' feelings, rather than appear intrusive about their personal loss experiences. Much depends on the situation and the way the concern is addressed.

There are a number of exercises that can be used to help students to begin to discuss issues around death and dying, such as 'ice-breakers' that need to have a specific aim and be explained properly and given adequate time. Without these important prerequisites, students may perceive that the facilitator is just playing games. Many of these introductory exercises can be adapted to focus on specific areas relating to death and dying – for example, students can be asked to make their own living will or funeral plan. These can then be discussed within the group as a way of generating ideas and discussion about our own sense of mortality and how it may influence professional practice.

TEACHING AND LEARNING ABOUT THE MANAGEMENT OF DEATH IN HOSPITAL

There are a number of interesting and creative ways of learning about death and dying in a hospital context. Much depends on the facilitator's confidence, ability and experience (Costello 2006). Discussions about self-mortality, which can involve disclosure of personal and professional hospital experiences, are extremely useful and can help to develop group cohesion and stimulate thinking about key issues. Group discussions, like any teaching and learning activity, need to be planned and have a clear aim. The challenge for the facilitator is to provide structure and enable the entire group to make a contribution, avoiding the situation where one or two talkative students dominate the discussion. There are a number of ways of doing this. The discussion needs to be planned and students given advance notice and time for discussion, as well as being informed if they are required to do some work in advance. Two discussion-based approaches will be described:

➤ using case studies as a basis for discussion
➤ role-play.

Case studies

The use of case studies to promote teaching and learning about managing death in hospital is an excellent way of ensuring credibility or, as one of my students pointed out, 'keeping it real'. In preparation for the discussion, students can be asked to select a case study with which they are familiar (either from the past or a current case) and in advance to give some thought to the impact it had on them, their role and what they have learnt from it. The group will be invited to present their case study and, having negotiated ground rules, students are invited to ask questions for clarification and to promote discussion. The facilitator's role is to ensure equity in allowing time, so that all students have the opportunity to present their case study. At the same time, it is important that the student explains the impact the case study had on them and for the group to consider the wider implications. Below is an example of a case study taken from my hospital research that summarises the nurses' responses to the inappropriate admission of a dying patient to an acute ward (Costello 2004).

Case study: Mrs Brown

Mrs Brown (aged 75) had a brain stem CVA and was transferred to the ward from the intensive care unit of an outlying hospital because of a bed shortage. Mrs Brown had originally been put on a ventilator but was extubated on the instructions of both

---

a physician and a neurologist who, following tests, determined that she was brain dead. On the day of her admission to the elderly care ward, her daughter (Sandra) was informed that the hospital was going to take her mother off the ventilator and that she would almost certainly die shortly afterwards. Subsequently, this did not happen and Mrs Brown, following extubation, continued to breathe without assistance and showed no immediate signs of dying. Instead, after being admitted into the side room that had been prepared for her, she was hydrated via an intravenous infusion, with a naso-gastric tube in situ and a urinary catheter on free drainage. She was deeply unconscious, unresponsive to stimuli of any kind and breathing by herself, although her breathing pattern was erratic and noisy.

In summary, the case study highlights how Mrs Brown was being nursed out of context. In other words, as a dying patient, she should not have been transferred to a ward where active curative treatment was the main focus. It was also clear that despite the predictions of medical staff, Mrs Brown did not die as they anticipated. This had a significant impact on the ward staff, who were given to understand that she was admitted with a view to dying in hospital a few days after transfer. Mrs Brown had a range of life-sustaining aids – such as a naso-gastric tube, intravenous infusion and an indwelling urinary catheter – all of which were removed over time. Eventually after a period of six weeks, she developed pneumonia and sadly died with her daughter at the bedside.

Mrs Brown's death, on reflection, raises a number of practical and ethical implications. One source of contention identified by students was the distress of her daughter, who felt let down by poor communication. The nurses on the ward felt guilty for not being able to do more for her mother and were saddened by what was felt to be a bad death. Further, it was an inappropriate referral, due to a political decision that was outside the nurses' control. This reflects the view that, in some cases, patients die in acute hospital settings when they should never have been there in the first place. Deaths such as this often involve healthcare professionals experiencing stress because of their lack of control over the circumstances. This is compounded by the frustration felt by relatives who look to nurses for guidance. Case studies have enormous potential for enabling nurses to reflect on practice, gaining greater insights from sharing their experiences in a group. As a teaching and learning tool, case studies can allow students to develop a sense of objectivity about their practice, while receiving support from their colleagues.

Enabling patients to experience a good death in hospital

The aim of much palliative care in hospital is to enable the patient and family to experience a *good death*. Often, as the literature points out, good death in a hospital setting is problematic because of organisational issues associated with power relations between staff (Porter 1998), the dominance of ward routine and the lack of individuality afforded to patients and their families. Good practice in contemporary care for dying hospital patients often involves the use of integrated care pathways (ICPs), in the latter stages 'preferred place of death' documents identifying patients' wishes, and much greater emphasis on healthcare professionals meeting the needs of patients' healthcare.

This can include enabling patients to make a living will and to discuss the things they would like to take place and happen. The latter can, of course, include patients and families becoming involved in discussion about 'do not resuscitate' (DNR) orders. Many of these initiatives contribute towards patients and their families experiencing a good death, a major component of which is control over the events leading up to and including the death itself (Kellehear 1990). As a way of clarifying how nurses and others can help patients to experience a good death, the following case study of an authentic patient experience illustrates some of the difficulties that can take place when a patient comes into hospital for terminal care. Read the scenario and then consider the care plan to assess the extent to which it helps Grace to experience a good death, within the constraints of an acute hospital ward. Remind yourself that the quality of care is as much, if not more, about how you provide the care itself in terms of effective communication, the available resources and the impact that treatment has on managing the patient's symptoms. Consider how you may have added to or deleted some of the care being provided.

Case study: Grace

Grace was a 58-year-old lady with advanced colo-rectal cancer. She was admitted to the medical ward in pain and acute distress resulting from a prolonged period at home where her symptoms became out of control. Her husband Bill was her primary carer and they received help from friends, neighbours and their daughter who lived 60 miles away. Grace did not want to die in hospital and was hoping to be cared for at home, with possibly respite care in a local hospice. On admission, she was found to be in pain, distressed and tearful. After being settled into the ward and medically examined it was confirmed that Grace was in pain, dehydrated, constipated and had been experiencing nausea and vomiting for two weeks. As a consequence of her symptoms, she had not been eating well, had lost weight, and her heels, sacrum and hips were red from prolonged periods in bed. She also had what appeared to be a urinary tract infection. Psychologically she felt frustrated at having to be admitted to hospital and acknowledged that in the last few weeks she had become quite depressed.

Role-play

Role-play is an important strategy for enabling healthcare professionals to critically examine the way end-of-life care is provided to patients in hospital. It provides students with opportunities for learning about themselves and about how others respond when faced with difficult, emotionally sensitive situations. Role-play enables simulation of interactions (that would normally be very difficult because of their emotional intensity) to take place in a safe and controlled setting. The aim of role-play in a palliative care context is often to limit the impact that a life-threatening medical illness has on the patient and family. Good experiences often take place when the facilitator has been sensitive and where timing and feedback to participants are consistent and clearly understood by all involved.

Preparation

It is important to discuss previous role-play experiences and to invite the group to share any anxieties about role-play in advance, by exploring helpful or unhelpful experiences and why these occurred. In this way the facilitator is aware of and prepared to deal with apprehensions about taking part in role-play. Providing clear ground rules helps to address and overcome anticipated problems, such as individuals being 'spotlighted' (being made to 'perform' in front of a large group). Highlighting safety issues, such as avoiding students' 'getting stuck' for what to do and say, can alleviate anxieties about role-play. The facilitator may be confident in their role-play skills, but needs to be mindful of the many perceived anxieties about role-play.

A gentle way to introduce role-play as a teaching strategy is to provide a scenario for students to role-play in pairs or as a threesome. Each person plays the role of patient, nurse or observer. Providing feedback or debriefing role-play participants is an important way for the facilitator to achieve a balanced, fair evaluation and for participants to encourage less self-confident members of the group to contribute.

Patient interviews

The *Cancer Plan* (DoH 2000) highlights the need to improve services for cancer patients in the UK, with more effective communication being raised in the report as a major issue. The provision of quality palliative care hinges on health professionals providing effective communication. Nurses and others able to communicate effectively with patients and their colleagues are likely to influence the rate of recovery, to limit distress from pain and other symptoms and to ensure greater concordance with treatment (Fallowfield and Jenkins 1999). Research suggests that nurses have a number of difficulties communicating emotional issues with patients who have cancer (Wilkinson 2002), which challenges educators to address communication as an integral part of teaching and learning. A common area for concern among health professionals is their ability to conduct interviews with patients and carry out an accurate assessment of needs. Patients' and relatives' complaints about healthcare often focus on a lack of communication or poor communication (Rogers *et al.* 2000).

Enabling students to become effective communicators when assessing patients can help them to develop the necessary skills required to create therapeutic relationships, and to gain a fuller understanding of patients' feelings, worries and concerns. Patients are likely to respond to nurses who enable them to disclose their concerns and feelings, especially when discussing emotional issues. Health professionals need to feel confident in their abilities to engage in interaction of this kind. The degree of self-confidence required to engage meaningfully with patients about emotionally sensitive topics can be gained through the appropriate use of guided role-play scenarios identified from previous group work discussions. The scenarios can be based on student practice experiences or typical examples. Effective role-play can take place when in small or large groups. I invite students to initially role-play in pairs, then threes, and when confidence has built up, in a larger group with students playing the role of patient and interviewer. The rest of the group observe, but take an active part in providing feedback.

The facilitator's role

The facilitator needs to make the task clear as well as the benefits. Most students asked to take part in role-play are apprehensive. Many are surprised by how much they learn just by looking at what they do. Students should be reminded that they learn more by doing than observing. It is useful to remind students that particular health areas (such as spiritual care or sexual problems) in clinical practice are often referred to as being problematic. When nurses complete assessment documents, for example, these areas are often incomplete. It is useful to ask for volunteers from the group to play the role of interviewer and patient. The chosen scenario can be based on areas of concern previously highlighted. The chosen scenario may well be one that a student found difficult in practice or one that reflects previous experience. This can lead to a realistic role-play, with the facilitator's being sensitive to potential difficulties such as the student's 'getting stuck' (getting tongue-tied, or losing their chain of thought). It is explained that if this happens, 'time out' strategies can be applied. When the role-play stops, participants can take a breather, to consider what to do next. In groups with a mature level of cohesion, students can act as 'stand-ins' and take the volunteer's place or provide a statement that they could use to help with a patient assessment, such as: 'Can you help me by explaining what you think is wrong with you?' This is referred to as *shaping* or *moulding* the role-play (Gibbs 1988). The facilitator needs always to carefully explain the particular situation. State clearly what the scenario is, for example: 'This role-play is to do with a 55-year-old man with bowel cancer (stage one tumour with possible nodal involvement).' Actors are assigned roles and timing is included, with five-minute role-plays often being more than sufficient.

Part of the facilitator's skill in preparation for role-play is to monitor the group's non-verbal cues – for example, when asking for volunteers, invite those whose body language suggests that they would like to give it a try. Conversely, the facilitator should avoid putting someone in a difficult position if they can tell that the student is very reluctant. I have yet to encounter a situation where no one volunteered. Being optimistic, once volunteers have come forward, remove them from the group and brief them for the scenario.

Briefing

Carefully brief the interviewer away from the group. Check out their previous experiences of this kind of scenario and ask them to think of an authentic experience from their not-too-distant past. Ask them what they found difficult about it and what they think they did wrong. Check that they are comfortable with the prospect of doing this 'for real' with a patient. If they cannot think of a scenario from practice, a written sheet with a basic scenario gleaned from typical examples of practice can be provided. The interviewer will have attended formal presentations based on patient assessment and be aware and have knowledge of how to structure an assessment focusing on the patient's agenda. The scenario will be carefully explained, timed (for about 10–15 minutes), with an end point and time for evaluation (debrief).

Example: briefing for role-play

You are in the outpatient's clinic and a patient (woman with breast cancer) attends for her first chemotherapy treatment. It is useful to provide an opening, such as introducing yourself – 'I am Susan, the breast care nurse specialist.'

Then ask the patient to provide an account of their problems (ascertain the patient's awareness of diagnosis and history of current problems) from the time they first felt that there was a problem. You, as the breast care nurse, carry out an initial assessment to discover what has been happening from the patient's perspective by setting the scene and using the patient's agenda, thereby attempting to establish a therapeutic relationship (Fallowfield and Jenkins 1999). This requires you to ascertain facts as perceived by the patient together with appropriate feelings. Empathic responses can be made by:

- supporting the patient and trying to prevent further anxieties being developed through blocking behaviours or superficial comments
- focusing on psychological aspects of care – that is, the feelings being expressed and not just the physical aspects of care (Wilkinson *et al.* 1998).

The facilitator reiterates the safety aspects, as well as the use of time out (by facilitator and participant), reminding the student who they are and the context of the role-play. Explain that you will be observing for any problems and ask them to get into role.

Patient briefing

The patient role may be played by a number of people including other students, real patients or simulated patients (SPs). The latter are actors used to play specific parts in a scenario. It may be useful to ask a student who has encountered a similar scenario to take on the patient's role as a way of learning more about the patient's perspective. Discuss their experiences in advance and check out if they feel comfortable with being in the patient's situation. Explain the safety strategies and how you will use them if you feel it is required. Ask them to try to keep the scenario specific to their experience and incorporate how their family may feel, if they were involved. Remind them not to 'play to the gallery' or embellish the situation too much by elaborating the details. Check their name and role-play biography and explain the context. Ask them to put themselves 'in role' and wait to be called in.

'Doing role-play'

The role-play scenario is explained to the rest of the group or a details sheet distributed explaining the scenario. The student group as observers can be structured so that they can take an active part in observing the role-play. Everyone is asked to 'catch people being good' by highlighting positive responses and communication strategies. Ask some to observe for verbal and non-verbal responses, making sure positive feedback comes first, before constructive criticism. Ensure that interviewer, patient and group are briefed about their role.

After the role-play, it is useful if the actors remain 'in role' for a while in order to enable the group to ask them questions, such as how they felt as (the patient), when they were asked about (a particular question). It is very useful to receive feedback about the role-play from the actors as they remain in touch with their feelings. Having invited questions, the actors can then be asked to come out of their role and become themselves again. Having done this, each should be asked to explain how it felt being in role and what feelings emerged from being the person. Feedback of this kind can be useful for each of the actors as well as allowing observers to gain insight into what it may be like to be in a similar situation. Positive feedback also involves constructive criticism to inform the actors how others may have handled the role-play or ways that could have helped the interaction go more effectively. This is difficult for students and often few students offer criticism of their colleagues. It needs to be explained by the facilitator that such feedback is useful as long as the aim is to look at ways to improve what was done. It is important not to underestimate the need for exercising sensitivity during role-play situations. Often it takes tremendous courage for students to take part in role-play. Students and facilitators need to focus on positive feedback after the role-play, to ensure that the scenario is a success.

Video role-play

To enable a greater degree of feedback to take place, a video recording can be made of the role-play. This requires greater preparation and discussion with a clear explanation and advance agreement. Video and audio-taped role-play offers a far greater scope for subsequent discussion and reflection, with the students having the ability to observe each other. Video role-play enables students to gain insight into their personal strengths and weaknesses when communicating with others. This particular approach is used extensively in the teaching I am involved with on all courses. Video role-play is a very powerful tool for reflecting on your performance, although many students dread this form of teaching. Interestingly, the vast majority of student evaluations of the video role-play scenarios state that, despite initial apprehension, the experience was very valuable. Video role-play is a difficult form of teaching and learning for facilitators, who need to be alert to individual and group needs, which may change from day to day. It is useful for facilitators to 'check out' volunteers who may have recently experienced a situation likely to trigger strong feelings and dissuade them from volunteering.

KEY POINTS

- ■ Effective communication has the power to influence patients', carers' and healthcare professionals' experience of death.
- ■ Notions of good and bad death are complex.
- ■ A range of teaching strategies in enhancing communication skills can be utilised.
- ■ Active participation in communication skills training requires the expertise of a skilled and sensitive facilitator.

CONCLUSION

This chapter has focused on a number of creative teaching and learning strategies designed to help healthcare professionals to manage death and to support patients and families at the end of life. Specifically, I have examined and described ways to improve communication with patients and families and to enable a good death to become a reality for patients and their families. It has become clear that death and dying are difficult subjects for some practitioners to discuss. Group discussion and role-play, despite being ideal ways of learning, are often difficult to initiate and sustain and can challenge facilitators to use the range of their communication skills. The use of case studies to develop learning is an excellent and creative way for practitioners to not only share their experiences and disclose their fears of difficult experiences, but also to enable others to learn from these critical incidents. The chapter has focused, as well, on the management of difficult ethical situations, for example when DNR orders are being considered. Essentially, healthcare practitioners need to develop their communication skills to a point where, rather than telling a patient what they can and cannot do in hospital, they consider what feelings underlie requests and negotiate how individual and family needs can be met. Such skills are best learnt in a group setting, with the facilitator adopting a more generic, enabling role to ensure that teaching and learning about death and dying is a positive experience.

IMPLICATIONS FOR THE READER'S OWN PRACTICE

1 When considering good and bad deaths, are there other creative ways that you could use to educate hospital staff?
2 How might you incorporate 'life lines' into your teaching sessions?
3 Many educators use the 'fear in a hat' exercise in different ways. How might you utilise this activity in relation to managing death in a hospital context?
4 How might you evaluate the success of your teaching and possible improvements to care in practice?

REFERENCES

Bradbury M (2000) The good death. In: Dickinson D, Johnson M, Katz S, editors. *Death, Dying and Bereavement*. London: Sage Publications: 59–63.

Clark D (2002) Between hope and acceptance: the medicalisation of dying. *BMJ*. **324**: 905–7.

Costello J (2004) *Nursing the Dying Patient: caring in different contexts*. London: Palgrave.

Costello J (2006) Teaching small groups and individuals. In: Wee B, Hughes N, editors. *Learning and Assessment in Palliative Care*. Oxford: Oxford Medical Publications.

Department of Health (2000) *The NHS Cancer Plan: a plan for investment, a plan for reform*. London: DoH.

Emanual EJ, Emanual LL (1998) The promise of a 'good death'. *Lancet*. **251** (5): 21–9.

Fallowfield L, Jenkins V (1999) Effective communication skills are the key to good cancer care. *European Journal of Cancer*. **35**: 1592–7.

Gibbs G (1988) *Learning by Doing: a guide to teaching and learning methods*. London: Further Education Unit.

Hopkinson JB, Hallett CE, Luker KA (2003) Caring for dying people in hospital. *J Adv Nurs*. **44** (5): 525–33.

Keizer B (1996) *Dancing with Mr D: notes on life and death*. New York: Doubleday.

Kellehear A (1990) *Dying of Cancer: the final year of life*. London: Harwood.

Kristjanson LJ (2001) Palliative care nurses' perceptions of good and bad deaths and care expectations: a qualitative analysis. *Int J Palliat Nurs*. **7** (3): 67–75.

Lawton J (2000) *The Dying Process: patients' experiences of palliative care*. London: Routledge.

McNamara B (2001) *Fragile Lives: death dying and care*. Buckingham: Open University Press.

McNamara B, Waddell C, Colvin M (1994) The institutionalization of the good death. *Soc Sci Med*. **39** (11): 1501–8.

Payne S, Langley-Evans A, Hillier R (1996) Perceptions of a good death: a comparative study of the views of hospice staff and patients. *Palliat Med*. **10** (4): 307–12.

Porter S (1998) *Social Theory and Social Practice*. London: Macmillan.

Rogers A, Karlsen S, Addington-Hall J (2000) 'All the services were excellent. It is when the human element comes in that things go wrong': dissatisfaction with hospital care at the end of life. *J Adv Nurs*. **31** (4): 768–74.

Seymour J (1999) Revisiting medicalisation and natural death. *Soc Sci Med*. **49**: 691–704.

Taylor B (1993) Hospice nurses tell their stories about a 'good death': the value of storytelling as a qualitative health research method. *Annu Rev Health Soc Sci*. **3**: 97–108.

Taylor B (2001) Views of nurses, patients and patients' families regarding palliative nursing care. *Int J Palliat Nurs*. **7** (4): 186–91.

Wilkinson SM, Roberts A, Aldridge J (1998) Nurse–patient communication in palliative care: an evaluation of a communication skills programme. *Palliat Med*. **12**: 13–22.

Wilkinson S (2002) The essence of cancer care: the impact of training on nurses' ability to communicate effectively. *J Adv Nurs*. **40** (6): 731–8.

Wilkinson S, Mula C (2003) Communication in care of the dying. In: Ellershaw J, Wilkinson S, editors. *Care of the Dying: a pathway to excellence*. Oxford: Oxford University Press: 74–89.

21

'Children should be seen and not heard': ensuring that children are *heard* throughout loss and life-threatening illness of a loved one, via education

Janis Hostad and John Holland

'There are two lasting bequests we can give our children: one is roots, the other is wings.'

William Hodding Carter

AIM

To encourage the development of the teaching of cancer, palliative care, loss and bereavement in healthcare, education and in schools. This will better support children and young people in their understanding and coping with this difficult and sensitive area.

LEARNING OUTCOMES

By the end of this chapter, the reader should be able to:
- recognise the importance of this subject, and of an ongoing, integrated approach to this type of education
- provide the reader with examples of research, or audit tools, which could be utilised within their role
- highlight ideas relating to whom, where, when and how to teach
- identify different ways of 'packaging' the teaching material into useful sessions or programmes
- be aware of the effective exercises which the authors have found useful in their practice
- consider ways of evaluating and auditing the success of this training.

NB It was considered beyond the scope of this chapter and the authors' abilities to discuss children *with* life-threatening illnesses.

INTRODUCTION

This chapter is designed be useful to those who are already involved in this type of teaching, allowing them to reflect on their approach, and to compare these methods and approaches with their own.

Readers could be Macmillan nurses, hospice staff, university lecturers, school nurses, psychologists or teachers. The chapter is aimed at helping such individuals who have the capability and resourcefulness to transfer knowledge and awareness in this area to those who are working directly or indirectly with children and young people. It will also be useful to those who are new to this type of education, but who plan to be involved with it in the future. This chapter will look at teaching the staff in hospitals, the community and schools in order to help and support those children and young people who experience the effects of life-threatening illnesses.

The authors have spent many years working with children, both independently and jointly, and bring together both diverse and connected experience in health and education. One author has worked as an infant teacher, a special educational needs (SEN) teacher, an educational psychologist, and as an author and researcher in the field of education (John). The other author has worked as a Macmillan nurse in hospitals, and as a lecturer, an author and a researcher, both in a hospice setting and in the NHS (Janis).

Before working jointly, both authors were involved with teachers, health professionals and psychologists in raising the awareness of these issues, and they combine to provide a wealth of experience in this field.

Initially, action research was carried out in education, and a training gap was identified in schools, in that teachers valued the area of child bereavement support highly, but felt that they lacked the skills to help children.

A survey of nurses' needs revealed a similar requirement, and it was concluded that many professionals in both education and health may not be recognising, assessing or responding to the needs of bereaved children.

Ideally, children and young people need to be equipped with the skills to enable them to be as resilient as possible and to cope as well as possible with life's losses.

WHO NEEDS TO KNOW WHAT?

To help children to cope with life-threatening events is not new. However, it is necessary that all the professionals encountered by the children are aware of how the children might be affected, and how they as professionals can help (Thomas 1997). Therefore, it is important for those embarking on this type of teaching to identify the different professionals within their own locality and context who could help.

The authors have found it particularly beneficial to work together across professional boundaries. Therefore, as a clinical nurse specialist or lecturer (health professional), or hospice staff member, you may be able to find a local educational psychologist with an interest in this area. Equally, as a teacher, a school nurse, or psychologist, you might find a suitable health professional to support you in your endeavours. The sessions or courses could be conducted at the local hospice, primary or secondary NHS trust, or young persons' services provider, or in specific schools.

Experience of involvement in many training courses, in all of the above settings, has indicated that there are generic training needs for all staff, regardless of profession or context. For example, all professionals need to have some understanding of bereavement theories and processes, for both adults and children; and how to respond to children before and after a death. In addition, professionals need to understand the various coping mechanisms used by children and their families, and to be able to overlay developmental issues on the tapestry of interventions and understanding. They also need to know how best to interact, support and help their clients. Another consideration is the effect on the facilitator of teaching such an emotive topic, which leads to issues around the concept of 'caring for the carers'. (Due to space constraints, this cannot be discussed here but is covered in Chapter 17.)

This chapter will also look at the variety of educational opportunities, first in regard to schools and second, in a healthcare context.

WORKING WITH SCHOOLS

Seventy per cent of schools have a bereaved pupil at any given time (www.childbereave ment.org.uk/for_schools), which illustrates that there is an educational need to be met. Even though there are many demands on a school teacher's time, the needs of these vulnerable children and young people cannot be overlooked or ignored. Over 90% of a sample of secondary schools could identify the number of children on their roll who had suffered a bereavement. On average, a secondary school could expect to have around eight children bereaved within the past two years (Holland and Ludford 1995).

There has been much activity in this subject area by Janis and John in their locality over the years. Some of this information might be useful to the reader if he (or she) was planning to set up similar programmes. After initially preparing and running a number of courses, it was obvious that it would be more beneficial to do a needs analysis, or some sort of comprehensive survey.

This initial research by John, which took place in Humberside schools, revealed a 'training gap' in the area of child bereavement (Holland 1993; Holland and Ludford 1995). This was action research, carried out in connection with an educational research project in the County of Humberside. Questionnaires were sent to all the schools in the county; the initial one to primary schools, and a second one to secondary schools. Teachers were asked a variety of both open and closed questions, in order to gain a measure of how they rated the area of child bereavement, about their current provisions, and whether they had a policy in place and individuals taking the lead in the area. The reason for asking schools how they respond to a bereaved child is so that a profile of training needs can be established, and a baseline obtained for future research to evaluate whether the training is having the desired and intended effect on school practice. It also provided 'food for thought' for those schools, which, for example, currently did not have a policy in place.

This type of questionnaire could easily be adapted to use with a targeted group in the context of the health service, by researching what is happening in this area, identifying issues and training needs, and then looking to respond to those needs. A questionnaire is always a very quick and useful way to gain this type of data. Its relative simplicity as a research tool (provided that it does not have too many questions and has a reasonable mixture of open, closed and scaling questions) makes it useful to the busy health professional or teacher. The danger, as with any research, is that respondents answer by predicting what the researchers would expect, or perhaps they exaggerate their practice in order to be well perceived. A mixture of other research tools such as interviews and statistics gained by other means should help to validate the results, through triangulation.

The results of this research showed that teachers value the area of child bereavement support relatively highly, but that they lacked the necessary skills to work in this area, and considered that they needed more training opportunities. John found that schools tended to rate the area higher if they had had a recent experience of bereavement than if they had not, which suggests that schools perhaps are more comfortable with the reactive, rather than proactive, role (Holland and Ludford 1995). This has also been the experience of Janis, and that probably of many other healthcare readers.

At the time of this research, there were no educational training opportunities in the area of child bereavement for teachers in this region, and so this was quite a novel initiative.

A book entitled *Wise Before the Event* (Yule and Gold 1993) had previously been provided for schools in England to help them to support their pupils, after the occurrence of a series of high-profile disasters – for example, the sinking of the ferry *Spirit of Free Enterprise* (Yule and Gold 1993). However, the book was a 'stand-alone' response, with no complementary training or support.

The research also showed that there were no educational staff who had received education-based bereavement training, although a very small minority of teachers had received training through a previous career in the health sector, or through their involvement in the voluntary sector.

The initial research, and the demand for training, led to the development of a series of training courses which were provided for teachers. The idea emerged of producing a training pack, and time was devoted to its development, eventually leading to the 'Lost for Words' project. A formal package was produced, and the training was trialled in schools. After initially being published locally, it was then published by Jessica Kingsley (Holland *et al.* 2005) and is now available both nationally and internationally.

The project is based on the results of the initial research, as already described, and also on research by Holland (1999), developed at the University of York. Project Iceberg looked into the experiences of bereaved children, and this ensured the inclusion of their voice in the project.

This research was carried out by a semi-structured interview (and a questionnaire) with adults who had been bereaved of a parent when they were children. The interviews took about an hour, and those involved were asked about their experiences at the time of the death, such as their feelings and their understanding of the issues, and whether they had been involved in the rites after the death, and how well they felt supported at school. An important element was to find out from the subjects which actions that they felt could have helped them at the time (Holland 2001).

Generally, children and young people reported that their schools had not been particularly helpful after the death of a parent, and there tended to be a poor response by school when they returned after the death (with some notable exceptions). Children mostly valued choice in connection with involvement in the rites after death, and many had felt quite isolated, and had no one to talk with about the events on a deep level. Children particularly valued non-patronising empathy, such as acknowledgment of their loss, and explanations in terms which they could understand. These findings, as with other research, suggested that for most children, they began to develop a 'close to adult' understanding of death at around the age of seven or eight years old (Safier 1964; Zach 1978; Slaughter *et al.* 1999). The potential emotional isolation of children is an important concept, because if the home is in emotional turmoil, with the surviving parent grieving, then school could provide an important element of support for the child.

> 'Many families can be supported in the community by drawing on their own social networks. Also, teachers, chaplains and volunteers who regularly work with children and can be equipped to support them through their loss.' (Kennedy et al. 2008)

However, schools do need to be able to organise an effective response to support bereaved children.

The results from both the action research project and the Iceberg research were integrated into the *Lost for Words* training programme, which is therefore underpinned with a research base (regarded as crucial). Without a foundation of research, the pack would have been a series of 'nice ideas' by the authors, with no substantive support. Lessons were learnt from both items of research, which are passed on to those attending the course.

Courses such as this one, developed from the research and the collective feedback from children, young people and teachers, seem to be the most effective in ensuring that all learning needs are met. Janis has found over the years that this seems to be a unique topic, in which teachers and pupils can learn together.

Indeed Leaman (1995: 117) supports this when he says:

> 'We have seen how death, risk and loss are topics around which teachers and pupils can unite in their ignorance. That is, there are no experts on what our attitudes to these topics ought to be, and teachers have much to learn from their pupils, and vice versa.'

When starting to prepare a useful training package, it is worth considering designing it so that it can be used in a variety of ways – for example, as a training resource taken as a whole, or with facilitators dipping in and out of relevant parts.

The *Lost for Words* package covers many topic areas which are considered important in terms of the knowledge needed by staff in schools, to both understand and support children who have experienced loss. There is a menu of topics which can be mixed and matched to provide suitable training, depending on the context and needs.

These include the broad models of loss, children's understanding of death (sudden or anticipated), helping children after a bereavement, the effect of a death on the school community, and changes in behaviour and learning.

Children's behaviours away from their home need to be observed for signs of distress due to the trauma (Randall 1993). There is a need to reflect on what school staff have noticed about children who have experienced a loss, and on how their learning and behaviour may have been affected.

This could be identified and discussed in an exercise.

Exercise 21.1 Signs of distress in bereaved children

In groups, the school teachers are asked to identify and agree on signs which might suggest that a bereaved child is distressed. These are brought back to the main group, and written on the flip-chart for group debate.

This list could include:

- lack of concentration
- decreasing attention span
- being withdrawn from friends
- becoming angry easily
- becoming upset easily
- getting quite panic stricken
- not responding to questions
- seeming sometimes vacant or dreamy
- no change in behaviour at all.

This often produces a healthy debate, discussing how much should be tolerated, when to discuss it with the child, and when to involve the parent.

This activity can be adapted for different groups of health professionals.

Risk assessment procedures should be taught and used to identify needs, both in schools and in healthcare (Kennedy *et al.* 2008). Aranda and Milne (2000) produced useful guidelines on identifying bereavement risk. However, this is really just a framework, and each of their points could be broken down to make it much easier for the practitioner.

Models of loss are always useful, and are included in order to give a theoretical framework on which to hang ideas and concepts. Ideally all courses should incorporate a number of models of loss, including stages, phases, tasks and the continuing bonds model. (These will be mentioned in the next chapter.) All the models seem to contain some elements which resonate with the bereaved. They can also strike a chord with the participants on courses, who have usually had some major loss in their own lives. This means that they can be engaged with their own losses through general discussions and through techniques such as 'life lines', which is often useful at this stage. (This approach is covered in more depth in Chapter 20 and Chapter 22.)

Research looking at the understanding of death and dying at differing ages dates back many decades. For example, Zach (1978) took the view that even at an early school age, children begin to grasp the meaning and fear of death. By the time children enter secondary school, most will have an adult concept of death. Kane (1979) postulated that even by the age of three years old, many children would have gained the realisation of death, though it would be an embryonic understanding of the concept. Lansdown and Benjamin (1985) reported that by the age of five years, around one-third of the children in their sample had acquired quite a good comprehension of death, including the idea that death is irreversible. By the time that most children reach the age of twelve years, they will probably have an understanding of death similar to that of adults. This theory does again link in with the Piagetian concept of children achieving 'formal operations' (Lovell 1973). In terms of quality of thinking, this is a 'conceptual leap' and is achieved by many children by around the age of twelve years. While this may be of only limited use when teaching, if teachers tend to underestimate the understanding of children regarding the area of death, they are less likely to provide a matched and appropriate intervention. Rather than the recognised five major aspects of children's understanding of death, the authors have simplified the scheme. In view of the fact that this understanding varies so much from one child to another, Table 21.1 provides just a simple framework that serves as a rough guide.

TABLE 21.1 Children and the concept of death (Holland and Hostad 2009)

Baby: 0–2 years	No concept of death, but awareness of loss of carer
Infant age: 2–7 years	Notion of death, although seen as a reversible state
Junior age: 8–11 years	A concept of death is developing (although accompanied by some strange ideas)
Secondary age: 11 years +	An adult concept of death

Children will have an understanding of events, both before and after a death, in terms of their own experience and their cognitive ability, maturity and development. Rather than specifically being concerned with the age of a child, a teacher needs to be alert to their interactions – best appreciated by listening to them, asking them to draw or paint, and questioning their carers – in order to know how to frame appropriate answers and assist with their understanding. Children need to be supported and helped, but may well have a greater understanding and awareness than they are given credit for by adults.

The picture given in Figure 21.1 was drawn by Evie, an eight-year-old girl, and depicts her thoughts on the meaning of death.

Children often do not have the expressive language to reflect on their emotions and to tell others what is on their mind. This applies to all age groups, for example very young children will often say that they are 'sad', and little more. The sadness is all too apparent in the drawing by Evie, where the bereaved person appears to be in a flood of tears. Older children, such as those in their teens, may also be reluctant to express their thoughts verbally.

One strategy is to ask children to draw their thoughts, and then to engage them in

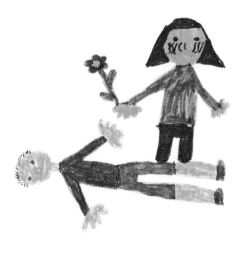

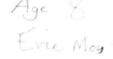

FIGURE 21.1 Eight-year-old Evie's depiction of her thoughts on the meaning of death

discussion about what they have drawn. Clearly, this needs to be done in a sensitive manner – not as an interrogation.

Children could also be observed at play, and again this may give clues as to their feelings.

Policies can be important drivers of awareness and change in schools, and hence they are included in the training. Schools can often feel overrun by policies in many forms, but actually planning what to do after the death of someone in the school community, or of a child's parent, can mean that things are less likely to be missed at a future time of crisis. A simple checklist, as suggested in Holland (1997), could suffice to ensure that nothing is overlooked, but it is also important to evaluate such events and try to refine procedures further where needed.

This approach could equally be adapted for use within the health service. An effective way of using teaching sessions is to have individuals work with others to create policies applicable in their own contexts, and this seems a productive use of the facilitators' time as well.

Janis has found that when health professionals attending a course have produced (with help) the rudiments of a protocol, or guidelines, or a policy for dealing with young people and children, it has altered their practice. However, this has only worked when the individual has experienced the need to put the protocol into practice, and has evaluated or audited its usefulness, as part of the course. (This has been used as a strategy both on the old ENB 931 course and as part of a 'stand alone' two-day children's bereavement course.) The second approach worked well, even though it was only a two-day course, because the two days were a month apart. This was deliberate, so that the participants could report back on their 'pitfalls and progress' in establishing this new working practice. All participants were informed before they attended the course about their 'homework', and asked to bring written consent from their manager that, under their supervision, these guidelines (or similar) could be piloted.

When developing any course, the importance of the language used when communicating with children about loss and death should be included. This is so as to minimise the confusion and fear that children will be feeling. An example of inappropriate language is saying that the dead person has 'gone to sleep', as this has the potential to frighten children at night.

Exercise 21.2 Language for communicating with a bereaved child

It can be useful to ask the teachers (or health professionals) to suggest all the different ways (including euphemisms) that they think of which are used to tell children that someone has died. These could be written on a flip-chart, and each one discussed in terms of its possible consequences to the child.

Participants usually produce a comprehensive list, which is often discussed at length. This list might include things such as:

- he has gone to be with the angels
- he has gone to be with Jesus
- he has gone to be a star
- he has gone to heaven
- he just went to sleep
- he is pushing up daisies
- he has popped his clogs
- he has kicked the bucket.

Often personal experiences are shared, which can be useful for the group in coming to realise the importance of honest plain-talking, provided with a gentle, caring voice and demeanour, which can achieve so much more than white lies and euphemisms.

Multicultural as well as faith issues are also often discussed, and again these are areas where a sensitive approach is needed, and an awareness of the needs of the local community.

An additional topic which is now included in the training relates to children attending funerals (Holland 2004a). This can be a very controversial area for teachers (with strong views held on both sides), although the Iceberg study suggested that the best option is to provide children with an informed choice and adequate information, such as visiting the church or crematorium prior to a funeral (Holland 2001). The teachers may be quite confused, too, if they have not attended a funeral before, and may not be sure exactly what happens. How much more might children be confused, when often the fantasies in their minds are much more real than reality? Sometimes they believe strange things, such as that the coffin will be burned in the open, during the funeral. Another misconception, which has been told in a number of ways over the years, concerns a child's voice heard to say at funerals:

'If my Daddy's body is in that coffin, what have you done with his head, arms and legs?'

It is easy to see how this might happen: due to the intense pressure on the adults trying to cope with the situation, none of them has stopped to explain simply and carefully to the child what they could expect.

This learning about funerals has been enhanced in East Yorkshire by teachers attending the regular funeral and crematorium visits organised by Janis (as detailed in the next chapter).

The teachers who have been on these visits have provided excellent feedback, and have reported that the experience has undoubtedly helped them to support their bereaved school children more effectively. An understanding of the importance of the rituals attached to these rites of passage enables them to interact with the child more appropriately, and not to perpetuate potentially disturbing myths.

The more children are able to exercise choice and be involved in what they are comfortable with, the less likely they will be to have regrets later in their life. A case study is also included in the training, and this helps to focus on the implications of loss for children after a significant death. However, the following example often works better.

Exercise 21.3 The implications of bereavement for the child

It can be useful to ask the teachers (or health professionals) to consider the implications for children after the death of a parent, and to ask for examples of children known to them who have been bereaved, along with their circumstances and the case's implications. By considering an example from their experience, rather than a fabricated case study, teachers and others can draw on their rich life experiences.

These could include such as:

- the child's new status as an orphan, or a 'half-orphan'
- changes in the child's learning which affect their behaviour
- the child's emotional responses
- the way school staff (or ward staff, or other healthcare group members) usually respond.

NB They will come up with a much longer list!

Then ask the group(s) to look at their list(s) and discuss ways they might best respond to each, and report back. Many really good ideas come out of this session. For example, one school gives children a coloured card to hold up if they need to leave the room due to their emotional state (if they think that would be helpful).

Children at this school report that this approach made them feel that their loss was being recognised: 'heard and seen'.

Course timing

These types of courses tend to be very interactive and thought provoking, because of the nature of the topics. Therefore, some serious preparation is needed before you teach the teachers. Often, one might be given an end-of-day slot, before the teachers are due to go home. Both Janis and John have found themselves in this situation, which needs to be avoided if at all possible.

The short lessons which Janis and John have facilitated often took place during the 'twilight' sessions, with the teachers attending training after a long day at school, and they were often very tired. At times, teachers could even be seen to be 'nodding off'! Holding the courses during the daytime helps those attending to arrive feeling fresh, and also implicitly raises the value and profile of the session by not holding it at the tail end of the day as a 'add-on' to other activities. However, sometimes the only opportunity available is to present a short 'taster' session at the end of the school day, and there will therefore be a need to adapt the material, rather than having no contact at all.

The effect of training has been carefully monitored and evaluated over a period of time in schools in the Hull area. Evaluation has taken place through questionnaires that are sent to schools every two years, in order to measure the effects of the training course. The results to date are quite optimistic, and progress has been made in some of the areas that are the focus of the project (Holland 2004b). This is a useful measurement, not only of the success of the teaching – and ultimately, helping children through these traumas – but also for providing feedback for the course reader's manager, illustrating effective use of time.

Within this project, schools still report a similar level of need for training in the area of child bereavement as they did in the initial research. However, significantly more schools have policies and systems in place to respond to a bereaved child, and there are now far more staff in schools who have received some sort of 'loss awareness' training, the substantial majority through *Lost for Words*. In some cases, whole services or schools have received training.

The questionnaire itself is a 'two-way' process. For example, schools have reported that the effect of parental separation is sometimes of even greater concern than parental bereavement and, as a result, the course has been fine-tuned to reflect these concerns.

John says that the idea of 'normalising loss' as a life experience is one of the aims of the course, and many of the schools are given opportunities to feed back through both the questionnaires and also through evaluations by those receiving training.

Janis says that this is just the same in the context of the health service. As well as researching and evaluating the training, the information should result in clinical practice changes and improvement, as a direct response to the feedback.

These courses run in schools are usually all basic 'loss awareness' sessions, and are not counselling courses, although most do include and encourage many of the skills relating to the counselling process, such as empathy and listening skills. The distinction is usually made between this type of training, and major critical incidents, where a more specialist approach may be necessary.

With the profile of child bereavement being raised in the Hull and Humberside area, this has led to the development of the 'Children and Loss: Time to Listen' series of conferences. These have been held every two years, and have attracted both national and international speakers. As with similar types of training, the core attendees are local and regional, but delegates often come from all corners of the UK. To date, there have been four conferences, with a fifth planned for 2010. It is the only one of its type, being solely dedicated to children, and attended by such a wide variety of professionals.

The view of the authors is that there is much to be gained by schools working towards joint multiprofessional training, as suggested at the beginning of the chapter. For example, specially trained educational psychologists, teachers or school nurses could deliver training, together with Macmillan nurses or paediatric oncology nurses, hospice staff or any other specialists from the health field with the relevant expertise. This brings together a much greater level of awareness, skills and knowledge of this important, multifaceted topic, rather than any individual professional or profession being responsible for delivering the training. This sits well with the idea of multi-agency cooperation and coordination, which should reduce duplication and the wastage of resources, as well as making links with the professionals and clients involved, who should receive a more seamless service. The information and training discussed so far has focused on preparing teachers to support children when coping with loss. Then, it is hoped, the teacher will feel comfortable and knowledgeable enough to address such issues with the child, or young persons. The next section will illustrate how these initiatives might also be led by health professionals, as well as focusing on actually *teaching* the children and young people about the effects that cancer (or any other life-threatening illness) might have on their family.

HEALTH PROFESSIONALS, SOCIAL WORKERS AND PSYCHOLOGISTS LEADING THE INITIATIVE

Health professionals working in the NHS (for example, Macmillan nurses) are well equipped with the knowledge and skills to run similar projects in schools. While they may need some 'topping-up' in specific child-related issues, such as developmental and cognitive implications, they are ideally placed to provide support for teachers; the option is there for them to develop one-off sessions, or a series of sessions, for staff in schools (as mentioned in the previous section). They could also respond to the ongoing requests from heads of schools, medical practitioners, and school nurses, to develop teaching resources to open up discussions and debates on issues which might confront the pupils' fears relating to life-threatening illness. This allows the pupils to gain support in coping with both the practical and the emotional realities of living with serious illness.

There is opportunity to either fully develop specific materials, or to utilise resources such as the *Cancer Talk* Macmillan teaching packs. These are excellent resources and work well, whether used in full, or in part, or adapted to a particular session. The packs come in both primary and secondary school versions. Both packs allow the facilitator to deliver effective personal and social health education lessons, by discussing cancer and associated issues (*see* Further information). Janis has worked with the local hospice, and latterly the hospital Macmillan team, in this respect. On the last occasion, the case study used (and very well received) was developed on the theme of *The Simpsons* cartoon series, which the pupils really enjoyed and related to easily. Pleasingly, it did not stop them also focusing on their own feelings and emotions. If the reader decides to use the Macmillan packs, and does not have a lot of time to prepare or deliver the material, then the sessions 'What Is Cancer?' and 'Anna's Story' are likely to be the most useful.

Janis has also used topical issues as addressed on soap operas, or raised by celebrities, or when someone 'famous' has died (for example, Princess Diana, or more recently Jane Tomlinson and Jade Goody). These types of stories often provide a way of raising the issue with a local school, and gaining access to the local classroom.

The St Christopher's Schools Project is another excellent tool, which hospices can use to bridge the gap in public education. This four-week project offers an innovative approach to dealing with the taboos, and negative attitudes, related to dying. It promotes awareness of hospices, and end-of-life care, and is given a high priority by the Department of Health (DoH 2008). While public education has been on the agenda for many years, over time it seems to have lost its impetus (Hostad *et al.* 2004). In the past many eminent palliative care authors have identified the importance of this type of education (Wilkes 1980; James and Field 1992; Clark 1997), and it is hoped that now it is back on the agenda, it is here to stay.

WHAT ABOUT THE CHILDREN AND YOUNG PEOPLE WHO ARE OFTEN NEITHER SEEN NOR HEARD?

These is another very important category requiring help: that of children and young people who have adult relatives being cared for in the healthcare system. Adults who have life-threatening illness are seldom asked by health professionals how the illness is affecting their loved ones, particularly the children in their families. Yet in the UK, approximately 135,000 children each year suffer the death of a parent. There have been suggestions that short-term skilled support and interventions prior to the parent's death could considerably benefit the child and their family (Christ 2000). If children are at school when the district nurse visits the family, or if they are not present during visiting time at hospital, then the health professional is unlikely to know how these children are coping unless they specifically ask. This means that there is a need to find out about the son, or daughter, or grandchild, who might be struggling to adapt. This is especially relevant when studies illustrate that those children of dying parents manifest significant distress, but despite a greater understanding of their parent's illness than is usually suspected, they are not handling the situation well. Also, it has been shown that timely intervention by competent health professionals can help to ameliorate the process of bereavement (Estela *et al.* 2004).

This might then enable the health professional to pick up the cues, and to recognise when to listen, intervene, or refer on. Often in healthcare, the role is one of enabling and empowering the family to support their children, so some of the work is done directly, and some indirectly. It is necessary for health professionals to realise that it is their responsibility to be prepared and ready to help. This is in order to support parents, grandparents and others, in many ways – for instance, when breaking bad news to children (Elsegood 1996; Sweetland 2005).

It is believed that a parent's death causes considerable distress, leading to possible depression in the first year, and an increased risk of developing a psychiatric disorder later in life (Wilkinson 2001). It has been known for many years that the family is an interactive entity, in which all members affect each other. Family dynamics can hinder adequate grieving (Worden 1983). It has also been suggested that the strongest predictor of risk to the child, in terms of psychological well-being, is the ability to adequately adjust shown by the surviving parent (Silverman and Worden 1993). Recognising this dynamic social structure and the relationships which define each unique family, and the major adjustments in coping with a life-threatening illness, prepares the health professional to offer effective help (Firth 2007). Staff need to be taught the importance of gently encouraging children to be there, if appropriate, when their family member is dying (Haas 2003).

When teaching this type of healthcare group, it is important to ensure that participants have some awareness of family dynamics – for example, the role that the dying (or deceased) patient played. This will in turn help the health professional to help the family in their grief. Burnham (1999) provides some useful exercises on how to achieve this in the classroom, via sculpting and other techniques.

In her chapter on family care, Firth (2007) probably provides the most helpful ways of deciding what to teach, and what not to teach, regarding families and life-threatening diseases. It is not unusual for children to know far more than their parents are aware of, or to worry unnecessarily. Many children are anxious about catching cancer, so health professionals need to be taught the importance of listening intently and attentively to discover the children's fears and concerns. This awareness-raising can be accomplished through both role-play and sculpting. (Role-play has been discussed in more detail in the previous chapter, and sculpting is discussed by Firth 2007.)

WHOM TO TEACH, WHERE, WHEN AND HOW

This education could happen in a variety of settings – hospital, hospice or community. Ensuring that the individual is competent to teach is most important.

The 'how' has been discussed as much as it can be in one chapter. All activities suggested so far work with all the above groups, with an occasional minor adjustment. However, both of the authors enjoy using other creative approaches, too, such as having participants put together workbooks for children, or treasure troves to help children remember their loved one.

Exercise 21.4 Making memories
- One group makes a treasure trove. This involves the participants bringing an item from home, and discussing why they would want the object to be something by which other people remember them.
- The other group makes a workbook, 'Memories of Me and My Life', with pens,

glue, poems, thoughts, questions, letters, photos etc. (This would relate to a fictitious person and family.)

● Then the groups change projects.

This usually takes some time to complete, but is worthwhile in terms of the discussions as to how they can help parents and children to achieve such goals. (Often they comment on how they might use this personally too.)

Janis says that the 'Treasure Trove' activity is sometimes referred to as 'Memory Box', and in her experience children often prefer one description over the other, so it is worth asking them which they prefer.

Readers can consult the Further reading and Useful websites sections for even more material to develop this type of educational session.

The 'when' and 'for whom' aspects of this section really need to be tackled at many different levels. Consider what effect it will have when courses are held at differing times of day, when pre-qualification and post-qualification people are present, and when the audience consists of different specialities. This also needs to be an integral part of the training of students and then, once qualified, training appropriate to their speciality should be added. Kennedy *et al.* (2008) support this, suggesting that there really needs to be a wider menu of support options, which should be clearly signposted, drawing on national organisations as well as local ones.

The 'when' aspect would then mean that the staff can receive the right information and education at the appropriate level and at the right time, and in turn children and young people can then receive the same.

KEY POINTS

- ▨ It is important that all relevant professionals are adequately trained in this field.
- ▨ It is impossible to shield children from death and dying.
- ▨ Within both palliative care and in the oncology setting, the needs of children must be addressed.
- ▨ Knowledge of children's and young people's cognitive understanding of death is necessary to teach the topic.
- ▨ There seems to be a lack of 'joined-up' thinking, with some of the different professionals and agencies in the field not working together.
- ▨ There is no national strategy, and ways around this need to be found.

CONCLUSION

While so many authors recommend support and help for this vulnerable group, interestingly Wilkinson (2001) advises caution before committing too many resources. In fact, Harrington and Harrison (1999) state that there are no data which prove that bereavement work with children is effective, and they go further, suggesting that bereavement counselling might even be harmful.

The authors, on the other hand, would suggest that training which allows all those involved with children to be better equipped to interact with and support this group in open, non-threatening ways, providing appropriate information as and when it is needed, must be useful.

Providing adults (parents and other relatives) with information and support must surely help them to work together more effectively as a family. John's research to date seems to support this, and other eminent authors take a similar view. Goldman (2000) postulated that by not allowing a child to attend the funeral, an environment of denial is created which actually inhibits children's grieving. Kubler-Ross (1991) stressed the importance of involving children, and letting them talk about things openly with other family members, in order to help their own grieving.

Janis and John plan a large study in 2010, in which they will look at the training needs and endeavours of the staff of a new oncology centre, in trying to help children and young people with these issues. (This will also be compared with the findings of the teachers' research.) Through this initiative and those of others, progress will be made along the road towards eventually providing effective multi-agency working.

It is hoped that this chapter will motivate the reader to increase their use of this type of education, and encourage more action research.

As Wilkinson (2001) suggested:

> 'Children's grief is an emotive issue, which palliative care professionals must address. However, the lack of evidence on its effects and the most beneficial intervention needs to be addressed before a commitment and resources to develop new services are given.'

This is still largely uncharted territory, and while some inroads have now been made, there is much still to be accomplished before these children and young people can truly be seen and heard.

IMPLICATIONS FOR THE READER'S OWN PRACTICE

1 How well are children and young people assessed and supported in your area of work?
2 How would you go about planning, developing and implementing one of these types of educational initiatives in your locality?
3 What new creative exercises and methods could you devise and utilise to teach these topics effectively, and to maintain interest and ensure learning?
4 In what ways will you now audit or evaluate your educational sessions or programmes aimed at children and young people?
5 What types of research might you undertake in order to change or improve the education which is available, and add to the limited research which has been conducted in this area?

REFERENCES

Aranda S, Milne D (2000) *Guidelines for the Assessment of Complicated Bereavement Risk in Family Members of People Receiving Palliative Care.* Melbourne: Centre for Palliative Care.

Black D (1976) What happens to bereaved children. *Proc Roy Soc Med.* **69**: 841–4.

Bowlby J (1980) *Loss, Sadness and Depression. Vol. 3: Attachment and Loss.* London: Hogarth Press.

Brown E (2007) *Supporting the Child and the Family in Paediatric Palliative Care.* 2nd ed. London: Jessica Kingsley.

Burnham J (1999) *Family Therapy.* New York: Routledge.

Christ GH *et al.* (1993) Impact of parental terminal cancer on latency-age children. *Am J Orthopsychiatry.* **63** (3): 417–25.

Christ G (2000) *Healing Children's Grief: surviving a parent's death of cancer.* Oxford: Oxford University Press.

Clark D (1997) Public education: a missed opportunity? *Prog Palliat Care.* **3**: 189–90.

Department of Health (2008) *National Implementation Advisory Board on End of Life Care.* London: DoH.

Elsegood J (1996) Breaking bad news to children. In: Linsey B, Elsegood J, editors. *Working with Children and Loss.* London: Ballière Tindall.

Estela A, Beale E, Silvesind D, Bruera E (2004) Parents dying of cancer and their children. *Pall Supp Care.* **2** (4): 387–93.

Firth P (2007) Family care: sensitive and dynamic approaches to teaching. In: Foyle L, Hostad J, editors. *Innovations in Cancer and Palliative Care Education.* Oxford: Radcliffe Publishing.

Goldman L (2000) *Life and Loss: a guide to helping grieving children.* 2nd ed. New York: Routledge.

Haas F (2003) Bereavement care: seeing the body. *Nurs Stand.* **17** (28): 33–7.

Harrington R, Harrison L (1999) Unproven assumptions about the impact of bereavement on children. *J R Soc Med.* **92** (5): 230–3.

Holland J (1993) Child bereavement in Humberside. *Educational Research.* **35** (3): 289–97.

Holland J, Ludford C (1995) The effects of bereavement on children in Humberside secondary schools. *Br J Spec Educ.* **22** (2): 56–9.

Holland J, Dance R, MacManus N, Stitt C (2005) *Lost for Words: loss and bereavement awareness training pack for adults.* London: Jessica Kingsley.

Holland J (1997) *Coping with Bereavement: a handbook for teachers.* Cardiff: Academic Press.

Holland J (1999) *Children and the Impact of Parental Death.* Doctoral Research Project at the University of York (Operation Iceberg).

Holland J (2001) *Understanding Children's Experiences of Parental Bereavement.* London: Jessica Kingsley.

Holland J (2004a) Should children be attending their parents funerals. *Pastor Care Educ.* **22** (1): 10–14.

Holland J (2004b) Lost for words in Hull. *Pastor Care Educ.* **22** (4): 10–14.

Hostad J, Macmanus D, Foyle L (2004) Public information and education in palliative care. In: Foyle L, Hostad J, editors. *Delivering Cancer and Palliative Care Education* Oxford: Radcliffe Publishing: 37–51.

James N, Field D (1992) The routinization of hospice: charisma and bureaucratisation. *Soc Sci Med.* **34**: 1363–75.

Kane B (1979) Children's concept of death. *J Genet Psychol.* **1**: 134–41.

Kennedy C, McIntyre R, Worth A, Hogg R (2008) Children and families facing the death of a parent. *Int J Pall Nurs.* **14** (40): 162–8.

Kubler-Ross E (1991) *Life After Death.* Berkeley, CA: Celestial Arts.

Lansdown R, Benjamin G (1985) The development of the concept of death in children aged 5–9 years. *Child: Care, Health and Education.* **11**: 13–20.

Leaman O (1995) *Death and Loss: compassionate approaches in the classroom.* London: Cassell.

Lovell K (1973) *Educational Psychology and Children.* Sevenoaks: Hodder and Stoughton.

Monroe B, Krauss F, editors (2005) *Brief Interventions with Bereaved Children.* New York: Oxford University Press.

Randall P (1993) Aspects of bereavement: 4. Young children grieve differently from adults. *Profess Care Mother Child.* **3** (2): 367.

Safier G (1964) A study in relationships between the life and death concepts in children. *J Genet Psychol.* **105**: 283–94.

Sheldon F (1994) Children and bereavement: what are the issues? *Eur J Palliat Care.* **1**: 42–4.

Silverman P, Worden W (1992) Children's reactions in the early months after death of a parent. *Am J Orthopsychiatry.* **62** (1): 93–104.

Silverman P, Worden JW (1993) Children's reaction to the death of a partner. In: Stroebe MS, Stroebe W, Hansson RO, editors. *Handbook of Bereavement Theory, Research and Intervention.* Cambridge: Cambridge University Press: 300–16.

Slaughter V, Jaakkola K, Carey S (1999) Constructing a coherent theory: children's biological understanding of life and death. In: Seigal M, Peterson C, editors. *Children's Understanding of Biology, Health and Ethics.* Cambridge: Cambridge University Press: 71–98.

Sweetman C (2005) The palliative care nurse's role in supporting the adolescent child of a dying patient. *Int J Palliat Nurs.* **11** (6).

Thomas J (1997) The child bereavement trust: caring for bereaved families. *Br J Midwifery.* **5** (8): 474–7.

Wilkes E (1980) *Report of the Working Group on Terminal Care Standing Medical Advisory Committee.* London: DHSS.

Wilkinson S (2001) How best to support bereaved children. *Int J Pall Nurs.* **7** (8): 368.

Worden JW (1983) *Grief Counselling and Grief Therapy.* London: Tavistock.

Worden W, Silverman P (1996) Parental death and the adjustment of school-age children. *Omega: J Death Dying.* **33** (20): 91–102.

Yule W, Gold A (1993) *Wise Before the Event.* London: Calouste Gulbenkian Foundation.

Zach H (1978) Children and death. *Soc Work Today.* **9** (39).

FURTHER READING

The authors of this chapter have chosen a number of resources and websites which they believe will be particularly helpful in responding to teaching this topic in your locality.

- Holland J (1997) *Coping with Bereavement: a handbook for teachers.* Cardiff: Academic Press.

     John, responding to the earlier research and to needs in schools, wrote this book specifically to provide teachers (and other staff) with an insight into how to plan both proactively and reactively, where young persons have been bereaved. The implementation of policies or procedures in schools seems a key element, and the book provides a specimen policy, and ideas for how schools can prepare.

Readers seeking more information on the research tools or methods are invited to contact John: john.holland@john-holland-ep.co.uk

- *Cancer Talk* (2001)

    Macmillan cancer relief offer two excellent teaching packages, one aimed for primary schools and the other for secondary schools (as referred to in the chapter). They are designed for direct teaching with pupils. The materials are certainly helpful to anyone new to this type of teaching, or with little time to plan activities. They also provide very useful websites to support these packs, which can be used in conjunction with the material or as independent resources for either teachers or children and young people (*see* Useful websites·below).

- St Christopher's Project (2006)

    This resource is designed to help hospices and schools to work in partnership. It provides guidance and information on how to run this type of project in your locality, with step-by-step instructions. This guide encourages hospices to work with their communities to start to integrate the concept of death into everyday lives, in a non-threatening way. (Brochures with CD are available from St Christopher's bookshop.)

- Good Grief series books, by Barbara Ward (Jessica Kingsley Publications): *Exploring Feelings, Loss and Death with Under Elevens* (Vol. 1, 1994), *Exploring Feelings, Loss and Death with Over Elevens and Adults* (Vol. 2, 1995).

    These books, while fairly old, are still excellent resources for preparing courses to teach about children and young people, or if working directly with them. These two books were designed with 20 educators contributing ideas, and piloted with children of different abilities and backgrounds in their care. They explore and demystify the experience of loss, in different contexts. They also work within the framework of the National Curriculum. These books are suitable for all professionals (including parents or other family members) who might be involved. They are activity based, facilitating the use of the children's own experiences, and they encourage improvisation. It is most definitely a useful resource for your toolbag.

- Goldman L (2000) *Life and Loss: a guide to helping grieving children*. 2nd ed. New York: Routledge.

    Goldman is well established as an author, child advocate and counsellor. This book is about life and loss, and about children. Goldman uses story, craft and feelings to guide children and parents. It is a complete teaching manual for everyone working and teaching in this field. Most of the suggested activities will not date, so the book will remain on your shelf, and be dipped in and out of for many years (as the authors have done).

- *Talking to Children when an Adult Has Cancer* (2002) Cancerlink, Macmillan Cancer Relief.

    This is a really useful, practical booklet which covers the questions that children might ask, their potential reactions and difficulties. Very helpful for parents and professionals.

USEFUL WEBSITES

- www.class-action.org.uk

    This Macmillan resource guide is for teachers and youth group leaders. Here you will find all the information, support and resources that you need to talk about cancer with children and young people. It works alongside the above Macmillan teaching resource, *Cancer Talk*.

- www.whybother.org.uk

    This website is particularly useful for helping and supporting children and young people, rather than health professionals. It is designed to help them answer the questions such as 'Why bother finding out more about cancer?' It explains that because there are over two million people in the UK who have been diagnosed with cancer, most children and young people will know someone affected by it. It provides the information in a fun way, with quizzes and video case studies.

- www.ncb.org.uk/cbn/

    The Childhood Bereavement Network (CBN) was established in 1998 to ensure that all children and young people receive information, guidance and support to enable them to manage the impact of death on their lives. CBN works in partnership with service providers to improve the range and quality of bereavement support for children throughout the UK and to increase access to information, guidance and support.

- www.riprap.org.uk

    Riprap is a website that can help the young to cope when a parent has cancer. There are stories from other young people going through the same situation. There is also information and there are tips to help understand and deal with what is going on in the family. Presentation is suitably youthful and colourful.

- www.childbereavement.org.uk

    The Child Bereavement Trust considers that grief that, if ignored, can harm us in countless ways. To support families at such difficult times and to limit the potential for psychological problems in the longer term, it is crucial that all professionals are able to recognise and respond appropriately to bereaved families' varied emotional needs. The charity's vision is for all bereaved children and grieving families to have access to relevant support and information from appropriately trained professionals.

- www.winstonswish.org.uk

    Winston's Wish is the leading childhood bereavement charity and the largest provider of services to bereaved children, young people and their families in the UK. They offer practical support and guidance to families, professionals and anyone concerned about a grieving child. The right support at the right time can enable young people to live with their grief and rebuild positive futures.

- www.royalmarsden.org.uk

    This website from the Royal Marsden Hospital, the UK's leading cancer centre, features 'The Adventures of Captain Chemo', which is a useful and fun way for young children to gain the information they might need about chemotherapy.

ACKNOWLEDGEMENT

Janis and John would like to thank Evie Elizabeth Moy for drawing the picture included in this chapter.

22

The graveyard shift: creative strategies for teaching bereavement and loss

Janis Hostad

'Death leaves a heartache no one can heal, love leaves a memory no one can steal.'

From a headstone in Ireland

AIM

This chapter aims to explore creative teaching strategies, to ensure that health professionals learn about the appropriate aspects of bereavement and loss, and to discuss the key issues and implications for providing this education, in order to improve clinical interventions.

LEARNING OUTCOMES

By the end of this chapter, the reader should be able to:
- explore ways of teaching some of the different theories and models, ensuring that they remain pertinent to the patient, family and student
- understand approaches to support individuals, both before and after bereavement, and how these might be best taught
- reflect on some of the creative ways in which the teacher might tackle the myths and taboos surrounding death, both within and outside the classroom
- demonstrate awareness of the consequences that different aspects of this topic could and should have regarding their own mortality
- recognise that loss is deeply personal to everyone, including students and the teacher
- reflect on their own personal vulnerabilities, and how these might affect them when teaching.

INTRODUCTION

Sessions on loss and bereavement, within course curricula on pre-registration and post-registration nursing courses, are not new. Indeed, they are now an integral part of educational programmes for a number of different disciplines. However, what is not clear is precisely what is included, for how long it is taught, and what rationale is used for its inclusion at a particular stage, or for teaching the topic in a particular way.

Loss, grief and bereavement affect the patient, family and the health professional, and each person experiences grief in their own way by utilising their own coping skills. For those health professionals who work in cancer and palliative care, loss, grief and bereavement become an everyday occurrence. The notion that health professionals grieve too has become more acceptable over the years, with a number of studies recognising their feelings of loss, and the impact that a patient's death may have on them (Saunderson and Ridsdale 1999; McIntyre 2002; Pullen 2002). The educational activities in this chapter respond to this by, in the main, being experiential in nature. This experiential approach allows the participants to increase their self-awareness, and identify their limitations, as well as challenging their beliefs and attitudes.

When embarking on a course related to loss and bereavement, death cannot be viewed as likely to happen only to the patient, as it is inevitable for everyone, including the student, and could occur at any time. So, just by attending this type of course, the process of increasing the participant's self-awareness will begin and, as a result, so will the preparatory work of coming to terms with their own mortality. (This will be discussed further, later in this chapter.)

Ideally, support for those affected by death should commence when the illness is found to be incurable, as this is the point at which death is first faced and the consequences dealt with on a daily basis.

Kinghorn and Duncan (2005: 303) state: '*Living with loss is therefore a constant companion for those patients and carers confronted by a life threatening illness.*'

Teaching bereavement and loss should mirror this, by beginning at the same point when the illness is found to be incurable, so that the health professional is ready to deal with the anticipatory loss issues as soon as they occur.

Anyone who works in these specialist fields will be all too well aware of the constant struggles faced by those involved in coping with loss, both present and anticipated. What kind of struggles does each individual face? Often they are overwhelmed by pain, fear, guilt, anguish, anger and many other related emotions.

Given these devastating effects of loss, it is therefore essential that all health professionals (and clergy) are adequately trained to deal with them (Payne 2001; Greenstreet 2004; Lloyd-Williams and Cobb 2006). This includes becoming competent at facilitating the grief process, by assessing grief and assisting the patient, relative, carer and health professional to progress through their grief at their own pace (Sheldon 1998; Parkes 1998; Melliar-Smith 2002).

Given that a multi-disciplinary team is usually involved, it makes sense for each of these major disciplines to contribute their expertise to the training of others. This is not always possible, but it does allow different individuals from different professions to play to their strengths and provide insight into their roles with patient and family. This does usually evaluate well, and is appreciated by the participant or student group(s).

This chapter will endeavour to examine the strengths and inherent weaknesses of different methods and approaches, and how best to accomplish this facilitation role, so that the students might be more effective in clinical practice. Therefore, it will certainly be useful for those who are embarking for the first time on teaching about bereavement and loss.

It may also be useful for the 'expert educator', when they are short of time, but would like an alternative teaching activity to adapt or to complement their tried and tested methods. For those who are teaching bereavement and loss regularly, who find that they use many similar approaches, it will reinforce the efficacy and benefits of this type of teaching. The activities utilised are ones which have had the best evaluations for the author, and also by other educational colleagues.

The chapter is designed to be practical rather than theoretical. The theories and literature related to bereavement are readily available in books and articles. Therefore, the emphasis is on how to put these models and theories into context, so that the student can apply them in their workplace, having experienced suitable and effective teaching activities. If, as educators, we can get this right, then we can truly make a difference to the care of patients and relatives.

Bereavement and loss is indeed traumatic for those who face it. If supported and helped in appropriate ways, people are able to get back to 'normal' life. Often, the help they receive can be a turning point, when their emotions of grief are released. This is why loss and bereavement education is so vital.

THEORETICAL FRAMEWORKS AND MODELS

Education about the theoretical frameworks and models alone is not sufficient to equip health professionals to deal with all the traumas faced by their patients, carers, relatives and colleagues as a result of loss. It must be acknowledged nonetheless that the frameworks and models do go some way towards making sense of this complex process. However, as Kinghorn and Duncan (2005) warn, models should not be taken to extremes by teaching and advocating their use in a rigid and prescriptive fashion.

It is often useful to start with elements of the seminal work related to attachment by Bowlby (1969). The teacher may then choose to use the work of Erickson *et al.* (1986), or Freud (1917), or Lindemann (1944). Ensuring that students are aware of the research and the models relating to attachment between humans, and what happens when these bonds are lost, is crucial. It reminds students that before any loss, there will be affinity and attachment, and that the closest attachments are often the triggers of the deepest grief.

There are many exercises which can be utilised to generate discussion and raise awareness of attachment. The following exercise, or a similar one, is commonly used when teaching this aspect of the topic.

Exercise 22.1 Attachment and loss

Suggest that the participants think of an inanimate object which is important to them, and which they have possessed for a significant time. They should then close their eyes, and picture it mentally.

Ask them to remember what it looks like, what it feels like, and why it is important. Ask them to remember an occasion when they had that feeling of its great significance, value and importance, and how good that felt. Then ask them to imagine that the object has suddenly gone missing, and they have no idea where it is. At this point participants should write down immediately their psychological responses to this loss.

To do this, it would be helpful if participants could consider their responses under the following headings:
- emotional
- cognitive
- behavioural.

Do any of these responses change over time, say a week, a month, a year?

Now suggest that participants imagine buying something that they need, spontaneously, today. They get home and find that it is missing; it has been lost on the journey. Now ask them to write down their responses again, using the three headings above. They should consider if these responses change over time.

Participants can share these findings in their subgroup. Then, they can elect a spokesperson to report back to the full group.

Discuss the feedback, under the three headings above.

Useful talking points
- How different, or similar, were their individual responses in your group, and why might this be?
- How similar, or different, were the reactions to each object. Why might this be?
- Are there any similarities at all in terms of the emotional, cognitive, and behavioural responses to the death of a person?
- Were there any surprises?
- How do you become attached to something?

NB Always ensure at the outset that the student will be comfortable discussing the object which they have chosen.

This exercise is an excellent way of leading into attachment theory, and it generates much discussion. By now the participants are already bridging the gap, first to their own circumstances, and then to those of the patient and their family.

To lose someone close, within an established relationship, is to be dispossessed and separated from something which is vital to our well-being, and which in part has been taken for granted, hence causing the acute pain.

The premise of the work by Bowlby was that attachment is a protective biological mechanism, which comes from a need to be secure and safe. The attachment which is formed (usually with a few individuals) tends to endure for a large part of the person's life (Bowlby 1980). He postulated that the tendency of humans (as compared to animals) is to form strong emotional bonds with others, and this is considered as normal behaviour. However, he also suggests that humans do not take irretrievable loss into account. Much of his work was through observation of children's separation in stressful situations – this behaviour was thought to be the same for adults as well as children (Small 2001). Therefore, the simple conclusion is that human beings are essentially social beings, and need to have relationships with others, regardless of the possible painful consequences. Interestingly, it is suggested that social relationships, in the form of social support, may enhance health and recovery from bereavement (Lehman *et al.* 1986; Rosenblatt 1993; Walter 1999; Payne *et al.* 1999).

Bowlby (1980) considered that children who had ambivalent parenting were more likely, in later life, to be inhibited in their attachments. Those who were more self-reliant were more likely to delay the grieving process, causing strain, irritability and sometimes depression.

This seems to illustrate why it is has been suggested that those who experience a happy and fulfilling relationship may find it easier to adjust, compared with those who have not had such a rewarding relationship (Payne *et al.* 1999). On the other hand, it is also proposed that the closer and stronger the attachment, the more intense and enduring the distress of the grief (Bowlby 1980).

However, those people who don't commit to a relationship still may not avoid pain, as they may live a life of loneliness. If a long-term healthy relationship gives a life of happiness and deep meaning, the severance of this attachment is bound to cause misery and anguish, in the form of pain and grief (Weston *et al.* 1998). This pain comes from having to readjust; the person has been forced to separate from their loved one and to try to adjust, and to resume life without their loved one.

Before introducing the student to the variety of research and theories into bereavement, the author would suggest that having an understanding of both adjustment theory and family dynamics is vital. These topics then act as a precursor to the different models, and provide better insight into how to help. Family dynamics and support cannot be covered in this chapter due to space constraints, but the topic is referred to briefly in the previous chapter. However, Firth (2007) does this topic far more justice in her chapter 'Family care: sensitive and dynamic approaches to teaching', in the previous book in this series. It is quite clear from feedback from families going through this process that they value receiving comfort, support and honesty (Smith 2004). Helping relatives both before and after bereavement is a service whose importance that must not be underestimated (Costello 1995).

Over much of the last century, theorists and researchers continued to try to produce an all-encompassing model, and to try to make sense of this complex process. Many writers devised creative and different approaches to try to pin down this process. However, most have written about the same symptoms and manifestations, but in slightly different ways. These authors are trying to achieve the same outcomes, but with different approaches, techniques or methods. In this author's opinion, as bereavement is so complex, no one model will ever encompass all the kaleidoscope of its facets. However, a number of the models have elements which really offer a true insight into particular aspects of grief.

For example, in Parkes' 'Phases' (1998), he uses the word 'yearning'. There cannot be many people who have had the misfortune of losing someone close and yet fail to relate to that term. When teaching, the author has found that many students comment on how much the word 'yearning' resonates with the way they feel, that the separation is like a 'desperate pining' for another person. Another word used by Parkes which often brings about much discussion, is 'searching'. This usually results in discussion about how the bereaved person thought they saw their deceased loved one, only to realise almost instantly that it was not them. This then provokes further dialogue regarding other participants' similar experiences, discussing how over time these sightings diminish, and why that might happen. Another theorist whom the author often mentions when teaching is Lindemann (1944). In the classroom, the 'Coconut Grove' fire disaster is discussed, relating to the benefits and limitations of his research. However, it is useful to discuss the fact that Lindemann was the first theorist to propose that grief generally follows a recognisable pattern. The students are then asked to debate the advantages and disadvantages in having a recognised pattern of grief to follow. The next exercise offers a method by which a greater awareness of grief can be created and, depending on how it is run, greater insight into a specific model.

Exercise 22.2 Word workshop

This is a very useful exercise for the students wanting to continue gaining understanding of the different terms and definitions, and to help the group realise how differently everyone views these words, and indeed how individual the process can be.

Words involving loss and grief (or it could be all the words which describe, or are associated with, a particular bereavement model) are written on cards.

This exercise works best in small groups, each assisted by a facilitator, in a circle.

Each participant takes a card. If a participant does not like the word, or it is 'too close to home', they can exchange it.

Each person then tells the group what the word is, and what it means to them, then the rest of the group can add their comments.

The exercise carries on until all the cards have gone.

If this 'word workshop' exercise has focused on words such as 'grief', 'mourning', 'bereavement' and 'loss', it can be helpful to provide the students with a dictionary definition of these words, as they are often misused.

Usually when providing a history of the development of the bereavement theories and their impact, most educators start with Freud (1917), and progress to Lindemann (1944), Engel (1961), Bowlby (1980), Parkes (1998), Worden (1991), Stroebe *et al.* (1993), and Walter (1996). Other authors are often included, but the previously

mentioned theorists seem to be referred to the most. There are a number of different aspects from each of these approaches which the teacher can use. For example,
Worden's (1982) work echoes and connects with the bereaved, they hear the word
'task' which confirms that the process will be hard work. (This aspect is important to
convey when teaching.) Worden talks about people having to 'work' through their
reactions, so that they can make a complete adjustment. Worden's 'Tasks' is one of the
most commonly referred to models in the English-speaking world (Walter 1999), and
certainly has much to offer. In the classroom, Clingerman (1996) adapted Worden's
work to use 'tasks for the student nurse' as a useful approach to teaching student nurses
about bereavement. Parkes' model is useful in that it conveys that the grieving process
gets worse before it gets better. Parkes' later work (1993, 2001) also addresses loss in
relation to psychological transitions such as divorce and redundancy. When focusing
on this type of loss, the 'lifeline' exercise described by Costello in Chapter 20 might be
useful. The author of this chapter tends to do the exercise slightly differently to Costello,
as seen in Exercise 22.3. The participants plot all the different types of 'losses' or 'life
transitions' in their life so far, on the graph included as Figure 22.1, marking their age
and the severity of loss as felt at the time.

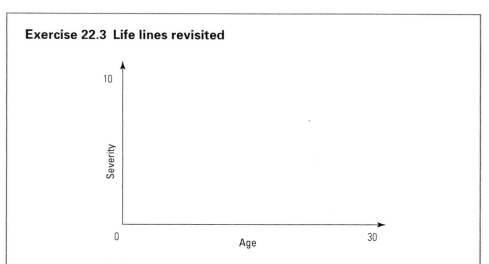

Exercise 22.3 Life lines revisited

FIGURE 22.1 Life lines graph

This exercise helps students to see how frequently loss affects their lives, and how
random it can be. Sometimes the rating they have allocated in this exercise turns out
not to be what they thought at the time of their loss, or not how they think it ought to
be, given the relationship with the person. For example, a student might have rated
their dog's death higher than when their mother-in-law died. This can be referred back
to the bereaved. How easy is it for patients or relatives to be honest and share similar
thoughts if they think they might be judged for this? This exercise also has the potential
to examine coping strategies. For example, do they always employ the same one? Are
there other variables, which affect which strategy they use? Could this exploration prove
useful when working with the patient, family and the bereaved?

While the many theorists and authors have explained the process in different ways, all would agree that grief does not progress in an orderly manner (Parkes 1998; Stokes *et al.* 1997; Stroebe *et al.* 1993; Martin and Weston 1998). When Stroebe *et al.* (1993) introduced their well-received dual process model, it was particularly acclaimed because it describes individuals oscillating from loss-orientation to restoration-orientation. This illustrates that individuals swing backwards and forwards as they learn to cope, and get back on with life. This diminishes some of the criticism with regard to the 'orderly process' which some models appear to suggest. In the classroom, a short case study is very useful for illustrating this, by having the participants place the reactions and emotions into the dual process model, and then discussing when the participants felt that the individual in the case study 'oscillated', what caused it, why, and whether it helped or not.

In 1996, Walter provided a new model of grief, which while based on a personal bereavement, offers much in terms of illustrating the importance of telling the story or biography. This validates the bereaved person to talk and share their feelings. His later book (1999) was also unique in applying sociological insights to this complex personal process.

This proves to be valuable material in a classroom, raising the awareness of students and highlighting the fact that bereaved people do not live in a social vacuum, but instead struggle with expectations of self, of others and maybe even of the academic theorists. Some of these researchers are in either the 'letting go' or the 'keeping hold' camp (as Walter terms them), however, the 'continuing bonds' case is becoming more and more established (Klass *et al.* 1996). This needs to be explored, and the implications discussed with students.

These models and guidelines do offer useful frameworks to direct how the health professional might interact more productively with the patient and family (Kinghorn and Duncan 2005).

However, the student needs to be aware of the many limitations of the research. To date, most models fail to unite the family, social, cultural, environmental and gender contexts that influence the process (Miles and Demi 1984; Stroebe *et al.* 1993). In earlier days, the research base was lacking, with studies having many methodological limitations (Payne *et al.* 1999). In most cases, the research fails to recognise the diversity and individuality of loss. The clinical models and research models are significantly different, with the former addressing manifestations of grief and the differing bereavement responses, and the latter identifying key variables. The search to find the answers continues.

When educating health professionals on bereavement theories and models, the message is that people do need to know what to expect when they or others are grieving. However, if a person-centred approach is also encouraged, taught and developed, connecting with the bereaved person in his or her own 'total uniqueness' might perhaps not be as hard as Walter contends. While he suggests it with some scepticism, it would be pleasing to think that:

> 'Individualism in mourning, as in so much else, may after centuries a-growing at last have come of age.' (Walter 1999: 208)

Many of the individuals working as cancer and palliative educationalists do so after working at a senior level as practitioners. Equally, practitioners who teach regularly do so usually with a sound knowledge base and a good grounding in practice. This means that it is much easier to illuminate the session with stories from the clinical setting, thus contextualising and interweaving the theory with real life.

Stories are dealt with by Foyle in detail, in Chapter 3. However, it is worth mentioning that there are many stories in the guise of television dramas or films, which can be very valuable in supporting your message in the classroom. It might be useful to play an excerpt, or ask the group to watch a certain programme before attending. With a little forward planning, this can be an excellent tool. For example, the film '*Tuesdays with Morrie*' is one in which Albom (1997) tells the story of a university professor who dies from an aggressive neurological illness. This story is informative and useful regarding the preparatory grief work which his friend does, with Morrie's help. It provides lessons about how much can be achieved *before death*, and reminds us that often not only are families (and in particular, children) sometimes forgotten mourners, but also that those *significant* others can be similarly overlooked.

There are other older films, such as CS Lewis' '*Shadowlands*', which would be a most constructive teaching tool. This story (for the readers who do not already know) is about Lewis' wife who died of cancer, and his attempts to cope, and to look after her two sons (Lewis 1961). He keeps a diary, in which he candidly pours out his emotions in a very articulate and eloquent manner. This poignant story captures the essence of what most families feel and go through. There are many films that can be used in this manner, and it is often useful to have a 'swap shop' with other colleagues, providing the specific aim of the film, and expected learning outcomes, and the exercise which you would use.

Another approach, discussed in the previous chapter by this author, was the use of drawing as a medium via which to work with children. This can also be used as a valuable teaching tool with adults. The rationale for using this approach with children is that often they do not have the expressive language required to reflect on their emotions, and to tell others what is on their mind. This, the author would suggest, can also apply to adults: some students find it difficult to articulate their feelings or may be reticent, or hesitant, in expressing these types of thoughts verbally.

One strategy which seems to work really well is to ask the participants to draw, using coloured pens, 'what bereavement looks like'. This has been a fascinating exercise when engaging them in discussions about what they have drawn and what it means to them. (Clearly, this cannot be achieved easily in a large group.) This can be most useful when teaching students to work with the families, and with children in particular. By completing this exercise, the health professional experiences this process for themselves. It is hoped that they then take away the message that it is *not* for the health professional to make these 'interpretations' with patients (that is, unless they have been trained and are qualified to do so). Nevertheless, this can be a useful way of 'connecting' with some individuals at a deeper level, enabling them to feel safer and more comfortable when engaging in a dialogue regarding their feelings and emotions (Kearney 1996). The arts and literature, too, can be an excellent resource, to give sorrow words (and pictures), and for this reason both are useful in the classroom, and with the bereaved.

As Bertman suggests, there is a need to 'explore the universal experiences which underlie these traditional and not-so-traditional expressions, to examine the truth that lies past the smart of feeling' (1991: 318). She also quotes that famous Shakespearean line 'Give sorrow words; the grief that does not speak, whispers the o'er-fraught heart and bid it break' (1991: 1334). This is a most eloquent and expressive illustration of the value of words and how suppressed emotions can be released by talking.

Much emphasis must be placed on the importance of preparatory grief work care. If this is not given the credence it deserves, this might lead to prolonged grief work, or an individual's getting stuck and requiring psychiatric intervention. Further ways of achieving this through education need to be explored, identified and accomplished in partnership with managers in the clinical setting. To reflect during a teaching session, using a case study, on what could have been done to prevent various aspects of grief is a helpful (but crude) way of achieving this; sometimes this is all that time constraints allow. Guidance must also be given with regard to risk assessment, so that health professionals will be aware which individuals might need more support, or referral to other agencies. It can be helpful to ask a group to identify what they think the risks might be, and then compare this with what the different theorists say. A useful, very simplistic, table is provided by Greenstreet (2004), adapted from the work of Sheldon (1998), which could be used as a straightforward checklist.

Another approach which the author uses is to ask the participants to read an article, or a brief case-history, or a short story, and then to get them to offer their help (and/ or advice) given the particular circumstances. A really useful article for doing this is in the *British Journal of Healthcare Assistants* (in their Open Forum), and is written by Wilson (David) and responded to by Becker (Bob) (2007). David tells the story about his two children, who died tragically in an accident, and then Bob provides a commentary and advice about caring for parents in this situation. In the classroom, the students are only given the account, not the commentary. The students are then asked to write their own commentary and response to David's story (in small groups). These are then discussed in the main group, and their answers are compared to the response from Bob. This article is useful with all types and levels of participants. However, as it was written for healthcare assistants, so it can be used to explore their role and reaffirm the importance of the part they play in supporting the bereaved.

To support families who are preparing for the forthcoming death of a loved one, it may be necessary to help them to think about the funeral arrangements, and the choice about cremation or burial. The health professional would be ill-equipped to do this if they had not first ensured that they knew the necessary facts, so they could assist the family to make the correct, informed, decision for them.

TACKLING TABOOS AND MYTHS

There are many taboos and myths related to death and bereavement. Because the subject of death is such a taboo, the public and health professionals alike do not have a clear picture of what is myth and what is fact.

Nurses are sometimes encouraged to follow 'traditions' relating to death in the workplace, like opening the window to let the soul out when someone has died.

Some nurses place a rose in the hand of the deceased, or lay one on the body. These practices, if observed by the relative, might well offend them. It is the teacher's role, therefore, to challenge and debate such practice. This is so that students will see that practices such as these should be fully discussed with the relatives, and only be carried out if this choice is acceptable to the patient's loved ones, and with their full permission.

The significance and value of funeral rites is irrefutable, however the inadequacies of these rituals have only recently been highlighted (Walter 1990; Durston 1998) and very rarely discussed or debated as part of educational programmes for health professionals.

A survey, carried out by the author almost twenty years ago, illustrated that those health professionals who had never attended any training had many misconstrued views about proceedings at the funeral directors, and at the crematorium.

Another small-scale survey in 2009 produced almost the same results. This illustrates that, without training, health professionals are often ignorant of the facts.

As many NHS Trusts are looking at reconfiguring their bereavement services, they would do well to look at the educational needs of their staff. Ignorance cannot be an excuse for poor practice.

Many years ago, there were only a small number of bereavement practitioners and educators who were raising awareness of what to do after death, about the funeral process, and the role of the funeral directors. However, more recently, the situation is changing and innovative and entrepreneurial funeral companies have started running courses for health professionals (free of charge). These do need to be regarded with a slight element of suspicion; after all, they are in business! The reader needs to be reminded of documentaries and of news items on television, and in the newspapers, which have uncovered unscrupulous business practices. They have highlighted high-pressure selling techniques, making sure that the bereaved had 'tears in their eyes', in order to sell the more expensive funeral packages.

If NHS Trusts, hospices, educational units or establishments send their staff on such seminars or visits, they must consider the ethics of doing so, and ensure that the information is beneficial to improved care. This is not meant to criticise or invalidate the excellent work carried out by most funeral directors and crematorium staff. In fact, such partnership working can be most useful. Asking local funeral directors if they want to take part in a joint venture, and choosing the one(s) with the best knowledge, practice, premises, service and humanitarian approach, (against your own pre-determined criteria), can be most beneficial. This ensures that health professionals can find out what is achievable, and what is available at an acceptable cost. The author has spent almost twenty years running well-evaluated trips to funeral directors and crematoria. However, this has not always been with the same companies. Only the ones who are committed to being involved, have the right attributes, and provide the highest quality services are considered.

By running such ventures as an educationalist or facilitator, your overseeing of the proceedings means that you can ensure that the participants are given the information which they require to improve their clinical practice for the patient and the family. The facilitation of this event by the educator or health professional also means that you can observe the group for any adverse emotional reactions triggered (perhaps by previous elements of unresolved grief) during the day.

The following example illustrates one approach to a funeral director and crematorium visit, which might prove useful to those planning similar trips.

Funeral director and crematorium visit

The day is open to anyone who is in some type of caring or helping role with patients who are dying, or who is working with the bereaved. (This often includes school teachers, as mentioned in the previous chapter.) Axiomatic to this arrangement is ensuring that the funeral director, as well as having the desired premises, also has the appropriate qualities to connect with the participants. The author would suggest that these qualities need to convey the caring ethos and philosophy that should be inherent in this industry. The funeral director and crematorium superintendent who were chosen provided a subtle blend of kindness, empathy, compassion, warmth and genuineness, coupled with great passion for their jobs.

Example: funeral director's visit

Beyond death, working together: the individual's continued pathway

The Programme

9.00 a.m. – Introduction
This section is led by the educationalist. The following issues are covered:
- introductions and welcome
- setting the scene
- ground rules
- learning outcomes and workbook.

9.30 a.m. – Exploration of funeral director's role
This section is led by the funeral director. The following issues are covered:
- history of the funeral director, explaining the development of the role
- the first call and building rapport with the family
- bringing the deceased person into the funeral director's care
- statutory procedure and documentation (doctor, coroner, registrar etc.)
- providing individualised care, looking for the best fit for everyone concerned
- options and decisions, including how to help the family make the right choice (type of funeral, flowers, songs, coffin, readings and much more)
- embalming, including the process, when it might be helpful and when it is not
- what happens at the funeral director's premises, from receiving the deceased until the day of the funeral
- how all the different professionals can work together to improve and individualise the care (and prevent things going wrong which might cause heartache to the relatives)
- discussion of what is deemed good practice, possibly followed by debate and dialogue.

There are questions and answers during and at the conclusion of this section.

The first part of the above section is led by the educationalist, the second part mainly by the funeral director, with the educationalist pointing out in context how the information might be used back in the students' workplace.

The educationalist will also start to challenge gently some of the students' thoughts, as well as conceptualising the theory as appropriate. This illustrates the useful symbiotic relationship of the funeral director and educator, who work together to ensure that the participants have all the information, and the theories, and know how to apply them in practice.

The group then has a detailed tour of the building and grounds. The tour of the premises includes:

- visitors' waiting rooms
- interview room
- looking at the different types of coffins, caskets and shrouds available
- the fleet of cars (and a discussion of why they are not black in this particular case)
- the chapel of rest (and a discussion of why viewing rooms were designed in this way, and why that makes them so efficient, functional and fit for purpose).

11.30 a.m. – Questions and answers and close

During the morning, participants are reminded that they can opt out anytime (as discussed during the ground rules session).

Before and during the tour of the premises, they are warned about what they will see. The sight of caskets or coffins, and the knowledge that someone is inside (even if they are not visible) can upset some participants, even though the majority will have seen many dead bodies in the past.

An effective funeral director and educationalist partnership means that they can keep a check on the participants, and the educationalist can deal with any problems as they occur.

11.30 a.m. to 2.00 p.m. – Lunch

This period involves travelling to the crematorium, with lunch taken on the way. The lunch venue is chosen because of its location close to the crematorium, and because it is quiet and private (as well as the excellent, reasonably priced food). The privacy aspect of the venue does need to be stressed, as at a previous venue, the session had to be curtailed when a group of very elderly people sat at the next table, and it seemed rather inappropriate to continue discussing funerals and different rites of passage! After lunch is finished, a short seminar is delivered.

Lunch seminar

This session allows the educator to continue with any unfinished business from the morning, and to check that everyone is alright.

Its aim is to explore how the participants might address the issues concerning the situation which arises after a loved one has died. Discussions relating to interactions with the patient before they have died, as well as with the relatives, are covered too.

The session includes different ways they might broach these issues sensitively and interact with the patient and relatives more successfully.

2.00 p.m. – The crematorium
This is run using the same format as the morning. Elements include:
- welcome by the crematorium superintendent and educationalist
- ground rules and learning outcomes for the visit
- history of the crematorium
- bringing the deceased into the care of the crematorium staff
- the role of the crematorium staff
- statutory procedures and documentation (funeral directors, coroners, doctors, etc.)
- providing individualised care and looking for what is the best fit for everyone concerned
- consideration of what is possible with respect to relatives being involved in the funeral service.

Tour of the premises
Participants are reminded of the ground rules, so that anyone who does not want to see a particular aspect of the visit can sit in the visitors' room until they wish to rejoin the tour.

Inside
Participants look in the visitors' waiting room and the separate quiet room. They then view the chapel and receive information about the service.

Such information might include whether the music should be played on an organ or from a compact disc, the choice of leaving the coffin on the catafalque, the curtains being drawn or left open, and any other aspects regarding the conducting of the service.

The group then follows the journey of the deceased, by visiting the operational cremation room, including the machinery which powers the cremators, witnessing the cremator and the crimulator (which grinds the remains into ashes) in action, and sees the ashes at the end of the process.

One of the students attending the 'Care of the Dying Patient and His Relative' course had studied a particular dying patient. By coincidence, after this patient died, his body was at the funeral directors on the morning of our visit, and was then taken to the crematorium, arriving at the same time as we did.

The student was able to see the 'behind the scenes' cremation, and followed the process until her former patient ended up in a casket. While a little upset by the experience, she regarded this as total holistic care, and was quite proud that she had managed to be there. As an unexpected bonus, the former patient's family were surprised but pleased to see the student present and they gained solace from this.

This is usually a most beneficial part of the day for dismissing many strongly held views. There are always many questions, with those listed below being the most common. They might sound a little macabre, but it is surprising what patients and their families do want to know. When the health professional is more knowledgeable, and feels comfortable and confident, they can offer answers to the most difficult questions in the most appropriate and sensitive manner.

As an educator in palliative care, or a practitioner, there is a need for you to be free of these myths, so that you can pass on the correct information when it is required.

Questions commonly asked

- They don't burn people individually, do they?
- When do they take them out of their coffins?
- Isn't it true that you always get more than one person's ashes back in the pot?
- How do you know that you have the correct person during the process?
- When do the handles get removed?
- How long does it take for someone to burn?
- How fat do you have to be not to fit in the average cremator?
- What happens to the jewellery?
- What happens to all the different prostheses?
- Can a member of the family come round the back if they want to?
- Do thin people burn faster than fat ones?

If the reader finds themselves wondering about the answer to some of these questions, maybe it is time for them to go on this type of visit.

This part of the visit is not suitable for everyone, so again participants are warned of what they might see, in order that they can make an informed decision before entering this room.

The group then visits the flower room, which is open to all visitors, and they find out what happens to the flowers after the ceremony.

Outside

The group makes a tour of the gardens, and sees where the ashes are scattered. They also see the visitors' remembrance room, visit the columbarium wall and see the photographs and personalised inscriptions.

Time is set aside to talk about the inscriptions and personalisation of the columbarium niches, and what this means in terms of the grief process.

Back inside, in the hospitality suite

Some of the initial session may have to be curtailed, because of funerals that are being conducted on that day, so any information which has not been given is provided at this point. It also allows the group to see a hospitality suite, which is a fairly new addition to the facilities of a crematorium. This can be an opportune time to discuss the vast array of memorial artefacts which families often wish to purchase, and why families feel this to be so important. Often the question of DIY funerals is raised by the students, and it helps them to know something of the issues involved so that they are able to pass on this knowledge to anyone else who might also be considering this possibility. With a thorough understanding of how complex a funeral is, the group can now appreciate that whilst attending a funeral is one thing, for a bereaved family actually to put one together and completely run it themselves is quite another, especially when family members are all grieving. Cardboard coffins are also usually mentioned at this point (if they have not previously been mentioned at the funeral director's premises). This is an opportunity to ensure that students know that anyone who chooses this option may well be sacrificing the dignity of their loved one. Suffice to say that such coffins do not always stay in shape and that they can leak. If it is a 'green' issue, then chipboard serves as a good solution, which will maintain the dignity of the deceased without costing much more than the cardboard option.

This final session provides an opportunity for more questions, as well as finding out what each participant will be putting into practice as a result of this visit, and checking that everyone is bearing up.

Choosing the crematorium

The crematorium the author uses for these visits (East Riding Crematorium, Octon, near Driffield) is chosen because it is one of only a few of its type in Britain, providing an exceptionally high standard of care with a most superior establishment. It is a privately run enterprise, but it has been very carefully designed to meet the needs of its client group, with a well organised chapel (with excellent acoustics), outstanding landscaping and beautiful gardens, as can be seen in Figure 22.2 and Figure 22.3.

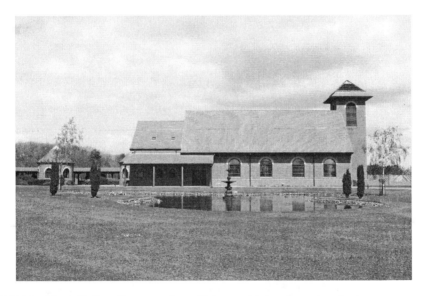

FIGURE 22.2 East Riding Crematorium, Octon, with landscaping features

Every detail of this venture has been carefully planned, including extended times for the funeral service and individualised care. It is pleasing to be able to illustrate best practice to the participants and, whilst not all council-run crematoriums might reach this standard at present, the bar is raised for all to aim at. The other reason for the visit to this particular crematorium is that a small (but increasing) number of individuals prefer to have their funerals away from where they live. The thought seems to be that the bereaved are thereby spared from the unacceptable level of grief caused to them by having to pass close to the crematorium on a regular basis. It means that they only need to visit when they want to, and this appears to provide a little extra control in a difficult situation. (For whatever reason, this particular crematorium has run funeral services for families who live not just twenty or thirty miles away, but sometimes from across the whole of the country.) If the reader does not have a crematorium like this one fairly close by, then they might try visiting the local council-run crematorium, as the staff are usually most helpful, welcoming, and keen to be involved.

The course participants usually travel about thirty to fifty miles to go on this particular visit, and often complain about the distance before attending. They never complain after the visit! A workbook has been developed for participants to complete during the day, in order to collect and document relevant information.

It is important that all those involved in providing the pre-bereavement and post-bereavement care are given enough information regarding funerals and other rites of passage. The information needs to be delivered in a style which stimulates critical thinking, encourages learning and, it is hoped, promotes attitudinal change.

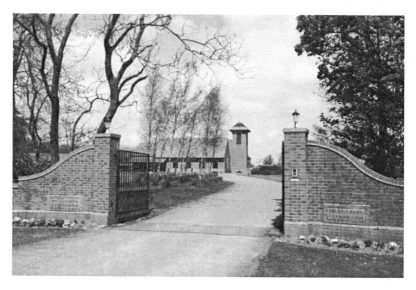

FIGURE 22.3 East Riding Crematorium, Octon, viewed from the front gates

CHANGING DEATH RITUALS

Cremation was illegal in Britain before 1884, but as recently as 1940 only a mere 9% of funerals ended in cremation. In 1968, for the first time, cremations exceeded burial and today cremation is chosen by more than 70% of the population in Britain.

The rise in cremations seems to have now levelled out, and there seems to be a slight trend back towards burial. However, cemeteries have reached or are reaching capacity, which will reduce choice in the future (House of Commons 2001).

As the rituals change, very few families have their loved one at home the night before the funeral anymore. In a practical sense, this has become less manageable due to the smaller size of houses, and to central heating! The rituals have also changed in terms of mourning dress (which is now seldom worn) and cars (which are no longer always black), and there has been a decline in the numbers of family members wishing to see the deceased. Views on all this vary, with some believing that while the meaning and significance of the rituals remains indisputable, these emotionally charged events can be commandeered for purposes other than the releasing of sorrow and grief (Payne *et al.* 1999; Litten 2002). In 1995, the National Funerals College was set up to work towards providing better care for the bereaved, which they so richly deserve (Johnson 1996; National Funerals College 2002). While funeral directors, on the whole, seem to be improving their services, providing what is required at a more realistic cost, there is still a long way to go. As Litten (2002: 4) says:

> *'If we want to rescue the funeral from the quicksand of commercialism, we need to ensure that we, the clients, get what we want: a wider choice of merchandise, a better funeral, a proper cremation format (rather than a poorly doctored version of the 1662 Order for the Burial of the Dead) and a latitude to express our grief openly without fear of criticism.'*

The cemetery is a public space for the collective disposal of the dead. However, it tells much about the local community and about the relationship between the deceased and the bereaved, their wealth and their grieving. The need for the bereaved to visit such burial grounds does support the continuing bonds theorists, who hold that bonds do not end with death, but continue in memories and actions (Walter 1996; Francis *et al.* 1997).

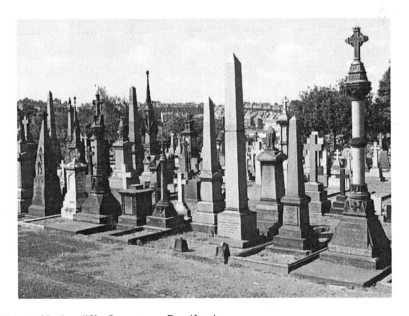

FIGURE 22.4 Undercliffe Cemetery, Bradford

Another useful exercise relating to cemeteries is to ask students to visit one in their locality, and to see what they can glean, bearing in mind the above points. It is also useful for the facilitator to be aware of all the local cemeteries, and to be able to signal those which it might be particularly useful to visit. For example, a well-known cemetery, and one which is frequently seen in Victorian dramas on television, is the Undercliffe Cemetery in Bradford (*see* Figure 22.4 and Figure 22.5).

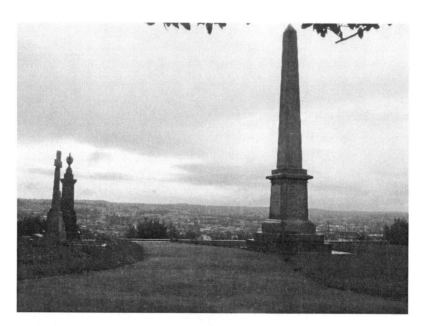

FIGURE 22.5 Undercliffe Cemetery, Bradford

Undercliffe Cemetery has been described as one of the most striking achievements of Victorian funeral design. It illustrates the social class system, with the rich wool merchants at the top of the hill with views across Bradford, and the poor at the bottom (Clarke and Davison 2004). It is full of extravagant mausoleums, huge obelisks and high columns, as well as pathways where the Victorians used to promenade.

Finding cemeteries such as this one allows the student to discuss the changes in society, and the bereavement theory in context, and perhaps even their own epitaph. It is also interesting to ask students to note different examples of funeral art and then to explain what the various symbols usually mean. In a local cemetery, the author has seen many striking symbols and inscriptions, such as a gravestone which depicts the Starship Enterprise, whose memorialised subject is apparently now 'Boldly going where no man has gone before'!

Another exercise is to have the group compare the epitaphs they have seen, interpreting what they mean, and deciding what makes a pleasing and appropriate one. Sometimes you might get them to prepare their own, and to discuss what they have included and why.

A further discussion might be related to whether burial or cremation is best, and can take the form of debating teams (if possible, with those who have a strong opinion trying to argue for the opposite side). This is what the author's students used to refer to as the 'compost or toast' debate. It is surprising how this debate can change people's minds, or leave them less sure of their opinions. This is an excellent way of illustrating how important it is for individuals, and society, to have all the facts in order to make informed choices. Ideally then, these mourning rituals need to meet the needs of the individual family members, as well as the wider family and society, as funeral rites characteristically encourage group cohesion.

Personal mortality

These exercises with inbuilt elements of self-awareness can be helpful in leading health professionals to face their own negative feelings and attitudes to death (Martin and Weston 1998; Farley 2004). When working with those facing such terrible loss, it is not surprising that the health professional's capacity to face their own mortality might be tested. There is a need to truly support these individuals who reach out with great compassion to help others. On the other hand, there is a need also to encourage them to examine their own losses and experiences of bereavement. It is essential to know that they can cope with the strong feelings of grief and loss which have been described throughout this chapter. Educational strategies need to be developed which are accepting of the student in sharing these difficult feelings (Durlak 1994). Farley (2004) suggests that students be allowed to share their anxieties, and that they be supported in doing so, so that in turn they are encouraged to share, work and learn together. However, it is also important to recognise the boundary between education and therapy; as Weston *et al.* (1998) comment, '*It is a thin one, but it is one to be respected.*'

The bottom line

The section above begins to illustrate the importance of raised self-awareness; the other vital component is to provide high-quality bereavement care by learning good communications.

As the founder of the modern-day hospice movement believed:

> '*Good communications can facilitate unexpected sharing and responses, and develop the growth through loss, we see so often.*' (Saunders 1994)

The bottom line is that communications must be an integral part of bereavement education. How can the health professional respond to the patients' or relatives' concerns if they have not heard them? In Chapter 1 of this book, 'Teaching communication skills to cancer and palliative care professionals: questions, challenges and debates', Fellows eloquently demonstrates from the research that health professionals often overestimate their own skills. She also suggests that the facilitator should have 'highly developed listening and facilitation skills which encourage participants to share rather than act out anxieties'. The importance of ensuring that the healthcare professional is equipped with good communications skills and is supported in practice with effective clinical supervision must not be underestimated.

KEY POINTS

- Bereavement is a vast topic, which requires the allocation of enough time for the necessary fundamentals to be taught.
- 'Change is loss and loss is change.' If this premise is accepted, how prepared are cancer and palliative care health professionals to do their job in this ever-changing health arena, especially in this demanding speciality?
- The theories identify the individuality and varying components of grief, which in turn has implications for the type of education, care and support offered.
- Coming to terms with death is not the same as coming to terms with your own personal mortality. The implications of this should be addressed when teaching this topic.
- Any education offered needs to be creative and flexible enough to engage staff members, in order that they might learn and ultimately improve practice.
- Educational strategists and clinical organisations need to work in partnership, and then education can guide practice and practice can guide education.

CONCLUSION

This chapter has explored some of the theories and models from the perspective of the educator, sharing different methods of teaching this complex topic, as well as introducing other contemporary ideas and approaches. The study of bereavement seems to be almost boundless, when considering all the facets which affect someone who is going through this process. So much more could have been written, including details of many other bereavement learning exercises. The limited space means that risk assessment has not been covered fully, and bereavement support has not been addressed; however, it must be acknowledged that these are crucial aspects of this topic. They do warrant being taught to all health professionals working with cancer and palliative care patients and their families. The author would suggest that this topic, given its magnitude, diversity, multi-dimensional nature and implications, must be addressed appropriately and taken seriously, as this is absolutely essential education. It must not be taught as an 'add on' to other cancer and palliative care topics, nor must it be simply included as part of some 'graveyard shift'; instead it needs to be seen as a subject in its own right and given the credence it requires.

Martin and Weston (1998: 17) talk of the importance of gaining true insight, knowledge and understanding into the experience of loss, including relevant ideas from all the different traditions, such as social, psychological and psychodynamic traditions. They say that, by understanding all these concepts,

> 'They illuminate the emotional cost of reorganising our inner world in response to uninvited changes in the external world as we attempt to provide the much needed continuity of coherence and meaning around which we organise our lives.'

By taking this perspective within education, and ensuring that this topic is taught effectively, it will also illuminate the cancer and palliative care educator's inner and outer worlds, allowing them to provide original, meaningful and resourceful educational initiatives.

Armed with a tool bag of teaching methods and approaches, and a caring, compassionate and empathic nature, the health practitioner can achieve the correct balance of theory, knowledge, self-awareness and practical guidance.

IMPLICATIONS FOR THE READER'S OWN PRACTICE

1 What aspects of bereavement and loss do you currently deliver? How might this be different as a result of this chapter?
2 How can you continue to increase your own self-awareness, and that of the student, in relation to this topic?
3 'You can only really, truly understand and support someone who is bereaved if you have also lost someone close.' What are your opinions on such a statement?
4 What would be the benefits (or limitations) associated with inviting someone who has lived through their loss to share their story in the classroom?
5 Could you develop an innovative method of teaching bereavement that would have a lasting effect on the student and, as a result, improve care?
6 Bereavement education lends itself to creative teaching methods, so what new creative approach will you try in the future?

REFERENCES

Albom M (1997) *Tuesdays with Morrie*. London: Sphere.

Bertman S (1991) *Facing Death: images, insights and interventions: handbook for educators, healthcare professionals and counsellors*. Washington, DC: Hemisphere Publishing.

Bowlby J (1969) *Attachment and Loss. Vol. 1. Attachment*. London: Hogarth.

Bowlby J (1980) *Attachment and Loss. Vol. 3. Loss: sadness and depression*. London: Hogarth.

Clarke C, Davison R (2004) *In Loving Memory: the story of Undercliffe Cemetery*. Stroud: Sutton Publishing.

Clingerman EM (1996) Bereavement tasks for nursing students. *Nurse Educ.* 21 (3): 19–22.

Costello J (1995) Helping relatives cope with the grieving process. *Prof Nurse.* 11 (2): 89–92.

Durlak JA (1994) Changing death attitudes through death education. In: Neimeyer RA, editor. *Death Anxiety Handbook: research instrumentation and appreciation*. Washington, DC: Taylor & Francis.

Durston D (1998) Community rites and the process of grieving. In: Weston R, Martin T, Anderson Y, editors. *Loss and Bereavement: managing change*. Oxford: Blackwell Science.

Engel GL (1961) Is grief a disease? A challenge for medical research. *Psychosom Med.* **23**: 18–22.

Erickson E, Erickson J, Kivnick H (1986) *Vital Involvement in Old Age*. New York: Norton.

Farley G (2004) Death anxiety and death education: a brief analysis of the key issues. In: Foyle L, Hostad J, editors. *Delivering Cancer and Palliative Care Education*. Oxford: Radcliffe Publishing.

Firth P (2007) Family care: sensitive and dynamic approaches to teaching. In: Foyle L, Hostad J, editors. *Innovations in Cancer and Palliative Care Education*. Oxford: Radcliffe Publishing.

Francis D, Kellaher L, Lee C (1997) Talking to people in cemeteries. *J Instit Burial Cremation Admin.* **65** (1): 14–25.

Freud S (1917) *Mourning and Melancholia. Collected papers Vol. 4.* New York: Basic Books.

Greenstreet W (2004) Why nurses need to understand the principles of bereavement theory. *Br J Nurs.* **9**: 590–3.

House of Commons (2001) *Select Committee Inquiry into Cemeteries.* London: Department of Transport and Regional Affairs.

Johnson M (1996) *The Dead Citizens Charter.* Stanford, CA: National Funerals College.

Kearney M (1996) *Mortally Wounded: stories of soul pain, death, and healing.* New York: Scribner.

Kinghorn S, Duncan F (2005) Living with loss. In: Lugton J, McIntyre R, editors. *Palliative Care: the nursing role.* London: Churchill Livingstone.

Klass D (1988) John Bowlby's model of grief and the problems of identification. *Omega.* **18** (1): 13–32.

Klass D, Silverman PR, Nickman SL, editors (1996) *Continuing Bonds, New Understandings of Grief.* Philadelphia, PA: Taylor & Francis.

Lehman DR, Ellard JH, Wortman C (1986) Social support for the bereaved: recipients' and providers' perspectives on what is helpful. *J Consult Clin Psychol.* **54**: 438–46.

Lewis CS (1961) *A Grief Observed.* London: Faber.

Lindemann E (1944) Symptomatology and management of acute grief. *Am J Psychiatry.* **101**: 141–8.

Litten J (2002) *The English Way of Death: the common funeral since 1450.* London: Robert Hale.

Lloyd-Williams M, Cobb M (2006) How well trained are clergy in care of the dying patient and bereavement support? *J Pain Symptom Manage.* **32** (1).

Martin T (1998) Personal mortality. In: Weston R, Martin T, Anderson Y. *Loss and Bereavement: managing change.* Oxford: Blackwell Science.

Martin T, Weston R (1998) A theoretical framework for understanding loss and the helping process. In: Weston R, Martin T, Anderson Y, editors. *Loss and Bereavement: managing change.* Oxford: Blackwell Science.

McIntyre R (2002) *Nursing Support for Families of Dying Patients.* London: Whurr.

Melliar-Smith C (2002) The risk assessment of bereavement in a palliative care setting. *Int J Palliat Nurs.* **8** (6).

Miles MS, Demi AS (1984) Sources of guilt in bereaved parents: towards the development of a theory of bereavement guilt. *Omega.* **14** (2): 299–314.

National Funerals College (2002) *Funeral Advisers: is there a need?* Bristol: National Funerals College.

Parkes CM (1993) Bereavement as a psychosocial transition. In: Stroebe M, Stroebe W, Hansson RO, editors. *Handbook of Bereavement: theory, research and intervention.* Cambridge: Cambridge University Press.

Parkes CM (1998) *Bereavement: studies of grief in adult life.* 4th ed. London: Tavistock.

Parkes CM (2000) Bereavement as a psychosocial transition: processes of adaptation to change. In: Dickinson D, Johnson J, Katz JS, editors. *Death, Dying and Bereavement.* London: Sage/ Open University Press.

Payne S (2001) Bereavement support: something for everyone. *Int J Palliat Nurs.* **7**: 108.

Payne S, Horns S, Relf M (1999) *Loss and Bereavement.* Buckingham: Open University Press.

Pullen ML (2002) Joe's story: reflections on a difficult interaction between nurse and patient's wife. *Int J Palliat Nurs.* **8**: 481–9.

Rosenblatt P (1993) Grief: the social context of private feelings. In: Stroebe M, Stroebe W, Hansson RO, editors. *Handbook of Bereavement: theory, research and intervention.* Cambridge: Cambridge University Press.

Saunders C (1994) Foreword. In: Inge B, Corless BG, Pittman M, editors. *Dying, Death and Bereavement: theoretical perspectives and other ways of knowing.* Boston, MA: Jones and Bartlett.

Saunderson EM, Ridsdale L (1999) General practitioners' beliefs and attitudes about how to respond to death and bereavement: qualitative study. *BMJ.* **319**: 293–6.

Sheldon F (1998) Bereavement. In: Fallon M, O'Neill B, editors. *ABC of Palliative Care.* London: BMJ Books: 63–5.

Small N (2001) Theories of grief: a critical review. In: Hockley J *et al.*, editors. *Grief, Mourning and Death Ritual.* Buckingham: Open University Press.

Smith P (2004) Working with family care givers in a palliative care setting. In: Payne S, Seymour J, Ingleton C, editors. *Palliative Care Nursing: principles and evidence for practice.* Buckingham: Open University Press.

Stokes J, Wyer S, Crossley D (1997) The challenge of evaluating a child bereavement programme. *Palliat Med.* **11**: 179–90.

Stroebe MS, Stroebe W, Hansson RO (1993) Bereavement research and theory: an introduction. In: Stroebe MS, Stroebe W, Hansson RO, editors. *Handbook of Bereavement.* Cambridge: Cambridge University Press.

Walter T (1990) *Funerals and How to Improve Them.* London: Hodder and Stoughton.

Walter T (1996) A new model of grief: bereavement and biography. *Mortality.* **1** (1): 7–25.

Walter T (1999) *On Bereavement: the culture of grief.* Buckingham: Open University Press.

Weston R, Martin T, Anderson Y (1998) *Loss and Bereavement: managing change.* Oxford: Blackwell Science.

Wilson D, Becker R (2007) Coping with grief and advice on appropriate support. *Br J Health Ass.* **1** (5): 232–3.

Worden JW (1982) *Grief Counselling and Grief Therapy.* London: Routledge.

Worden JW (1991) *Grief Counselling and Grief Therapy.* 2nd ed. New York: Springer Publishing.

USEFUL WEBSITES

www.crusebereavmentcare.org.uk
www.bbc.co.uk/relationships/coping_with_grief/bereavement_index.shtml
www.cancer.gov/cancertopics/pdq/supportivecare/bereavement/HealthProfessional

FURTHER READING

- Kinghorn S, Duncan F (2005) Living with loss. In: Lugton J, McIntyre R, editors. *Palliative Care: the nursing role.* London: Churchill Livingstone.

  This chapter is recommended to any educationalist or facilitator of bereavement. It looks at many aspects of loss, which is useful, but what are most beneficial are the exercises peppered throughout the chapter, which could be easily used as activities in the classroom.

- Jacobsen F, Kindlen M, Shoemark A (1997) *Living Through Loss: a manual for those working with issues of terminal illness and bereavement.* London: Jessica Kingsley.

  This is a useful manual, designed as a course to train people to support or counsel the bereaved. There are activities which relate mortality, self-awareness and skills acquisition to enable the student to become more effective at supporting the bereaved. These could be adapted to suit the needs of the facilitator.

- Litten J (2002) *The English Way of Death: the common funeral since 1450.* London: Robert Hale.

  Julian Litten is one of the country's few funeral historians. His book is an excellent resource for anyone embarking on facilitating sessions related to rites of passage. It contains a wealth of information associated with funerals, burial and cremation.

Index

accountability 213–14
    and advanced nursing practice 122–7
action learning 23–6
    described 23
    methods 25–6
    models and cycles 25
    teaching and facilitating 24–5
actors in role play 33–4, 35, 36
adult learning theory 270–1
advanced nursing practice 120–30
    background and context 121
    changing professional boundaries 121–2
    implications for educators 129
    legal challenges and accountability 122–7
    professional regulation issues 127–9
albumin 233
'anchors' (memory) 78–9
anecdotes 43–4
anorexia 232
appetite loss 232–3
appraisal research 166–7
Assisted Dying for the Terminally Ill Bill-2004
    224–5, 226
associations 60
    and 'anchor' points 78–9
attachment and loss 367–9
auditory memories 61–2
autocratic leadership 297–9
autonomy
    and education 264
    group 275–6

Bandler, Richard 56–7
Bateson, Gregory 57
'being available' 103–4
Belbin's self-perception inventory (SPI) 321–2
beliefs, religious 90–1

bereavement
    children's experiences 356–7, 359
    and individualism 371–3
    and life lines 370
    teaching curricula 365–6
    theoretical frameworks and models
        366–73
    use of teaching workshops 369–70
bibliotherapy 42–3
Black, James 155
blood urea nitrogen (BUN) levels 233
body image 30–1
body language 46–7
    matching and mirroring techniques
        63–5
Bristol diet 234
burials 80
burnout 284–91
    prevention 288–90
    signs and symptoms 285–6

Cable, Paul 331
Cancer Networks 20
cancer services
    background and contexts 135–6
    challenges and need for change 136–8,
        178–81
    change design 138–40
    key change lessons and guidelines 148–9
    palliative philosophy 211–12
    patient feedback 138–40, 147–50
    practical experiences of relocation 150–2
    role of the design team 146–7
    staff rotations and placements 140
    strategy development 140–6
    use of focus groups 147–8
    word changes 139

'Cancer Tales' communication teaching tool 18–37
  background and inspiration 19–20
  context and policy drivers 20–1
  development and approaches 21–2
  integrating into teaching sessions 30–2
  marketing and showcasing 34–6
  role of action learning 23–6
  use of chapter meetings 26–9
  use of role play 32–4, 35, 36
  use of workbooks 29–30
care services *see* cancer services
care standards 124–5
carer education *see* patient and carer education
case stories 43
case studies 201–2, 223
Castle, Roy 30–2
cemeteries 381–3
change processes
  key lessons and guidelines 148–9
  learning from feedback 147–50
  strategic development theories 141–2
  understanding design team role 146–7
Changing Patients' Worlds through Nursing Expertise (Manley *et al.*) 92
chapter meetings 26–9
chemotherapy, and body nutrition 232–3
children 344–59
  concepts and understandings of death 350–1
  how much to tell them 345–6
  implications of bereavement for child 353
  language use 352–3
  recognising distress 349–52
  suffering bereavement 356–7
  teaching methods 357–8
  types and timing of courses 354–5
  working with schools 346–53
  working within teams and with other professions 355–6
civil law 213
clinical supervision
  role of critical companionship 85–93
  role of neurolinguistic programming 67–71
Cochrane reviews 168–9
Codes of Conduct 127–9
  and professional boundaries 122
Codes of Practice, and critical thinking 114
communication skills
  benefits and importance 2, 5
  competency evaluations 13–14
  engaging an audience 50–1
  non-verbal 46–7
  patient priorities 5
  posture and expression 46
  problems and challenges 2
  qualifications and standards 12
  skills and training needs 6–9, 12
  training challenges and goals 3–5
  training facilitators 11
compassion 47–8
  challenges and conflict 178–81
  definitions and concepts 182–5
competence
  concepts and definitions 181–2
  vs. compassion 178–81
concept mapping 114–15
confused patients 49–50
'Connected' national communication skills programme 20–1
consent 216–17
coping theory 271–2
countertransference 3–4
Countess Mountbatten House Hospice (Southampton) 254
courage 200
Cowey, SR 83
crematorium and funerals 375–80
  choice of venues 379–80
  and commercialism 381–2
criminal law 213
critical appraisal skills 166–7
  learning progression 171
  see also research teaching and learning
Critical Appraisal Skills Programme Resource (CASP) 166
critical companionship 83–93
  described 85–90
  diagrammatic model 86
  domains and methods 86–9
  facilitation strategies 89–90
  practice 90–1
Critical Reasoning (Thompson) 115
critical thinking skills 110–18
  definitions 111
  development and skill acquisition 113–14
  importance and benefits 111–12
  introducing into curriculum 114–17
  measurement 112–13
  practice and exercises 115–16
Critical Thinking Skills (Cottrell) 115
cues, and reflection 101–3

Dalai Lama 177
databases, healthcare-related 163–4
death and dying (hospital settings) 331–42
    different experiences of death 322–3
    different rituals 380–3
    discussions and learning 333–5
    enabling patients to experience a good
      death 336–7
    teaching aspects 335–6
    traditions and rites 373–5
    use of role play 337–41
decision-making in end-of-life care 209–11
    moral and legal doctrines 217–18
    see also legal issues
deletions 75–6
democratic leadership 299–300
Dewey, John 95
Dickinson, Emily 195, 196
diet and nutrition
    background and approaches 230–1
    as causes of disease 230
    loss of appetite 230–1
    multiprofessional implications 233–4
    as possible protective measures 231
    teaching approaches 232–3
    therapies and management 234–8
    Bristol diet 234
    Gerson diet 235–6
    Gonzalez therapy 238
    macrobiotic diet 236–7
dignity of patients 114, 115–16, 224–5
Dimond, Margaret 270
dissociation 60–1
distortions 75–6
Dunn, Nell 18–20
duty of care 123
dysphagia 232

education theory 270–1
electronic databases, healthcare-related 163–4
emotional impact of disease 3–4
    exploring through role play 7–8
emotional memory 61–2
empathy
    barriers to 32
    and compassion 183–4
    definitions 183–4
    skills development 8, 58
    use of metaphor 77–8
    use of role play 32–4
    see also neurolinguistic programming
      (NLP)

empirical knowledge 6
End of Life project (EOL 2006) 206
euthanasia 224–5
evidence hierarchies 168
evidence-based practice 3, 21, 157, 158–9
    definitions 158–9
existential knowledge 9
expert practitioner 84–5
Expertise in Practice Project (RCN) 84–5, 86
eye movements 46, 61–3

facial expressions 46
facilitated skills practice session 7–8
fatigue 233
focus groups 147–8
framing perspectives 103–4
    for 'being available' 103–4
funerals and crematorium 375–80
    choice of venues 379–80
    and commercialism 381–2

generalisations 76–7
Gerson diet 235–6
Gonzalez therapy 238
Gordon, Suzanne 188–91
'graceful care' 87
Grinder, John 57
group autonomy 275–6
group learning 222–3
    topics for study 224–5
group support 275

hallucinations 49–50
healthcare policies 20–1, 136–7
    on leadership 293–4
    on teamworking 308
    on user involvement 245
healthcare professionals
    awareness of own limitations 126–7
    changing roles 121–2, 179–81
    coping with patient emotions 3–4
    knowledge requirements 6–9
    professional boundaries 121–2
    professional regulation 127–9
    self-care 281–91
    self-knowledge 6–9
    stress responses and burnout 284–91
healthcare services
    cancer care 133–53
    impact of policy changes 136–7
Herceptin 226
Herth's Hope Index 198

history of healthcare 185–8
    thirteenth-century 185–6
    eighteenth-century 186
    nineteenth-century 186–7
    swinging sixties 187–8
    late twentieth century 188–92
homosexuality 31–2
hope 204–6
    definitions 196–8
    developmental tools and inventories 198
    teaching approaches 199
    teaching methods and exercises 199–204
Hospers, J 116
hospices, education and training courses 218
Hull and East Yorkshire Hospitals NHS Trust
    cancer care service development strategy
        135–53
    care challenges 136–8
Human Rights Act-1998 212–13
humour 46–7, 200

Improving Outcomes (DoH 1999) 165
individualism 371–3
information literacy skills 161–4
insights
    co-creating 105–6
    framing perspectives 103
integrity 47–8
internal dialogues 62
intuition 87–9
INTUTE 163–4

Johns, C 95–6, 100, 102
'journaling' 97–9
    significance 101

Kearney, M 60
kinesthetic memories 62
knowledge requirements (healthcare
    professionals) 6–9
    awareness of own limitations 126–7

laissez-faire leadership 300–1
latent learning 275
leadership 293–304
    characteristics 296–7
    concepts and definitions 294–5
    development history 293–4
    functions and roles 295
    importance 302
    styles 297–302
    training and programmes 302–3

Leading an Empowered Organisation (LEO)
    programmes 302–3
lectures 221
legal issues
    accountability 122–4, 213–14
    after death 214–15
    consent 216–17
    decision-making doctrines 217–18
    important areas 212–13
    relating to treatments 215–16
    sources of information 218
    standards of care 124–5
    training and education 218, 219–27
letting go 200
liability and negligence 123–4
life lines 370–3
life stories 40
    see also storytelling
listening 99
literature reviews 167
        systematic reviews and meta-analysis
            167–70
litigation 123
    culture of 210–11
Living with Cancer project (Sargent *et al.*)
    57–8
loss lines 333–4
    see also bereavement

macrobiotic diet 236–7
malnutrition 233
market forces 137
matching behaviours 63–5
'meaning', and hope 197
medical research teaching *see* research
    teaching and learning
medical treatments
    legal issues 215–16
    patient consent 216–17
meditation 100–1
memory
        associations and 'anchor' points 60, 78–9
        cues and signals 61–2
Mental Capacity Act-2005 222
meta-analysis 169–70
metaphors 40, 41–2
    and empathy 77
    and neurolinguistic programming 77–8
the Milton Model (neurolinguistic
    programming) 77
mindfulness 95–6
Mintzberg, H *et al.* 141–2, 153

mirroring techniques 63–5
model for structured reflection (MSR) 100, 106
moral guidance 210, 211–12
mortality 383
Mortally Wounded (Kearney) 60
MSR *see* model for structured reflection
multidisciplinary teams
    defined 308
    see also team working
mutuality 86

narrative
    about hope and suffering 200
    see also storytelling
National Cancer Action Team (NCAT) 20
National Library for Health *see* NHS Evidence
National Service Frameworks, critical
    evaluations 166–7
nausea 233
negligence 123
neurolinguistic programming (NLP) 45, 55–81
    background and development 56–8
    concept described 58–9
    current applications 57–8
    evaluation 57–8
    methods and systems 59–67
        dissociation techniques 60
        evaluation of the 'well-formed
            outcome' 73–4
        eye movement analysis 61–3
        'opportunity' skills 69–71
        pacing 57–8, 66–7
        rapport development 59, 63–7, 69
        reframing 71–3
    the Milton Model 77
    origins and pioneers 56–7
    outcomes evaluations 73–4
    recognising deletions, distortions and
        generalisations 75–7
    use of anchors 78–9
    use in clinical supervision 67–73
    use of metaphor and story 77–8
    use in phobia management 79–80
NHS Evidence 162–3
NHS services *see* healthcare services
NICE Supportive and Palliative Care Guidance
    (2004) 20
Nightingale, Florence 186–7
non-verbal communication skills 46–7
North Devon Hospice 253–4
Now and Then (Castle 1993) 30–2
nurses *see* healthcare professionals

nursing practice
    accountability issues 122–4
    changing professional boundaries 121–2
    competence vs. compassion challenges
        178–81
    descriptions of integrated care 188–92
nutrition *see* diet and nutrition

O'Donohue, John 99
'opportunity' techniques and skill 69–71

pacing 57–8, 66–7
Paley, John 116–17
palliative care, concepts and philosophy
    211–12
participation 255–6
particularity 86–7
passion 47
patient briefings 340–1
patient and carer education 262–78
    background and contexts 262–3
    benefits and rationale 263–6
    coping theory and stress management
        271–2
    course delivery models and approaches
        266–70
    education theory 270–1
    facilitation processes 272
    potential problems and concerns 274–7
    topics and content 272–4
patient consent 216–17
patient dignity 114, 115–16, 224–5
patient interviews 338–40
patient involvement 243–58
    benefits 248–50
    context and policy background 244–5
    in education 246–58
    frameworks and guidelines 252–3
    problems and barriers 250–1
    stages and levels 253–5
    and user participation 255–6
patient–healthcare professional relationship 5
    impact of role expansion 179–81
patient-centred care 4–5
person-centred helping relationship 85
personality 320–1
Petrone, Michele 255–6
philosophy 113
phobias, use of neurolinguistic programming
    79–80
'Pit head time' 68
professional accountability 122–7, 213–14

professional boundaries 121–2
professional networks 219
professional regulation 127–9
professionals *see* healthcare professionals
psychologists 355–6

qualifications, counselling 12
question techniques, to maintain rapport 63

rapport 44
    exercises 65–6
    meta-frames and models 69
    methods and techniques 59, 63–7
    observation sheets 66
reciprocity 87
reflection within/on practice 95–6
reflective effort 96
reflective practice 42, 94–108
    background 94–5
    concepts and descriptions 95–6
    dialogical movements 97–107
    effectiveness and patient outcomes 103
    framing perspectives 103
    key features 96–7
    narrative construction as educational
        process 97–107
    practitioner performance 103–4
    template for being available 104
reframing techniques 71–3
relaxation techniques, visualisation and
    dissociation 60–1
religious beliefs 90–1
research teaching and learning 155–72
    attitudes towards 156–9
    background and context 156–9
    contemporary focuses 159–61
    evidence hierarchies 168
    evidence sources 167–70
    impact of evidence–based practice 157
    information literacy skills 161–4
    skills development 170–2
    stepped approaches 160–1
    systematic reviews and meta-analysis
        167–70
    uses and applications 166–7
Rinpoche, Songyal 100
risk, identification and recognition 125–6
role play 32–4, 337–41
    developing self–knowledge 7–8
    use of actors 33–4
    use of health professionals 32–3
    use of video 341

Royal College of Nursing, Expertise in Practice
    Project 84–5
Rushworth, Claire 57

St Christopher's Education Advisory Group
    254
Saint Francis Hospice (Essex) 254
St Wilfrid's Hospice (Chichester) 255
Sargent, P *et al.* 57–8
Saxe, John Godfrey 133–4
Schon, D 95
SCONAL Seven Pillars model for information
    literacy 161–2
self-care 281–91
    concept of the 'wounded healer' 283–4
    definitions 282–3
    lack of care problems 282
    stress and burnout 284–91
self-awareness 290
    of mortality 383
self-disclosure by teachers 46
self-knowledge, healthcare professionals 6–9
self-learning, use of workbooks 29–30
self-perception inventory (SPI) (Belbin) 321–2
self-reflection exercises 202–4
    see also reflective practice
seminars 221–2
sexuality and intimacy 30–1, 104–5
Shadowlands (CS Lewis) 372
short stories 200–1
    see also storytelling
situational leadership 301–2
social workers 355–6
spirituality 201
staff support, role of clinical supervision 67–71
standards of care 124–5
Stanislavski, C 34–5
storytelling 39–52
    background and definitions 41–4
    benefits of using 44–5
    disadvantages 51
    delivery techniques 46–7
    effectiveness and impact 45–8
    engaging an audience 50–1
    functions and characteristics 49
    generalisation potentials 49
    models 47–8
    and neurolinguistic programming 77–8
    passion, compassion and integrity 47–8,
        51
    on subject of dying 45
strategy development theories 140–6

stress management 271–2
stress responses, health professionals 284–91
suffering 196, 198, 204–6
  developmental tools and inventories 198
  teaching approaches 199
  teaching methods and exercises 199–204
supervision *see* clinical supervision
systematic reviews 167–9
Szasz, Thomas 55

teachers
  self-disclosures 46
  vulnerability 46
team working 306–29
  background and policy contexts 307–8
  dealing with differences 328
  developing effective working models
    310–14
  ground rules 314
  and personality 320–1
  planning stages 323–4
  qualities for effectiveness 309–10
  setting agendas 315–16
  team activities 316–23
  types of team 308–9
technology and nursing care, conflicts and
  resolutions 188–92
thinking skills *see* critical thinking skills
touch 99
training and education
  developing critical thinking skills 110–18
  formal teaching settings 221–2
  group work 222–3
  in death rites and practices 364–85
  in legal aspect of care 218, 219–27
  in nutrition and diet 232–40
  in strategic planning 143–6
  importance of communication skills 1–15
  multi-professional vs. uni-professional
    courses 10
  opportunities and courses 218–19
  qualifications and standards 12
  in research skills 155–72
  role of intensive courses 9–10, 22

structure and length of courses 9–10, 22
teaching challenges of advanced nursing
  practice 120–30
tutorial sessions 224
use of 'Cancer Tales' communication
  approaches 18–37
use of case studies 201–2, 223
use of neurolinguistic programming
  (NLP) 45, 55–81
use of reflective practice 94–108
    self-reflection exercises 202–4
use of storytelling 44–52
user involvement 246–58
web-based learning 224
see also clinical supervision; patient and
  carer education
treatment legal issues 215–16
  and consent 216–17
  and decision-making 217–18
trust issues 179–80
tutorials 224

user involvement 243–58
  context and policy background 244–5
  in education 246–58
  patient benefits 248–9
  and patient participation 255–6
  problems and barriers 250–1
  stages and levels 253–5

values, and team work 322–3
vicarious liability 124
video role plays 341
visualisation techniques
  coping with fear 60
  relaxation purposes 60
vitamin supplements 231
voice, tone and rhythm 50, 64
vulnerability 46, 88–9, 90

Wardle, J 243
web-based learning 224
weight loss 232
workbooks 29–30